PRENATAL DIAGNOSIS
& REPRODUCTIVE GENETICS

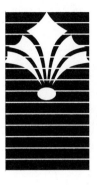

PRENATAL DIAGNOSIS & REPRODUCTIVE GENETICS

JEFFREY A. KULLER, M.D.
Assistant Professor of Obstetrics and Gynecology
Director of Reproductive Genetics

NANCY C. CHESCHEIR, M.D.
Associate Professor of Obstetrics and Gynecology
Director, Prenatal Diagnosis Program

ROBERT C. CEFALO, M.D., Ph.D.
Professor of Obstetrics and Gynecology
Director of Maternal-Fetal Medicine

University of North Carolina School of Medicine
Chapel Hill, North Carolina

With 32 illustrations

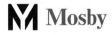

St. Louis Baltimore Boston Carlsbad Chicago Naples New York Philadelphia Portland
London Madrid Mexico City Singapore Sydney Tokyo Toronto Wiesbaden

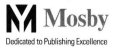

Mosby

Dedicated to Publishing Excellence

A Times Mirror Company

Editor: Susie H. Baxter
Developmental Editor: Ellen Baker Geisel
Project Manager: Mark Spann
Production Editor: Melissa Martin
Designer: David Zielinski
Manufacturing Supervisor: Betty Richmond

Printed in the United States of America
Composition by Shepherd, Inc.
Printing/binding by R.R. Donnelly & Sons Co.

Mosby–Year Book, Inc.
11830 Westline Industrial Drive
St. Louis, Missouri 63146

International Standard Book Number 0-8151-5209-4

96 97 98 99 00 / 9 8 7 6 5 4 3 2 1

Foreword

Most textbook authors underestimate the amount of time and effort necessary to complete their task. The writing of this focused textbook was accomplished within the context of another important challenge—the goal of transforming complex subjects into "user-friendly" chapters by presenting most of the teaching material in a question and answer format. Obviously, complex issues are easier to master when the subject matter is divided into many smaller segments. I commend the authors of *Prenatal Diagnosis & Reproductive Genetics* for achieving their goal of writing a practical textbook for the clinician.

The ever-increasing importance of genetics and prenatal diagnosis is reflected in our peer-reviewed literature and in clinical practice. I compliment the authors on this timely addition to the obstetric literature. The authors should begin preparing immediately for the next edition of this text because of the exponential growth rate of new knowledge in this field. However, the last three chapters are intended to compensate for the rapid acquisition of new scientific information by predicting the directions research will take in the immediate future.

William Droegemueller, M.D.
Robert A. Ross Distinguished Professor and Chairman
Department of Obstetrics and Gynecology
University of North Carolina School of Medicine
Chapel Hill, North Carolina

Preface

Prenatal diagnosis and reproductive genetics are integral components of obstetric and gyne-cologic practice. Fetal sonography has revolutionized our ability to diagnose congenital anom-alies; most clinicians have now incorporated obstetric sonography into their practices. Maternal serum screening is an increasingly effective tool for the detection of aneuploidy and fetal struc-tural abnormalities. The field of genetics has become the newest frontier in medicine. Through the Human Genome Project, our genetic constitution is currently being mapped. Reproductive genet-ics is an important component of residency training; each year more obstetrician-gynecologists enter medical genetics training programs. Six of the contributors to this textbook are obstetrician-gynecologists who are board certified in medical genetics in addition to their own specialty certification.

This textbook was written with the goal of being both accessible and practical. A wide variety of pertinent topics in prenatal diagnosis and reproductive genetics is covered in a conversational format. Our contributors are primarily obstetrician-gynecologists and genetic counselors skilled in prenatal diagnosis, medical genetics, or management of high-risk pregnancies. We have strived to present clinically relevant material to residents in training, practicing obstetrician-gynecologists, maternal-fetal medicine specialists, and geneticists interested in prenatal diagnosis.

We gratefully acknowledge the excellent clerical efforts of Jane C. Mitchell and the superb editorial assistance of Melissa Martin and Ellen Baker Geisel.

Jeffrey A. Kuller
Nancy C. Chescheir
Robert C. Cefalo

To Barbara, for her unwavering support, and to Max and Isabel, who help me maintain my perspective about what's important.

J.A.K.

To Chip, whose constancy supports me, and to our sons, Alex and Stuart, who daily remind us what life is all about.

N.C.C.

To my entire family, who tolerated my reading of the chapters while on the beach.

R.C.C.

Contributors

DIANA W. BIANCHI, M.D.

Chief of Perinatal Genetics

Associate Professor of Pediatrics
  and Obstetrics and Gynecology

Tufts University School of Medicine

Boston, Massachusetts

MICKI L. CABANISS, M.D.

Associate Professor of Obstetrics
  and Gynecology

University of North Carolina
  School of Medicine

Mountain Area Health Education Center

Asheville, North Carolina

CHRISTINE R. CADRIN, M.D.

Assistant Professor of Obstetrics
  and Gynecology

University of Montreal

Montreal, Quebec, Canada

NANCY P. CALLANAN, M.S.

Clinical Assistant Professor

Genetic Counselor

Department of Pediatrics

Division of Genetics and Metabolism

University of North Carolina
  School of Medicine

Chapel Hill, North Carolina

ROBERT C. CEFALO, M.D., Ph.D.

Professor of Obstetrics and Gynecology

Director of Maternal-Fetal Medicine

University of North Carolina
  School of Medicine

Chapel Hill, North Carolina

NANCY C. CHESCHEIR, M.D.

Associate Professor of Obstetrics
  and Gynecology

Director, Prenatal Diagnosis Program

University of North Carolina
  School of Medicine

Chapel Hill, North Carolina

CAROL C. COULSON, M.D.

Assistant Professor of Obstetrics
  and Gynecology

Pennsylvania State University
  School of Medicine

Hershey, Pennsylvania

MELISSA H. FRIES, M.D.

Clinical Geneticist

Department of Medical Genetics
  and Obstetrics and Gynecology

Keesler Medical Center

Keesler Air Force Base, Mississippi

MITCHELL S. GOLBUS, M.D.

Professor of Obstetrics, Gynecology,
  and Reproductive Sciences

Reproductive Genetics Unit

University of California–San Francisco
  School of Medicine

San Francisco, California

WENDY F. HANSEN, M.D.

Assistant Professor of Obstetrics
  and Gynecology

University of North Carolina
  School of Medicine

Chapel Hill, North Carolina

JENNIFER HELWICK SHAFER, M.S.

Clinical Instructor and Genetic Counselor
Department of Obstetrics and Gynecology
University of North Carolina
    School of Medicine
Chapel Hill, North Carolina

STEPHEN K. HUNTER, M.D., Ph.D.

Fellow Associate
Division of Maternal and Fetal Medicine
Department of Obstetrics and Gynecology
University of Iowa School of Medicine
Iowa City, Iowa

VERN L. KATZ, M.D.

Associate Professor of Obstetrics
    and Gynecology
University of North Carolina
    School of Medicine
Chapel Hill, North Carolina

JEFFREY A. KULLER, M.D.

Assistant Professor of Obstetrics
    and Gynecology
Director of Reproductive Genetics
University of North Carolina
    School of Medicine
Chapel Hill, North Carolina

STEVEN A. LAIFER, M.D.

Associate Professor
Department of Obstetrics, Gynecology,
    and Reproductive Sciences
University of Pittsburgh
    School of Medicine
Magee-Womens Hospital
Pittsburgh, Pennsylvania

BETH LINCOLN-BOYEA, M.S.

Clinical Instructor and Genetic Counselor
Department of Obstetrics and Gynecology
University of North Carolina
    School of Medicine
Chapel Hill, North Carolina

M. CATHLEEN McCOY, M.D.

Assistant Professor of Obstetrics
    and Gynecology
University of North Carolina
    School of Medicine
Chapel Hill, North Carolina

MICHAEL J. McMAHON, M.D., M.P.H.

Fellow, Maternal-Fetal Medicine
Department of Obstetrics and Gynecology
University of North Carolina
    School of Medicine
Chapel Hill, North Carolina

MARY E. NORTON, M.D.

Assistant Professor of Obstetrics
    and Gynecology
Harvard University School of Medicine
Brigham and Women's Hospital
Boston, Massachusetts

**DONNA JEANE HITCHCOCK
PAPPAS, M.Ed.**

Grief Counselor
Perinatal Grief Support Program
Department of Obstetrics and Gynecology
University of North Carolina
    School of Medicine
Chapel Hill, North Carolina

KATHLEEN W. RAO, Ph.D.

Associate Professor of Pediatrics
  and Pathology
Director, Cytogenetics Laboratory
University of North Carolina
  School of Medicine
Chapel Hill, North Carolina

MYRA I. ROCHE, M.S.

Clinical Instructor and Genetic Counselor
Department of Pediatrics
Division of Genetics and Metabolism
University of North Carolina
  School of Medicine
Chapel Hill, North Carolina

THOMAS W. SADLER, Ph.D.

Professor of Cell Biology and Anatomy
Director, North Carolina
  Birth Defects Center
University of North Carolina
  School of Medicine
Chapel Hill, North Carolina

CARLA BOOR SMITH, M.S.

Clinical Instructor and Genetic Counselor
Department of Obstetrics and Gynecology
University of North Carolina
  School of Medicine
Chapel Hill, North Carolina

WILLIAM J. SWEENEY, M.D.

Assistant Clinical Professor of Obstetrics
  and Gynecology
University of North Carolina
  School of Medicine
Coastal Area Health Education Center
Wilmington, North Carolina

BARBARA A. WEDEHASE, M.S.W.

Genetic Counselor
Department of Pediatrics
Division of Genetics and Metabolism
University of North Carolina
  School of Medicine
Chapel Hill, North Carolina

STEVEN R. WELLS, M.D.

Assistant Professor of Obstetrics
  and Gynecology
University of North Carolina
  School of Medicine
Chapel Hill, North Carolina

JOSEPH M. WILEY, M.D.

Associate Professor of Pediatrics
Director, Division of Pediatric Hematology
  and Oncology
Co-Director, Program in Bone Marrow
  Transplantation
University of North Carolina
  School of Medicine
Chapel Hill, North Carolina

JEROME YANKOWITZ, M.D.

Assistant Professor of Obstetrics
  and Gynecology
University of Iowa School of Medicine
Iowa City, Iowa

Contents

PRENATAL DIAGNOSIS
& REPRODUCTIVE GENETICS

PART ONE

PERICONCEPTIONAL COUNSELING AND INTERVENTION

CHAPTER 1

Prevention of Neural Tube Defects

ROBERT C. CEFALO

Neural tube defects (NTDs) are one of the most common congenital malformations, with an estimated worldwide annual incidence of 400,000 births. The incidence of NTDs varies geographically; Wales and Ireland have the highest incidence, with 8 per 1000 births in Northern Ireland. For couples of Irish descent who have migrated to the United States, the risk is approximately halved. In the United States, the geographic and race-specific prevalence of spina bifida alone is estimated to be a high of 8 per 10,000 total births for Caucasians in southern Appalachia and a low of fewer than 1 per 10,000 for blacks in the Pacific Northwest.[9] Neural tube defects are more common in first born than in later born children, with a male-female ratio of 0.7:1 for spina bifida and 0.45:1 for anencephaly.[13]

Neural tube defects follow a multifactorial pattern of inheritance; the recurrence risk is directly associated with the incidence of a disorder in a given population. In the United States, the risk of recurrence of a defect after one affected child is 1.5% to 2%, and the risk is 4% to 6% after two affected siblings.[23] In the United Kingdom, the recurrence risk is 4% to 5% after one affected child.[12]

❧ Patient Profile: Counseling for recurrence of a neural tube defect

The patient (gravida 1, para 0000) is a 20-year-old woman who at 16 to 17 weeks' gestation had an increased maternal serum α-fetoprotein (MSAFP) level of 4.7 multiples of the median. An ultrasound examination revealed a fetus with anencephaly. No other structural abnormalities were noted. After informed consent, the patient decided to terminate the pregnancy. A prostaglandin induction of labor occurred at 18 weeks' gestation. The fetus was confirmed by pathologic examination to have anencephaly. The patient requests further counseling concerning the risk of recurrence in a subsequent pregnancy.

QUESTION 1: WHAT ARE THE OCCURRENCE AND RECURRENCE RATES OF NEURAL TUBE DEFECTS?

In the United States, neural tube defects, including meningomyelocele, anencephaly, and encephalocele, occur in 1 in 2000 deliveries. The Centers for Disease Control and Prevention (CDC) reports that approximately 3000 to 4000 infants with NTDs are born annually in the United States.[3] About 95% of NTDs occur de novo as an isolated defect of unknown etiology; in the United States, the risk of recurrence is 1.5% to 2% the background risk. Couples with a sibling, niece, or nephew who had an NTD have a risk of approximately 0.3% to 1%; women with insulin-dependent diabetes mellitus (IDDM) have a risk of approximately 1%; women with seizure disorders who are being treated with carbamazepine or valproic acid have a risk of 0.6% and 2%, respectively.[1,18,20,21]

QUESTION 2: WHAT STUDIES RECOMMEND FOLIC ACID SUPPLEMENTATION TO PREVENT THE RECURRENCE OF NEURAL TUBE DEFECTS?

Lawrence and Smithells[14,24] published the seminal articles demonstrating the reduced incidence of recurrent NTDs when folic acid was administered before conception and during the first 3 months of pregnancy. Subsequently, the British Medical Research Council vitamin study, involving 33 medical centers in six European countries, followed 11,095 patients with a history of NTDs in their offspring. The researchers demonstrated that a dosage of 4 mg/day of folic acid alone or with other vitamins taken preconceptionally and through the twelfth gestational week resulted in a 1% recurrence rate, compared with a 3.5% recurrence rate for those taking other vitamins without folic acid or taking a placebo.[16]

The CDC subsequently recommended that women who had a prior pregnancy affected by NTD and who are planning conception should consume 4 mg of folic acid daily starting at least 1 month before conception and continuing through the first 3 months of pregnancy.[3]

In a case-control study, Milunsky and colleagues[17] assessed the dietary intake of folic acid as well as supplementation of the nutrient in 23,491 women undergoing MSAFP screening or amniocentesis at approximately 16 weeks' gestation; a substantially reduced risk of NTDs was found among women who took multivitamins with folic acid during the first 6 weeks of pregnancy. The prevalence of NTDs was 3.2 per 1000 pregnancies for women who began taking multivitamins containing folic acid after the seventh week of gestation and 1.1 per 1000 pregnancies for women who took multivitamins with folic acid during the first 6 weeks of gestation and beyond. The authors concluded that use of multivitamins containing folic acid during the first 6 weeks of pregnancy will reduce by more than 50% the occurrence of NTDs.

QUESTION 3: WHAT ARE THE RECOMMENDATIONS OF THE UNITED STATES PUBLIC HEALTH SERVICE AND THE AMERICAN COLLEGE OF OBSTETRICIANS AND GYNECOLOGISTS REGARDING FOLIC ACID CONSUMPTION?

It is well established that there is an inverse relationship between periconceptional and early pregnancy folic acid use and the recurrence of NTDs. To achieve a timely exposure to vitamin supplementation, a woman must receive appropriate advice before conception. Projecting a potential reduction of 50% of NTDs among American women, the United States Public Health Service recently made the following recommendation:

All women of childbearing age who are capable of becoming pregnant should consume 0.4 mg of folic acid daily for the purpose of reducing their risk of having a pregnancy affected with spina bifida and other neural tube defects. Women who have had a prior neural tube affected pregnancy are at high risk of having a subsequent affected pregnancy. When these women become pregnant, they should consult their physician for advice.

This recommendation is based on strong scientific evidence demonstrating that consumption of folic acid before pregnancy and during the first 12 weeks of gestation reduces the frequency of NTDs by 60% to 70%.[3] In 1993, the Committee on Obstetrics: Maternal-Fetal Medicine of the American College of Obstetricians and Gynecologists stated in a Committee Opinion: "Patients who have had a fetus with an NTD in a previous pregnancy should be offered treatment with 4.0 mg of folic acid, preferably starting one month prior to when they plan to become pregnant and then continu[ing] through the first three months of pregnancy."[1] Supplementation with folic acid will not prevent all NTD recurrences, possibly because some of these are genetic or are related to inherited metabolic disturbances, such as in patients with homocysteinuria.[26]

QUESTION 4: HOW CAN ADEQUATE INTAKE OF FOLIC ACID BE ENSURED IN ALL POTENTIALLY FERTILE WOMEN?

Naturally occurring folate as a B vitamin is found mainly in spinach, asparagus, broccoli, liver, collard greens, citrus fruit and juice, yeast, and beans. As a preventive therapy for recurrent NTDs, it is difficult to consume enough folic acid through diet alone. The recommended daily requirement for folic acid in all pregnant women is 0.4 mg. This compares with a recommended daily allowance (RDA) of 0.18 mg in nonpregnant women. The Food and Drug Administration (FDA) is currently exploring ways of meeting this recommendation: improvement of dietary habits, fortification of the U.S. food supply, and routine use of dietary supplements.[7]

Approximately 20% of American women now consume multivitamin preparations, which generally contain 0.4 mg folic acid. However, vitamins should not be considered a substitute for dietary intake of food containing folic acid, which is the preferred method of folic acid ingestion. Imbalances in women's diets do occur, however, and at times vitamin supplementation is a reasonable option. Prescribed multivitamin supplements for pregnant women usually contain 0.8 to 1.0 mg of folic acid. Because more than 50% of pregnancies in the United States are unplanned, it would be prudent for a woman to consume 0.4 mg of folic acid daily as long as she is capable of becoming pregnant.[10]

QUESTION 5: WHAT ARE THE COMPLICATIONS OF EXCESSIVE FOLIC ACID INTAKE?

The effects of high intakes of folic acid are not well known but include complicating the diagnosis of vitamin B_{12} pernicious anemia. Folic acid may improve the hematologic aspects of pernicious anemia but not the neuropathy, which may progress irreversibly. Only a small percentage of patients present with neuropathy; however, it is usually reversible with vitamin B_{12} treatment.[15] Thus, care should be taken to keep total folic acid consumption at less than 1 mg per day except in patients who have had a previous pregnancy affected with an NTD. Fortification of foods such as bread, flour, and breakfast cereals could increase the bioavailability of folic acid. Folic acid is a water-soluble vitamin; intake of large amounts would be rapidly excreted and probably nontoxic. Fortification of food should be limited to a level that would add 0.1 to 0.2 mg folic acid a day. The overall risk-benefit ratio favors fortification rather than excessive concern about masking the signs and symptoms of vitamin B_{12} deficiency.[28]

QUESTION 6: CAN ADDED FOLIC ACID PREVENT THE FIRST OCCURRENCE OF A NEURAL TUBE DEFECT?

Czeizel and Dudas[5] conducted a randomized, double-blind, controlled study in Hungary to define the extent to which preconceptional folic acid intake along with first-trimester nutrient supplementation with folic acid would reduce the incidence of first occurrences of NTDs among women intending to become pregnant. One group of 2104 received a supplement containing 12 vitamins, minerals, and trace elements, including 0.8 mg of folic acid. This group was compared with 2154 women who received vitamin and trace element supplementation without folate. The incidence of congenital malformation, with six cases of NTDs, was significantly more common in the group receiving no folate supplementation (22.9 per 1000), compared with an incidence of 13.3 per 1000, with no NTDs, in the group whose supplement included folate. A case-control study published in 1993 found a 60% reduction in NTDs among women who used daily vitamins containing folic acid during the periconceptional period; the study documented a significant protective effect of supplements containing 0.4 mg of folic acid.[29]

Like the reduction in the incidence of congenital malformation among diabetic patients whose disease is well controlled before pregnancy, folic acid supplementation is another example of primary prevention of a potentially lethal malformation. This is indeed good news.

QUESTION 7: ARE ANY PARTICULAR MINERALS NECESSARY IN THE DIET TO PREVENT BIRTH DEFECTS?

Considerable interest has developed regarding the significance of zinc deficiency and adverse pregnancy outcome. The RDA for zinc is increased during pregnancy from 3 to 15 mg/day. Like folic acid and iron, zinc must be supplied daily by the diet; it is excreted through the kidneys and sweat glands, so those who participate in strenuous exercise may be deficient in zinc. Because it is difficult to meet the RDA for zinc unless the diet contains some animal protein, vegetarians may be deficient in this mineral.

Zinc deficiency is teratogenic in nonhuman primates, and in Scandinavia, women with low serum levels of zinc had a high incidence of offspring with congenital malformations. Soltan and Jenkins[25] found low plasma zinc concentrations in 54 women who gave birth to malformed offspring. It appears that maternal zinc status may have a direct effect on pregnancy outcome and that information concerning dietary zinc intake should be an important part of a complete nutritional history.

Among poor urban women, marginal zinc intake during pregnancy may be associated with an increased risk of low birthweight and preterm delivery. Scholl and colleagues[22] recently reported that when zinc levels were assessed according to dietary recall, women who had consumed only 40% of the RDA for zinc during pregnancy doubled their risk of bearing a low birthweight or preterm infant, compared with those whose zinc intake was moderate. The investigators noted that the risk for a very low birthweight infant increased more than threefold.

QUESTION 8: CAN EXCESSIVE VITAMIN USE CAUSE ANY PROBLEMS DURING PREGNANCY?

When vitamin preparations are taken, hypervitaminosis can sometimes occur. In the case of water-soluble vitamins, such as folic acid, excess amounts are readily excreted in the urine, so there is not much cause for concern. Fat-soluble vitamins, on the other hand, are not so easily metabolized.

High doses of vitamin E have not been found to be teratogenic in humans.[19] During pregnancy, the RDA for vitamin A is 5000 IU; most prenatal vitamins contain 8000 IU or less. It is possible to increase the daily intake of vitamin A from 4500 to 5000 IU by increasing food intake of deep yellow or green vegetables and orange fruits. Research has shown that offspring of women who take 25,000 to 150,000 IU of vitamin A (retinol or retinyl ester) daily have an increased incidence of fetal growth retardation and urinary tract and central nervous system abnormalities.[2,8,11]

Vitamin A tablets of 25,000 IU are readily available as over-the-counter preparations. Isotretinoin (Accutane, Roche Dermatologics, Nutley, NJ) is an FDA-approved oral vitamin A isomer used in the treatment of severe acne. The drug has been assigned category X risk because it is highly teratogenic to the fetal central nervous system, heart, and skeletal system.[27] The obstetric patient should be advised to bring the multivitamins she is taking to her obstetrician's office so that the total dosage can be calculated and overdose avoided.

REFERENCES

1. American College of Obstetricians and Gynecologists Committee on Obstetrics: Maternal-Fetal Medicine: Committee Opinion 120, *Prevention of neural tube defects*, Washington, DC, 1993.
2. Bernhardt IB, Dorsey DJ: Hypervitaminosis A and congenital renal anomalies in a human infant, *Obstet Gynecol* 43:750, 1974.
3. Centers for Disease Control: Recommendation for the use of folic acid to reduce the number of cases of spina bifida and other neural tube defects, *MMWR* 41:RR-14, 1992.
4. Collaborative study of Down's syndrome using maternal serum alpha-fetoprotein and maternal age, *Lancet* 2:1460, 1986.
5. Czeizel AE, Dudas I: Prevention of first occurrence of neural tube defects by periconceptional vitamin supplementation, *N Engl J Med* 327:1832, 1992.
6. Elwood JM, Little J, Elwood JH: Monographs. In *Epidemiology and biostatistics*, vol 20, New York, 1992, Oxford University Press.
7. Food Labeling: Health claims and label statements; folate and neural tube defects, U. S. Public Health Service, 21CFR, part 101, Docket No. 91H-100H.RIN0905-AB67, 1993.
8. Geelen JA: Hypervitaminosis A induced teratogenesis, *CRC Crit Rev Toxicol* 6:351, 1979.
9. Greenberg F, James LM, Oakley GP: Estimates of birth prevalence rates of spina bifida in the United States from computer-generated maps, *Am J Obstet Gynecol* 145:570, 1982.
10. Grimes DA: Unplanned pregnancies in the United States, *Obstet Gynecol* 67:438, 1986.
11. Hick JB, Evans CA: Growth inhibition and occurrence of cleft palate due to hypervitaminatosis, *Experientia* 37:1189, 1981.
12. Holmes LV: Neural tube defects. In Gastelv-Haddow JE, Fletcher JC, editors: *Maternal serum alpha-feto protein: issues in prenatal screening and diagnosis of neural tube defects*, U.S. Government Printing Office, 1981.
13. Janerich DT: Anencephaly and maternal age, *Am J Epidemiol* 95:319, 1972.
14. Laurence KM, James N, Miller MH: Double blind randomized control study of folate treatment before conception to prevent recurrence of neural tube defects, *Br Med J* 282:1509, 1981.
15. Lindenbaum J, Healton EB, Savage DG, et al: Neural-psychiatric disorders caused by cobalamin deficiency in the absence of anemia or macrocytosis, *N Engl J Med* 318:1720, 1988.
16. Medical Research Council Vitamin Study Research Group: Prevention of neural tube defects: results of the Medical Research Council vitamin study, *Lancet* 338:131, 1991.
17. Milunsky A, Jick H, Jick SS et al: Multivitamin/folic acid supplementation in the earliest weeks of pregnancy reduces the prevalence of neural tube defects, *JAMA* 262:2847, 1989.
18. Robert E, Guibaud P: Maternal valproic acid in congenital neural tube defects, *Lancet* 2:937, 1983.
19. Roberts HJ: Perspectives on vitamin E as therapy, *JAMA* 246:129, 1981.
20. Roza FW: Spina bifida in infants of women treated with carbamazepine during pregnancy, *N Engl J Med* 324:674, 1992.
21. Saunders M: Epilepsy in women of childbearing age: if anticonvulsants cannot be avoided, use carbamazepine, *Br Med J* 299:581, 1989.
22. Scholl TO, Hediger ML, Schall JI, et al: Low zinc intake during pregnancy: its association to preterm and very preterm delivery, *Am J Epidemiol* 137:1115, 1993.
23. Simpson JL, Golbus MS, Martin AO, Sarto GE: Single anatomical malformations usually inherited in polygenic/multifactoral fashion. In *Genetics in obstetrics and gynecology*, New York, 1982, Grune & Stratton.
24. Smithells RW, Nevin NC, Seller MJ et al: Further experience of vitamin supplementation prevention of neural tube defects recurrence, *Lancet* 1:1027, 1983.

25. Soltan MH, Jenkins MH: Maternal and fetal plasma zinc concentrations and fetal abnormalities, *Br J Obstet Gynæcol* 89:56, 1982.

26. Steegers-Theunissen RPM, Boers GHJ, Trijkels FJM, Eskes TCAB: Neural tube defects and derangements of homocysteine metabolism, *N Engl J Med* 324:199, 1991.

27. The public affairs committee and the council of the Teratology Society: The recommendations for isotretinoin in women of childbearing potential, *Teratology* 44:1, 1994.

28. Wald MJ, Bower C: Folic acid, pernicious anemia and prevention of neural tube defects, *Lancet* 343:307, 1994.

29. Werler MM, Shapiro S, Mitchel AA: Periconceptional folic acid exposure and risk of occurrent neural tube defects, *JAMA* 269:1257, 1993.

CHAPTER 2

Diabetes Mellitus
and Pregnancy Outcome

ROBERT C. CEFALO

Much of the reduction in incidence of maternal and perinatal morbidity and mortality associated with insulin-dependent diabetes mellitus (IDDM) has been secondary to advances in antenatal and intrapartum maternal-fetal surveillance, ultrasonography, and neonatal care. This is welcome news, yet the incidence of congenital malformation in infants of insulin-dependent diabetic mothers remains two to three times that of nondiabetic mothers. In infants of mothers with IDDM, congenital malformation is the leading cause of perinatal death. Carbohydrate intolerance affects approximately 1.5 million women of reproductive age in the United States; about 90% of these patients have type II disease, and 10% have insulin-dependent diabetes. Many of the problems seen in infants of insulin-dependent diabetic mothers are the direct result of high maternal blood glucose levels, both during the prepregnancy period and throughout pregnancy.

✤ Patient Profile: Periconceptional glucose control

The patient is a 29-year-old (gravida 1, para 0000) who had her first prenatal visit at 17 weeks' gestation. She is a known type I diabetic who administers 20 units of neutral protamine Hagedorn (NPH) insulin with 5 units of regular insulin every morning. Her evening dose of insulin is inconsistent. Her physician checks her fasting and postprandial blood glucose level every 3 months. She reports that her range is 120 to 140 mg/dl fasting and 180 to 200 mg/dl postprandial. She has had irregular menses, and she did not report her missed menses to her physician, although the physician knew she was attempting to become pregnant.

On physical examination, her uterus was noted to be 18 weeks' size. Ultrasound examination indicated a single fetus with a large thoracolumbar meningomyelocele and fetal cardiac abnormalities suggesting a large ventricular septal defect and single auricle with abnormalities in the outflow tract. The patient's blood glucose level was 220 mg/dl, and her glycosylated hemoglobin was 18.1%. The patient declined a genetic amniocentesis. She was advised that the defects appeared to be incompatible with life, and she decided to terminate the pregnancy. At the patient's 6-week postdelivery check she inquires about what she can do to decrease her risk of having another child with severe malformations.

QUESTION 1: WHAT EVIDENCE EXISTS THAT CONTROL OF BLOOD GLUCOSE IN DIABETIC WOMEN BEFORE AND DURING THE FIRST TRIMESTER OF PREGNANCY IS IMPORTANT IN REDUCING THE CONGENITAL MALFORMATION RATE?

Women with IDDM have offspring with major congenital malformations at a rate two to three times that of women in the general population.[5] The most common types of abnormalities seen in infants of diabetic mothers include ventricular septal defects and neural tube defects; these malformations involve organs that are formed within the first 7 to 8 weeks of gestation, suggesting that preventive strategies must be employed either early in pregnancy or during the preconceptional period. Numerous studies have demonstrated that the increased congenital malformation rate of infants born to mothers with IDDM is significantly reduced when the women are euglycemic during organogenesis (days 17 to 56 postconception).[4,7,12] Because organogenesis begins around day 17 after fertilization, steps to provide the ideal environment for the developing pre-embryo and embryo must be taken before the traditional initiation of prenatal care.

Ideally, the patient's glycosylated hemoglobin (HbA_{1c}) level should be within normal limits for a specific reference laboratory, usually 4% to 8%; this level is generally achieved by maintaining a fasting plasma glucose level of 60 to 100 mg/dl and a 1-hour postprandial level of 120 to 140 mg/dl.[8] Measurement of HbA_{1c} provides a retrospective indication of the degree of hyperglycemia over the past 4 to 6 weeks and provides a tool for investigating the relationship between control of diabetes during early pregnancy and congenital malformation in the offspring.

Oral hypoglycemic agents are potentially teratogenic and should be discontinued before pregnancy and replaced by insulin. Most patients' diabetes can be controlled well using a regimen of 2 to 3 injections of insulin per day. A combination of strict adherence to a prescribed diet and use of NPH and regular insulin effects euglycemia in most patients.

In 1990, Steel and colleagues[12] investigated 143 insulin-dependent diabetic women attending a preconception clinic and 96 insulin-dependent diabetic women not receiving intervention. Compared with the control group, the women attending the preconception clinic had a lower HbA_{1c} concentration during the first trimester of pregnancy and had fewer infants with congenital abnormalities. The authors concluded that tight control of maternal blood glucose during the early weeks of pregnancy can be achieved through a prepregnancy clinic approach.

To determine whether intensive outpatient management of diabetes mellitus before and during early pregnancy would reduce the frequency of major congenital malformation, Kitzmiller and colleagues[7] studied 84 women, all of whom became pregnant, recruited from a preconception clinic and compared them with 110 women who were 6 to 30 weeks pregnant when they registered in the diabetes mellitus program. All women performed daily measurements of fasting and postprandial capillary blood glucose levels; the goals of therapy were to achieve postprandial capillary blood glucose levels of 120 to 140 mg/dl and fasting levels of 60 to 100 mg/dl. Only one major congenital malformation (1.2%) occurred in the group of infants of women treated before conception, compared with 12 infants (10.9%) in the postconception group. The difference was significant. In the latter group, the increased frequency of congenital malformation correlated with increased levels of glycohemoglobin. In the preconception group, 50% of women achieved their goal of euglycemia during the period of organogenesis and 90% had an average plasma glucose level of less than 150 mg/dl. The authors concluded that education and intensive treatment for glycemia control before and during early pregnancy reduce the frequency of major congenital anomalies in infants of diabetic mothers.[7]

QUESTION 2: HOW IS DIABETES MELLITUS CLASSIFIED?

The National Diabetes Data Group[9] introduced a new classification of diabetes in 1979. Among pregnant women, gestational diabetes, type III, constitutes 90% of all diabetic patients, while insulin-dependent diabetes mellitus, type I, and non–insulin-dependent diabetes mellitus (NIDDM), type II, constitute about 10%.

NATIONAL DIABETES DATA GROUP'S CLASSIFICATION OF DIABETES

Type I: insulin-dependent diabetes mellitus (IDDM)

Formerly called *juvenile-onset diabetes, ketosis-prone diabetes*, or *vascular-laden diabetes*.

Type II: non–insulin-dependent diabetes mellitus (NIDDM)

Formerly called *adult-onset diabetes* or *maturity-onset diabetes*. Subclassified as *obese type II* and *nonobese type II*.

Type III: gestational diabetes mellitus (GDM)

Subclassified as *obese type III* and *nonobese type III*.

Type IV: secondary diabetes

Conditions and syndromes associated with impaired glucose tolerance and drug-induced glucose carbohydrate intolerance.

QUESTION 3: WHAT LABORATORY AND DIAGNOSTIC STUDIES SHOULD BE INCLUDED IN THE PRECONCEPTIONAL EVALUATION OF A PATIENT WITH TYPE I DIABETES MELLITUS?

Preconceptional laboratory and diagnostic studies for a diabetic woman should include analysis of a 24-hour urine specimen for creatinine clearance and total protein concentration, an ophthalmologic examination with pupillary dilation, and an electrocardiogram to assess the prospective mother's risk and degree of end-organ damage. While pregnancy does not itself accelerate the natural course of diabetic nephropathy, the complications of pregnancy and the presence of retinopathy and hypertension are serious and potentially life threatening. The risk of pregnancy for diabetic patients who have reduced creatinine clearance and hypertension should be carefully reviewed before conception. Patients should be aware that diabetic retinopathy may either progress or regress during pregnancy, but that no controlled prospective study suggests that pregnancy permanently alters the natural course of the disease.[10] Patients should also be aware that many of the preconceptional tests will be repeated during pregnancy and that serial ultrasound examinations and fetal evaluation tests will also be needed to assess growth and well-being. Because of the increased incidence of neural tube defects in the offspring of diabetic mothers, patients should be started preconceptionally on a prenatal vitamin that contains 0.8 mg folate. Finally, the diabetic patient and her partner should understand that it is not possible to reduce the incidence of congenital malformation to zero, as there is still a 2% to 3% incidence of major congenital malformation in the general population.

QUESTION 4: WHAT ARE THE EFFECTS OF DIABETES ON PREGNANCY AND OF PREGNANCY ON DIABETES?

The fetus of a pregnant diabetic woman is likely to be larger than the average fetus; the cause of this macrosomia is still controversial, but it may be due to fetal hyperglycemia and fetal hyperinsulinemia, both caused by maternal hyperglycemia. Elevated levels of fetal insulin are associated with macrosomia, which may lead to increased maternal morbidity secondary to the more frequent need for cesarean delivery and to increased perinatal morbidity secondary to birth trauma caused by shoulder dystocia. Optimal maternal glucose control with insulin may decrease the incidence of macrosomia, but it is no guarantee.[3] In contrast, women with vascular disease caused by long-standing diabetes may have a higher incidence of growth-retarded babies.

Pregnant diabetic women have a higher incidence of preeclampsia, which may be secondary to a large placenta associated with macrosomia or to inherent vascular disease. They also have an increased incidence of urinary tract infections, which may be secondary to glucosuria. Although pregnancy does not accelerate the natural course of diabetic nephropathy, it is inadvisable in a diabetic patient who has the combination of a creatinine clearance rate $\leq$30 ml/min, a blood urea nitrogen (BUN) value $\geq$30 ml/dl, and hypertension. The course of proliferative diabetic retinopathy suggests that it may either progress or regress during pregnancy, but no controlled prospective study has suggested that pregnancy either permanently accelerates or retards the disease process.[10] Pregnancy does not interfere with laser photocoagulation treatment.[10] Patients with diabetic ischemic heart disease have a high maternal mortality rate, but the number of patients with this complication is small. Therefore, pregnancy is not recommended for a patient with diabetes mellitus and angina pectoris, a prior myocardial infarction, or coronary artery disease.

Because of the hormonally induced peripheral resistance of insulin, requirements for insulin are increased. Episodes of hypoglycemia are more frequent during pregnancy if the prescribed diet is not strictly followed.[1]

QUESTION 5: WHAT ARE THE COMPLICATIONS OF EXCESSIVELY TIGHT GLUCOSE CONTROL?

The couple should understand that proper care of diabetes before and during pregnancy, including extensive glucose monitoring, requires a very cooperative effort. All diabetic patients should adhere strictly to the recommended diet and insulin regimen. Frequently, telephone consultations as well as many visits are necessary.

Because tight control may cause episodes of hypoglycemia, the physician must teach the patient to recognize and treat this state. Mild hypoglycemia is easily treated by the patient and is of no serious consequence, but severe and prolonged hypoglycemia is potentially dangerous. Type 1 diabetics have a blunted adrenergic counterregulatory response to hypoglycemia.[1] A number of patients will have coma, seizures, or motor vehicle accidents. The peak incidence of hypoglycemia is in the first trimester. It is not known whether tight glucose control is additive to these defective counterregulatory mechanisms. The main potential adverse effect of hypoglycemia is maternal; the effect on fetal development is not known. Experimental rat and mice embryos have demonstrated an increased rate of congenital malformation when exposed to hypoglycemic media during critical periods of embryonic development.[11] Therefore, patients on strict caloric and insulin regimens must be especially careful to eat regularly and to learn to recognize hypoglycemic symptoms. Unfortunately, many type 1 diabetics report the peak incidence to be during sleep hours. Patient education includes the use of injectable glucagon and of D-glucose oral tablets; evaluation and, in particular, diet management require a coordinated team approach and continual surveillance. Patients who have repeated episodes of hypoglycemia should consider not driving a car, not operating moving machinery, and not working under conditions in which they could potentially harm themselves or those around them.

QUESTION 6: HOW GREAT IS THE RISK OF TRANSMITTING DIABETES MELLITUS TO ONE'S OFFSPRING?

The exact mechanism of inheritance of insulin-dependent diabetes is not known. It was formerly suggested that the risk of the offspring's inheriting diabetes with one affected parent is in the range of 1% to 6%. Based on more recent information, it has become clear that IDDM is transmitted less frequently to the offspring of diabetic mothers than diabetic fathers: if the mother has IDDM, the chance of her offspring's inheriting the disease is 1%, compared with 6% if the father has diabetes. The high preferential paternal transmission rate may be related to a higher rate of transfer of paternal *DR4* alleles to offspring than that observed in the offspring of *DR4* mothers. Family studies have estimated that the risk of recurrence of IDDM in offspring of families with one affected sibling and unaffected parents is 5% to 6%.[13] Warram and colleagues[14] have further refined the data to indicate a negative correlation between the risk of IDDM in offspring with maternal age at delivery. The author studied 103 families with 304 offspring followed up to the age of 20. These findings were combined with those of a 1984 study of 1391 offspring. The results indicated that the incidence of diabetes mellitus in offspring born to mothers over age 25 at the time of delivery was one fifth that in offspring born to younger mothers. The authors concluded that, in addition to genetic factors, there may be intrauterine determinants of susceptibility to diabetes.[14]

It was previously believed that the offspring of a diabetic mother was approximately three times more likely than a person in the general population to develop the disease at some time. Typing of human leukocyte antigens (HLAs) may allow a more accurate estimate of the risk of diabetes to an individual fetus; studies over the past decade have indicated that type I diabetes is on the major histocompatibility complex marker on chromosome 6.[2]

In contrast to IDDM, there does not appear to be a genetic heterogeneity in non–insulin-dependent diabetes mellitus. The genetic markers for NIDDM have not yet been defined, and there is a special subgroup of people with NIDDM in whom the disease develops not at midlife, but much earlier, in adolescence or young adulthood. Patients in this subgroup are referred to as having *maturity onset diabetes of the young*; this form is transmitted in autosomal dominant fashion, with as many as 50% of the offspring inheriting the disease and manifesting glucose intolerance. The empiric risk of NIDDM relatives' developing the disease is much higher than that of IDDM relatives. When both parents have type II diabetes, the chance of development of the disease is much higher, reaching 60% to 75%.[6]

REFERENCES

1. Bolli G, DeFeo P, Compognucci P et al: Abnormal glucose counterregulation in insulin dependent diabetes mellitus: interaction on anti-insulin antibodies and impaired glucagon and epinephrine secretion, *Diabetes* 32:134, 1983.
2. Cahil CH, McDevitt HO: Insulin-dependent diabetes mellitus: the initial lesion, *N Engl J Med* 304:1454, 1981.
3. Coustan DR: Management of the pregnant diabetic. In Warshaw JB, Hobbins JL, editors: *Principles and practice of perinatal medicine: maternal, fetal and newborn care*, Menlo Park, Calif, 1983, Addison-Wesley.
4. Fuhrman NK, Reiher H, Sennler K et al: The effect of intensified conventional insulin therapy before and during pregnancy on the malformation rate in the offspring of diabetic mothers, *Exp Clin Endocrinol* 83:173, 1984.
5. Gabbe SG, Lowensohn RI, Woo PK et al: Current patterns of neonatal morbidity and mortality in infants of diabetic mothers, *Diabetes Care* 1:335, 1978.
6. Ginsberg-Fellner F, Witt ME, Franklin BH et al: Triad of markers for identifying children at high risk for developing insulin-dependent diabetes mellitus, *JAMA* 254:1469, 1985.
7. Kitzmiller JL, Gabin AL, Gin GD et al: Preconception care of diabetes: glycemic control prevents congenital anomalies, *JAMA* 265:731, 1985.
8. Miller E, Hare JW, Cloherty JP et al: Elevated maternal HbA$_{1c}$ in early pregnancy and major congenital anomalies in infants of diabetic mothers, *N Engl J Med* 304:1331, 1981.
9. National Diabetes Data Group: Classification and diagnosis of diabetes mellitus and other categories of glucose intolerance, *Diabetes* 28:1039, 1979.
10. Singerman LH, Aiello LM, Rodman HM: Diabetic retinopathy: effects of pregnancy on laser therapy, *Diabetes* 29:1, 1980.
11. Smoak JW, Sadler TW: Embryopathic effects of short term exposure to hypoglycemia in mouse embryos in vitro, *Am J Obstet Gynecol* 163:619, 1990.
12. Steel JM, Johnston EFD, Hepburn DA, Smith AF: Can pregnancy care of diabetic women reduce the risk of abnormal babies? *Br Med J* 301:1070, 1990.
13. Warram JH, Karolewski AS, Gottlieb MS, Kahn CR: Differences in risk of insulin-dependent diabetes in offspring of diabetic mothers and diabetic fathers, *N Engl J Med* 311:149, 1984.
14. Warram JH, Martin BC, Karolewski AS: Risk of IDDM in children of diabetic mothers decreases with increasing maternal age at pregnancy, *Diabetes* 40:1679, 1991.

PART TWO

CLINICAL GENETICS
AND GENETIC COUNSELING

CHAPTER 3

Principles of Genetic Counseling

BETH LINCOLN-BOYEA
ROBERT C. CEFALO

Prenatal diagnosis has been called "one of the most powerful advances in medical technology."[7] To most patients, the concepts of mendelian and molecular genetics, cytogenetics, and prenatal diagnosis are foreign and overwhelmingly complex. In contrast, procreation is the most inherent, personal, and emotion-laden aspect of human existence.

To help patients integrate these diverse components in a meaningful way, master's-level genetic counselors combine the use of client-centered counseling techniques with a working knowledge of medical genetics and with extreme sensitivity to the psychosocial and cultural aspects of childbearing and genetic disease. Genetic counselors conduct sessions in a nondirective manner; they support the patient's autonomy by providing timely, accurate, and complete information that is relevant to the patient and her partner. An underlying assumption is that the patient's values, not the professional's, ought to guide decision making.

An important principle in genetic counseling is that genetic or prenatal diagnostic information should not be made available to third parties without the consent of the patient. In exceptional cases, however, the right of confidentiality may be overridden when the following criteria are met: (1) there is a strong probability that identifiable persons will suffer serious harm if the information is withheld; (2) the disclosed information will be used to avert harm; (3) reasonable efforts to elicit voluntary consent to disclosure have failed; and (4) only information necessary to prevent harm will be disclosed.

❧ Patient Profile: Previous child with a birth defect

The patient (gravida 2, para 1000) is 38 years old and reports 8 years of infertility before this pregnancy. She is referred at 18.5 weeks' gestation for counseling regarding the risk of chromosome abnormalities based on her age and for consideration of amniocentesis. At the time of scheduling, the family history was reviewed and was found to be noncontributory. During the genetic counseling session, a detailed three-generation pedigree was obtained. Only then did the patient disclose that her first child, born 22 years earlier, had died shortly after birth and may have had some type of birth defect.

QUESTION 1: WHO SHOULD BE REFERRED FOR GENETIC COUNSELING?

Patients should be offered genetic counseling for a variety of indications (Table 3-1), many of which are identifiable through a routinely applied family and pregnancy history questionnaire and biochemical or genetic screening tests. Among patients of certain ethnic origins, carrier screening for specific autosomal recessive diseases, such as Tay-Sachs disease, thalassemia, or sickle cell disease, is indicated. Patients at increased risk for having a fetus with an open neural tube defect, trisomy 18, or Down syndrome may be identified through maternal serum (MS) screening for α-fetoprotein (AFP), unconjugated estriol (uE_3), and human chorionic gonadotropin (hCG).

Table 3-1   Indications for referral for genetic counseling

I. Positive history

- Multiple spontaneous abortions
- Consanguinity
- Patient, partner, or family member has a birth defect, a known or suspected genetic condition, a chronic neuromuscular or neurologic condition, or abnormalities of physical sexual development
- Ethnic background of one or both parents suggests increased risk for recessive genetic disease

II. Positive screening

- Maternal age ≥35 years at delivery
- Paternal age ≥55 years
- Positive maternal serum screening test for Down syndrome or trisomy 18
- Positive maternal serum screening test for open neural tube defect
- Heterozygous for a recessive disease that is more common in certain ethnic populations

III. Teratogen exposure

- Exposure to a known or suspected teratogenic agent(s)

Chapters 1, 4, 6, 7, 9, and 10 explore these indications for genetic counseling and prenatal diagnosis in detail.

QUESTION 2: WHAT IS THE PURPOSE OF GENETIC COUNSELING?

The goals of genetic counseling have shifted dramatically throughout this century. In the 1910s, genetic "advisors" clearly had eugenic aspirations.[13] Over twenty years ago, Seymour Kessler[10] wrote:

The principal purpose of genetic counseling is the prevention of genetically determined disorders. This is usually accomplished by the provision of information concerning the risks of occurrence or recurrence.

In keeping with attitudinal shifts throughout the field of medicine, genetic counseling has moved away from paternalism and toward patient autonomy. Today, genetic counseling focuses not so much on disease prevention and the greater good of society as on the communication process itself. In 1975, the Ad Hoc Committee on Genetic Counseling of the American Society of Human Genetics agreed upon the following definition of genetic counseling:

> Genetic counseling is a communication process which deals with the human problems associated with the occurrence, or risk of occurrence, of a genetic disorder in a family. This process involves an attempt by one or more appropriately trained persons to help the individual or family (1) comprehend the medical facts, including the diagnosis, the probable course of the disorder, and the available management; (2) appreciate the way heredity contributes to the disorder; (3) understand the options for dealing with the risk of recurrence; (4) choose the course of action which seems appropriate to them in view of their risk and the family goals and act in accordance with that decision; and (5) make the best possible adjustment to the disorder in an affected family member and/or to the risk of recurrence of that disorder.[2]

This definition of genetic counseling evolved from the recognition that life experiences, values, cultural beliefs, and goals vary tremendously among individuals. Because of these differences, the perceived burden of a disease or condition and the perceived magnitude of risk are also highly variable.[3,6,9] For example, the woman described in the patient profile may be more concerned about the risk of miscarriage associated with amniocentesis than would someone who had conceived easily. Similarly, the neonatal death of her first child when the patient was very young may also influence her feelings about pregnancy termination.

QUESTION 3: WHEN SHOULD PATIENTS BE REFERRED FOR GENETIC COUNSELING?

Whenever possible, genetic counseling should be provided before pregnancy. This allows the greatest amount of time to obtain and review necessary medical records, autopsy reports, and other evaluations. In addition, DNA testing on family members can be performed if necessary (e.g., in Duchenne muscular dystrophy families) without the added stress of time limitations imposed by pregnancy. Preconceptional counseling also enables couples with a 25%, 50%, or even 100% risk of conceiving an affected fetus to choose from the greatest variety of reproductive options, including artificial insemination by donor, ovum donation, and adoption.

For some couples, preconceptional counseling and behavior or diet modification can prevent or substantially reduce the risk of birth defects. For example, preconceptional folate supplementation has been shown to reduce the risk of open neural tube defects among offspring of parents who have previously had an affected child (see Chapter 1).[14] In addition, folate supplementation also reduces the incidence of first occurrences of neural tube defects.[5] Abstinence from alcohol consumption during pregnancy eliminates the risk of fetal alcohol syndrome. Smoking cessation decreases the risk of fetal growth retardation, placental abruption, and fetal death. Women with phenylketonuria who resume a diet free of phenylalanine before pregnancy drastically reduce the risk of mental retardation in their children.[11] The ideal is for all patients who are contemplating pregnancy or who have a history of genetic disease to receive preconceptional counseling.[4] Unfortunately, this is not always possible or practical.

Efforts should be made to identify risk factors during a pregnant patient's first prenatal visit. Referral for genetic counseling during the first trimester allows time to perform any necessary additional testing and to obtain and review pertinent medical records. Even a patient for whom the only apparent indication for genetic counseling is increased maternal age benefits from early referral, during the time when she can choose between chorionic villus sampling (CVS) and amniocentesis. In addition, the most routine case can become complex unexpectedly when pedigree analysis reveals a previously unsuspected history of genetic disease.

Because targeted (level II) ultrasound and maternal serum screening for Down syndrome, trisomy 18, and open neural tube defects are performed during the midtrimester, many patients are referred for genetic counseling and consideration of prenatal diagnosis at 16 to 20 weeks' gestation. Regardless of the estimated numeric risk for fetal anomaly, patients whose increased risk was identified through midtrimester screening tests tend to be significantly more anxious than those who were aware of the risk early in pregnancy.[1] In general, genetic counseling and prenatal diagnosis should be timed such that results from prenatal diagnostic tests are available while pregnancy termination remains a legal option. The fetal karyotype determined through amniocentesis may be available in 7 to 14 days, while complex DNA or family studies can take up to 6 weeks. Furthermore, laws regarding pregnancy termination and the interpretation of those laws vary tremendously among states, institutions, and physicians.

Although this patient's referral at 18.5 weeks' gestation is clearly within the prenatal diagnosis "window," it leaves little time to obtain records on her first child. If that child had a neural tube defect, for example, the opportunity to administer effective periconceptional folate supplementation has passed. The option of CVS, which might have appealed to this patient, is no longer available. And finally, in the event of abnormal amniocentesis results, the patient may have little time to decide whether to terminate or to continue this pregnancy.

QUESTION 4: AFTER A PATIENT HAS BEEN REFERRED, WHAT IS THE USUAL PROCESS OF GENETIC COUNSELING?

Information gathering

Precise and useful genetic counseling depends heavily on the accuracy of the clinical diagnosis and screening test results. Before and during the prenatal genetic counseling visit, pertinent information is gathered from a variety of sources, including medical records, autopsy reports, and laboratory results (e.g., maternal serum screening, hemoglobin electrophoresis, and previous chromosome analyses). The pedigree remains one of the most widely used tools in medical genetics. Using fairly standardized notation, genetic counselors use pedigrees to record medical, pregnancy, and social histories for three generations, including siblings, parents, aunts, uncles, cousins, and grandparents. Paternity should be tactfully confirmed.

Risk assessment

The likelihood of conceiving or delivering a baby affected with the birth defect or genetic condition in question is estimated based on population data, pedigree analysis (bayesian analysis), empiric risk data, or some combination of these. This risk can often be mathematically modified by analysis of genetic or biochemical screening test results or detailed ultrasonography or both.

Maternal serum screening for open neural tube defects provides an excellent example of this risk assessment process. The general population risk for a Caucasian couple living in a given region of the United States may be 1 to 2 per 1000 liveborn babies. If the woman's sister had a child with a neural tube defect, that risk rises to 3% to 5%. A normal maternal serum α-fetoprotein (MSAFP) level can be used to adjust this risk downward, while an elevated MSAFP level suggests an even greater risk for an open neural tube defect in the fetus. With a 90% sensitivity and a very low false-positive rate for the identification of neural tube defects, targeted ultrasound examination provides additional data that can be incorporated into the risk estimate.

For patients referred for genetic counseling regarding a condition that has an unclear etiology or for which a diagnosis is uncertain, accurate risk assessment is virtually impossible. These families often must make decisions about pregnancy and invasive testing procedures based on very uncertain risk estimates or wide risk ranges (e.g., 0% to 25%). Prenatal diagnosis is often extremely limited in these cases.

Communication and decision making

After information gathering and risk assessment, genetic counselors focus on communicating this information to the patient in a meaningful way. The clinical aspects of the condition in question are reviewed in detail, including the range of physical and mental disability, life expectancy, and available treatment. This education process also includes actively soliciting and gently correcting misinformation, anticipating questions and concerns, and continually assessing the patient's level of comprehension. The patient is also educated regarding the etiology of the condition in question. This often necessitates a clear, concise explanation of molecular or mendelian genetics and chromosome analysis. Special care must be taken to alleviate any sense of guilt or abnormality that can result from a genetic diagnosis.

Numeric risk information, while crucial for informed decision making, can be very difficult for patients to understand. Genetic counselors often spend a considerable amount of time helping patients to comprehend and frame numeric risks in order to make them personally meaningful. One simple and helpful approach is to express the risk in a variety of ways. A 5% risk of an unfavorable outcome, for example, can also be expressed as a 95% chance of a good outcome or as 1 chance in 20. Representative drawings can also be helpful for patients who have difficulty comprehending risk magnitude. Numeric risks assume meaning to patients according to their own sense of vulnerability to risk, their level of risk taking, and their perception of the burden of the condition in question.[12]

The genetic counselor describes prenatal diagnostic procedures in detail. The risks, benefits, and limitations of diagnostic and screening tests must be explained in a way that enables the patient or couple to make appropriate decisions regarding further testing and to give informed consent. Not only should a patient understand the numeric risk of miscarriage associated with an invasive procedure, but she should also be encouraged to consider the potential emotional repercussions of miscarriage after a voluntary procedure. Decision making regarding invasive prenatal diagnostic testing often involves weighing the level of personal concern regarding the condition in question against the perceived risk of complications related to the procedure. The patient or couple must also consider the usefulness of prenatal diagnostic information: abnormal findings provide the opportunity either to prepare for the birth of a child with special needs or to consider pregnancy termination; normal results give the family tremendous reassurance that significantly reduces anxiety during pregnancy. Many couples who have had an affected child indicate that they would not have attempted a subsequent pregnancy if prenatal diagnosis had not been available. However, many patients have inappropriately high expectations regarding the information obtainable through prenatal testing. Therefore, the limitations and caveats of screening and diagnostic testing should be delineated.

At the time of prenatal diagnosis, the genetic counselor and the patient agree upon how diagnostic test results will be relayed. Although most patients receive reassuring news about the health of their baby, couples should be encouraged to consider what decisions they might make in the event of an abnormal result. Normal results are usually conveyed to the patient by telephone as soon as they are available. Care is taken to disclose results only to the patient, according to the previous agreement. Depending on the situation, the patient may not wish to have the results made available to her partner. Fetal sex, if determined through chromosome analysis, remains undisclosed unless the patient specifically requests this information.

When prenatal diagnosis reveals an affected fetus, the referring physician should be consulted before results are relayed to the patient. Most often, the genetic counselor calls the patient at home in the evening, when her partner is expected to be available. It is preferable to relay abnormal test results early in the week. This allows the patient to return to the medical center for further consultation or confirmatory testing with pertinent specialists within 1 or 2 days. Decision making regarding pregnancy termination or continuation is most effectively facilitated by involvement of several members of the prenatal diagnosis team, which can include the genetic counselor, social worker, clergy member, perinatologist, medical geneticist, cytogeneticist, pertinent pediatric specialists, and the referring obstetrician. The genetic counselor often acts as a liaison between the patient and other members of the team, coordinating consultations, anticipating the patient's questions and concerns, and translating technical or medical language. The counselor-counselee relationship established before the diagnosis becomes invaluable as couples are thrust into one of the most intense crises of their lives. At this point, the counselor's understanding of perinatal grief and appreciation of cultural and religious beliefs greatly enhance his or her effectiveness as a facilitator of decision making.

Follow-up

Regardless of the outcome of prenatal diagnosis or pregnancy, the final task of the genetic counselor is follow-up. This may include a follow-up genetic counseling session at a time when the patient is more able to absorb and understand the information, telephone consultation, and referral to additional medical, social, or counseling services. Every patient who receives genetic counseling should be given a written summary of the counseling session as well as any recommendations for the current pregnancy or for future pregnancies. Recommendations for other family members should also be provided in writing when appropriate, and the patient should be strongly urged to discuss these recommendations with pertinent members of her family. Patients are encouraged to keep this letter of summary with other important documents, since it may be instructive years later.

REFERENCES

1. Abuelo DN, Hopmann MR, Barsel-Bowers G, Goldstein A: Anxiety in women with low maternal serum alpha fetoprotein screening results, *Prenat Diag* 11:381, 1991.
2. Ad Hoc Committee on Genetic Counseling: Genetic counseling, *Am J Hum Genet* 27:240, 1975.
3. Black RB: The effects of diagnostic uncertainty and available options on perceptions of risk, *BD:OAS* XXVVV(5C):341, 1979.
4. Cefalo RC, Moos MK: *Preconceptional health care: a practical guide*, ed 2, St Louis, 1995, Mosby.
5. Czeizel AE, Dudas I: Prevention of the first occurrence of neural tube defects by periconceptional vitamin supplementation, *N Engl J Med* 327:1832, 1992.
6. Ekwo EE, Seals BF, Kim J-O et al: Factors influencing maternal estimates of genetic risk, *Am J Med Genet* 20:491, 1985.
7. Elias S, Annas GJ: Prenatal diagnosis: indications. In *Reproductive genetics and the law*, St. Louis, 1987, Mosby.
8. Hollerback P: Reproductive attitudes and the genetic counselee. In Shia YE et al, editors: *Counseling in genetics*, New York, 1979, Alan R. Liss.
9. Kessler S, Levine EK: Psychological aspects of genetic counseling IV: the subjective assessment of probability, *Am J Med Genet* 28:361, 1987.
10. Kessler S: Introduction to genetic counseling. In Kessler S, editor: *Genetic counseling: psychological dimensions*, New York, 1979, Academic Press.
11. Lenke RR, Levy HL: Maternal phenylketonuria—results of dietary therapy, *Am J Obstet Gynecol* 142:548, 1982.
12. Lippman-Hand A, Fraser FC: Genetic counseling: the postcounseling period: parents' perceptions of uncertainty, *Am J Med Genet* 4:51, 1979.
13. Lubinsky M: Scientific aspects of early eugenics, *J Genet Couns* 1:77, 1993.
14. Wald N: Prevention of neural tube defects: results of the Medical Research Council Vitamin Study, *Lancet* 338:131, 1991.

CHAPTER 4

Increased Maternal Age and Prior Aneuploid Conception

JENNIFER HELWICK SHAFER
JEFFREY A. KULLER

The most common method of genetic screening in pregnant women is assessing the patient's age-related risk for having a child with a birth defect. It has been well established that the risk for chromosome abnormalities in the fetus increases with increasing maternal age. The risk for birth defects other than chromosome abnormalities is fairly consistent regardless of maternal age. The association between increasing maternal age and chromosome abnormalities in the fetus is believed to be related to an increased risk for a nondisjunctional event in the ovum. Because eggs age as a woman ages, they are susceptible to a variety of exposures over a woman's lifetime. These exposures increase the risk for nondisjunction of the chromosomes during cell division and, thus, the risk for a conceptus with an abnormal number of chromosomes (aneuploidy). Genetic screening is also recommended to couples who have had a previous aneuploid conception.

The most common chromosome abnormality in liveborn infants is trisomy 21 (Down syndrome). Trisomy 21 comprises approximately half of all chromosome abnormalities in liveborn infants. Down syndrome is always associated with mental retardation, although the degree of retardation can range from mild to severe. In addition, approximately 50% of children with Down syndrome are born with a congenital heart defect. Mortality for Down syndrome children with congenital heart disease is highest during the first 2 years of life, and only 40% to 60% of these children live to the age of 10. However, especially when not affected by congenital heart disease, many live into adulthood and often past the age of 50.

Other chromosome abnormalities that are associated with increased maternal age are trisomy 18, trisomy 13, 47,XXY (Klinefelter syndrome), 47,XYY, and 47,XXX. Trisomy 18 and trisomy 13 are almost always lethal; babies with either of these chromosome abnormalities are often stillborn or die shortly after birth. However, approximately 10% of babies who are born with trisomy 18 will live past the age of 1 year, and there are a few reports of children with this condition living into their teens. The sex chromosome abnormalities are not associated with mental retardation, although learning disabilities and phenotypic abnormalities are observed in individuals with some of these conditions. Structural chromosome

23

abnormalities, such as deletions, translocations, and inversions, are not associated with increased maternal age.

❧ Patient Profile: Down syndrome recurrence

A 35-year-old woman (gravida 2, para 1001) and her 43-year-old husband seek preconceptional genetic counseling. The couple has a 5-year-old daughter who was born with trisomy 21 Down syndrome. The child is enrolled in an early infant stimulation program and is doing well. The patient and her husband are considering another pregnancy and are concerned about the risk for chromosome abnormalities in any of their future children. They are pleased with their daughter's progress and do not think that they would terminate another pregnancy if the fetus was found to have Down syndrome. However, they would like to be more informed about their risks.

QUESTION 1: WHAT IS THE CAUSE OF DOWN SYNDROME IN OFFSPRING OF WOMEN UNDER THE AGE OF 35?

Trisomy 21 is the most common cause of Down syndrome and occurs as a result of chromosomal nondisjunction in either the egg or the sperm. *Nondisjunction* is the failure of a pair of chromosomes to separate during meiosis. Chromosomal nondisjunction is a random event that occurs more frequently as women get older. However, since it can occur at any time, children with trisomy 21 can be born to women of all ages. The woman described above, for example, was only 30 years old when her daughter was born with trisomy 21. In fact, because most pregnancies occur in younger women, approximately 80% of all babies with trisomy 21 are born to women under the age of 35.

Down syndrome occurs due to trisomy 21 in approximately 95% of all cases. However, the extra number 21 chromosome in Down syndrome can occur as the result of a translocation (rearrangement) in the chromosomes. Translocation Down syndrome is usually inherited from one of the parents, who carries a "balanced" rearrangement in his or her chromosomes and passes it on to the child in an unbalanced form. Chromosome abnormalities other than Down syndrome can also result from translocations. Parents who carry balanced translocations have an increased risk of having children with unbalanced translocations (see Chapter 5). Therefore, it is imperative that the type of Down syndrome or other chromosome abnormality be determined before counseling a patient about her recurrence risk for chromosome abnormalities.

QUESTION 2: AT WHAT AGE DOES A WOMAN BECOME "AT RISK" FOR CHROMOSOME ABNORMALITIES?

The risk for chromosome abnormalities continually increases as a woman ages. This increase is gradual until about the age of 33, when the risk begins to rise at a faster rate (see Tables 4-1 and 4-2). There is no age at which a woman's risk increases considerably. The

Table 4-1   Regression-derived estimated rates per thousand of cytogenetic abnormalities by maternal age at the time of amniocentesis

Maternal age (yr)	47,+21*	47,+18	47,+13†	47,XXX	47,XXY	Other clinically significant abnormalities‡	All abnormalities§
33	2.4	0.3	0.4	0.4	0.4	1.1	4.6-5.4
34	3.1	0.8	0.4	0.5	0.5	1.2	5.8-8.5
35	4.0	1.0	0.5	0.6	0.6	1.3	7.4-8.0
36	5.2	1.3	0.6	0.7	0.8	1.3	9.5-9.9
37	6.7	1.8	0.8	0.8	1.0	1.4	12.1-12.2
38	8.7	2.1	0.7	1.0	1.2	1.5	15.4-15.2
39	11.2	2.6	0.9	1.2	1.5	1.6	19.6-19.0
40	14.5	3.3	1.0	1.4	1.9	1.7	25.0-23.8
41	18.7	4.2	1.1	1.7	2.4	1.8	31.9-29.9
42	24.1	5.2	1.3	2.0	3.0	1.9	40.7-37.8
43	31.1	8.8	1.5	2.4	3.8	2.0	51.9-47.5
44	40.1	8.4	1.8	2.9	4.7	2.2	68.1-80.0
45	51.8	10.8	2.0	3.4	5.9	2.3	84.3-78.0
46	68.8	13.3	2.4	4.1	7.4	2.4	107.5-98.5
47	88.2	18.9	2.7	4.9	9.3	2.6	137.1-122.8
48	111.2	21.3	3.1	5.9	11.7	2.7	174.9-155.9
49	143.5	26.9	3.8	7.0	14.8	2.9	222.9-198.6

*A value of 0.08 per 1000 should be added to this figure to allow for structural rearrangements associated with Down syndrome.

†A value of 0.06 per 1000 should be added to this figure to adjust for structural rearrangements associated with trisomy 13.

‡Includes structural rearrangements associated with trisomy 13 and Down syndrome.

§The first value of the range given is derived from a regression equation analysis on all abnormalities; the second, by adding values for all abnormalities. Including abnormalities of more questionable significance would result in addition of about 2.7 per 1000 at the younger ages (around 35 years) and about 2.1 per 1000 at the older ages to the second values given in the range.

Values extrapolated from regression equation derived for ages 35 to 39 years.

From: Hook EB et al: Chromosomal abnormality rates at amniocentesis and in live-born infants, *JAMA* 249:2034, 1983.

traditional age at which a woman is considered to be at high risk for chromosome abnormalities is 35. This cutoff of age 35 is somewhat arbitrary. It was originally considered to be the cutoff for considering a woman at increased risk for chromosome abnormalities because at the age of 35 the risk for Down syndrome is similar to the generally accepted risk of miscarriage from amniocentesis. However, there are several problems with this logic. First, the risk of miscarriage from amniocentesis can vary from center to center. In addition, it is expected that as a practitioner gains experience with amniocentesis this risk will decrease. Therefore, the risk of miscarriage from amniocentesis can vary even within the same center. Finally, even the risk of chromosome abnormalities in pregnancy can vary, depending on how the data are interpreted. For example, a 35-year-old woman's risk of having a Down

Table 4-2   Regression-derived estimated rates per thousand of cytogenetic abnormalities by maternal age at the time of expected live birth

Maternal age (yr)	47,+21*	47,+18	47,+13†	47,XXX	47,XXY	Other clinically significant abnormalities‡	All abnormalities§
33	1.6	0.2	0.2	0.4	0.4	0.8	2.9-3.5
34	2.0	0.2	0.2	0.5	0.4	0.8	3.7-4.2
35	2.8	0.3	0.3	0.5	0.6	0.9	4.7-5.2
36	3.4	0.4	0.3	0.8	0.7	0.9	5.9-8.4
37	4.4	0.5	0.4	0.8	0.9	1.0	7.8-7.9
38	5.7	0.6	0.4	0.9	1.1	1.0	9.7-9.8
39	7.3	0.8	0.5	1.1	1.4	1.1	12.3-12.1
40	9.4	1.0	0.5	1.3	1.7	1.2	15.7-15.2
41	12.2	1.2	0.6	1.6	2.2	1.2	20.1-19.0
42	15.7	1.6	0.7	1.9	2.7	1.3	25.9-23.9
43	20.2	2.0	0.8	2.2	3.4	1.4	32.8-30.2
44	28.1	2.5	1.0	2.7	4.3	1.5	41.8-38.1
45	33.7	3.2	1.1	3.2	5.4	1.8	53.0-48.2
46	43.4	4.0	1.3	3.8	6.8	1.7	67.8-81.0
47	58.0	5.1	1.5	4.8	8.6	1.8	98.2-77.5
48	72.3	8.4	1.8	5.5	10.7	1.9	109.9-98.5
49	93.3	8.1	2.0	8.5	13.4	2.0	140.1-125.3

*A value of 0.09 per 1000 should be added to this figure to allow for structural rearrangements associated with Down syndrome.

†A value of 0.03 per 1000 should be added to this figure to adjust for structural rearrangements associated with trisomy 13.

‡Includes structural rearrangements associated with trisomy 13 and Down syndrome.

§The first value of the range given is derived from a regression equation analysis on all abnormalities; the second by adding values for all abnormalities. Including abnormalities of more questionable significance would result in addition of about 2.7 per 1000 at the younger ages (around 35 years) and about 2.1 per 1000 at the older ages to the second values given in the range.

Values extrapolated from regression equation derived for ages 35 to 39 years.

From: Hook EB et al: Chromosomal abnormality rates at amniocentesis and in live-born infants, *JAMA* 249:2034, 1983.

syndrome pregnancy detected during the second trimester is approximately 1 in 270. This same woman's risk of having a child with Down syndrome at term is approximately 1 in 365. This is because approximately 30% of Down syndrome pregnancies will be lost between 16 weeks' gestation and delivery. Approximately two thirds of trisomy 18 pregnancies and one third of trisomy 13 pregnancies will be lost during this same time period.

Some investigators think that the risk for chromosome abnormalities other than Down syndrome should be considered when determining at what age a patient should be offered prenatal diagnosis. This method of calculation decreases the age at which a woman's risk of having a child with a chromosome abnormality becomes equal to the risk of amniocentesis. For example, a 33-year-old woman has a risk of approximately 1 in 400 of having a fetus with Down syndrome detected during the second trimester of pregnancy. The risk for any chromosome abnormality to be detected at this time in her pregnancy is approximately 1 in 200 (0.5%). If the risk of miscarriage from amniocentesis is considered to be approximately 0.5%, a statistic quoted by many centers in this country, then it seems reasonable to offer amniocentesis to this patient. However, others argue that the risk for other chromosome abnormalities should not be considered because these conditions are either lethal, such as trisomy 18 and trisomy 13, or relatively less severe than Down syndrome, such as the sex chromosome abnormalities.

Although the determination of age 35 has been arrived at somewhat arbitrarily, it is still the traditional age at which women are considered to be at increased risk for chromosome abnormalities. The American College of Obstetricians and Gynecologists (ACOG) recommends that all women who will be age 35 and over at the time of delivery be offered amniocentesis during pregnancy.

QUESTION 3: DOES HAVING A PREVIOUS CHILD OR FETUS WITH TRISOMY 21 INCREASE THE RISK FOR CHROMOSOME ABNORMALITIES IN FUTURE PREGNANCIES?

Whenever a couple has a child with trisomy 21 or another genetic abnormality caused by chromosomal nondisjunction, as does the couple described in this patient profile, they are at an increased risk over the woman's age-related risk of having another child with a chromosome abnormality if the woman is under 35. This risk is approximately 1% until she reaches the age of 35. The woman in the patient profile is 35 years old and, because of her age, already has approximately a 1% chance of having a child with a chromosome abnormality. The fact that she has a previous child with Down syndrome does not increase this risk. When the mother reaches the age of 35, the risk of aneuploidy increases with the mother's age-related risk.

If a couple has had a previous child with trisomy 21 Down syndrome, their risk for chromosome abnormalities in future pregnancies includes not only Down syndrome but also trisomy 18, trisomy 13, and various sex chromosome abnormalities. This is because such couples appear to have an increased risk for nondisjunction of any of the chromosomes in the egg or sperm.

QUESTION 4: WHAT EFFECT DOES PATERNAL AGE HAVE ON THE RISK FOR CHROMOSOME ABNORMALITIES?

It has been demonstrated that nondisjunction of the chromosomes can occur in either the egg or the sperm. This knowledge prompted researchers to study the possibility of an association between an increased risk for chromosome abnormalities and increased paternal age. A few studies have shown that there is a slightly increased risk for chromosome abnormalities in pregnancies in which the father is over the age of 55. Other reports have failed to confirm these findings. If such a risk does exist, it is likely to be small.

There are sufficient data to indicate that advanced paternal age is associated with an increased risk for new autosomal dominant mutations in the offspring. This risk is slightly higher in fathers over the age of 50 than in younger fathers. The large number of different autosomal conditions that can arise from these mutations does not allow for any specific prenatal diagnosis.

REFERENCES

1. Erickson JD: Down syndrome, paternal age, maternal age and birth order, *Ann Hum Genet* 41:289, 1978.
2. Erickson JD: Paternal age and Down syndrome, *Am J Hum Genet* 31:489, 1979.
3. Hook EB, Chambers GM: Estimated rates of Down syndrome in live births by one year maternal age intervals for mothers aged 20-49 in a New York State study—implications of the risk figures for genetic counseling and cost-benefit analysis of prenatal diagnosis programs. In Bergsma D, Lowry RB: The National Foundation March of Dimes *Numerical taxonomy of birth defects and polygenic disorders*, New York, 1977, Alan R. Liss.
4. Hook EB, Lindsjo A: Down syndrome in live births by single year maternal age intervals in a Swedish study: comparison with results from a New York State study, *Am J Hum Genet* 30:19, 1978.
5. Hook EB et al: Paternal age and Down syndrome in British Columbia, *Am J Hum Genet* 33:123, 1981.
6. Hook EB: Rates of chromosome abnormalities at different maternal ages, *Obstet Gynecol* 58:282, 1981.
7. Hook EB et al: The natural history of cytogenetically abnormal fetuses detected at midtrimester amniocentesis which are not terminated electively: new data and estimates of the excess and relative risk of late fetal death associated with 47,+21 and some other abnormal karyotypes, *Am J Hum Genet* 45:855, 1989.
8. Hook EB: Chromosome abnormalities and spontaneous fetal death following amniocentesis: further data and associations with maternal age, *Am J Hum Genet* 35:110, 1983.
9. Matsunaga E et al: Reexamination of paternal age effect in Down's syndrome, *Hum Genet* 40:259, 1978.
10. Regal RR et al: A search for evidence for a paternal age effect independent of a maternal age effect in birth certificate reports of Down's syndrome in New York State, *Am J Epidemiol* 112:650, 1980.
11. Stene J et al: Paternal age effect in Down's syndrome, *Ann Hum Genet* 40:299, 1977.

CHAPTER 5

Evaluation of Translocations, Inversions, and Markers Found at the Time of Prenatal Diagnosis

CARLA BOOR SMITH
JEFFREY A. KULLER
KATHLEEN W. RAO

Most couples who elect to have prenatal diagnosis do so because of concern about the more common chromosome abnormalities, such as Down syndrome. However, unexpected chromosome abnormalities are sometimes found, including structural rearrangements such as translocations and inversions. These structural rearrangements are detected in approximately 1 of every 300 amniocenteses.[12] Supernumerary marker chromosomes are found in about 1 in 1000 amniocenteses.[7] When a translocation, inversion, or marker chromosome is detected during prenatal diagnosis, it is imperative to rapidly perform parental chromosome analysis. This is because the risk for birth defects or mental retardation or both depends on whether a chromosomal rearrangement is familial or de novo (an event occurring for the first time in the patient or fetus being studied). This information is also important for appropriate counseling of patients and their families regarding future pregnancies.

❦ Patient Profile: Balanced reciprocal translocation discovered at amniocentesis

A 38-year-old woman (gravida 2, para 0010) seeks genetic counseling at 15 weeks' gestation for increased maternal age. She elects to undergo amniocentesis, and at 17 weeks' gestation the completed chromosome analysis indicates that the fetus has an "apparently" balanced reciprocal translocation. Subsequent parental chromosome analysis indicates that the pregnant mother carries the same translocation. The patient and her husband have many questions about the risks to the fetus in this pregnancy and in future pregnancies.

29

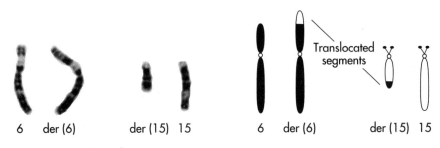

Fig. 5-1 A reciprocal translocation.

QUESTION 1: WHAT IS THE RISK TO THE FETUS WHEN A TRANSLOCATION IS DISCOVERED PRENATALLY?

The fetal and maternal karyotypes reveal reciprocal translocations (rcp's), which occur when two different (nonhomologous) chromosomes break and exchange material (Figure 5-1). A translocation is considered *balanced* when no apparent loss or gain of genetic material has occurred. Therefore, a balanced translocation carrier is usually phenotypically normal. When a reciprocal translocation is discovered prenatally, predictions about the risk to the fetus cannot be made until parental chromosome studies have been completed. If one parent carries the same translocation, the fetus is not at increased risk for abnormalities.[14] However, if the translocation is de novo, studies demonstrate that the risk for birth defects or mental retardation or both is in the range of 6% to 10%.[13] Although no genetic material appears to be missing on cytogenetic analysis, this risk still exists because of the inability to detect submicroscopic abnormalities that may have been caused by the new chromosome breakage. If a de novo reciprocal translocation involves more than two chromosomes, the risk to the fetus is probably even higher.[1]

QUESTION 2: WHAT IS THE RISK TO FUTURE PREGNANCIES WHEN A CHROMOSOME REARRANGEMENT IS DISCOVERED?

To determine the risk to future pregnancies, the specific rearrangement must be further evaluated. If one parent carries a balanced translocation, a variety of chromosomal outcomes are possible, depending on the results of segregation during meioses of the chromosomes involved in the translocation.[3] Generally, translocations in which the breaks occur close to the centromeres, causing the exchange of entire arms of each chromosome, are more likely to result in fetal or neonatal death or spontaneous abortion. In translocations in which at least one of the translocated segments is small, unbalanced viable pregnancy outcomes are possible. Therefore, it is necessary to search the literature to determine whether there have been reports of liveborn offspring who carry rearrangements similar to the one in question.

The mode of detection also is important. If a rearrangement was detected through the birth of a previous child with a chromosome imbalance, the family history alone proves that it could recur. In other cases, when a rearrangement is detected through recurrent miscarriage, infertility, or prenatal diagnosis, there may still be the possibility of having a liveborn child with an unbalanced karyotype.[6] Studies have shown that when a rearrangement is detected through chromosome analysis of a previous affected child, the risk of detecting an unbalanced karyotype through amniocentesis is higher than when a rearrangement is detected through recurrent miscarriage.[4]

A familial reciprocal translocation, then, must be extensively researched in order to appropriately counsel a couple and family members regarding the risk to future pregnancies. For a de novo reciprocal translocation, the risk for recurrence is small.[6]

QUESTION 3: WHAT ARE THE RISKS WHEN A ROBERTSONIAN TRANSLOCATION IS DISCOVERED AT THE TIME OF AMNIOCENTESIS?

Robertsonian translocations (rob's) result when two acrocentric chromosomes fuse (Figure 5-2). The acrocentric chromosomes, in which the centromeres are positioned near the ends of the chromosomes, include numbers 13, 14, 15, 21, and 22. In these chromosomes, the short arm (p) appears to carry no critical genetic information. Robertsonian translocations are among the most common types of chromosome rearrangements and are found in about 1 in 1000 amniocenteses.[8] These rearrangements can involve two different (nonhomologous) acrocentric chromosomes or two of the same (homologous) acrocentric chromosomes. Unlike de novo reciprocal translocations, de novo balanced Robertsonian translocations are not believed to increase the risk for abnormalities in the carrier fetus.[13] The risk to future pregnancies when one parent carries a familial Robertsonian translocation depends on which chromosomes are involved in the translocation and on which parent is the balanced carrier.

Of the Robertsonian translocations involving the nonhomologous chromosomes, the most common is the 13;14 translocation. In theory, a 13;14 translocation carrier has the potential for any one of three viable pregnancy outcomes: a child with normal chromosomes, a child who is a balanced carrier like the parent, or a child with translocation trisomy 13. There is, therefore, a theoretic 1 in 3 risk for an abnormal fetus. All other possible chromosome combinations are nonviable and result in spontaneous abortion. However, observation of pregnancy outcomes in many families in which one parent is a carrier of the 13;14

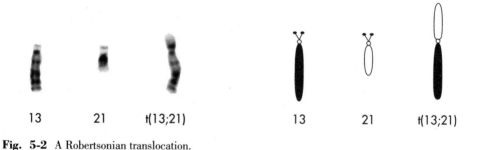

13   21   t(13;21)   13   21   t(13;21)

Fig. 5-2 A Robertsonian translocation.

translocation indicates that the actual (empiric) risk of having a liveborn child with translocation trisomy 13 is approximately 1%.[5]

When a fetus is diagnosed with Robertsonian translocation Down syndrome, it is imperative to differentiate between a familial and a de novo origin in order to determine risks to future pregnancies. With de novo translocation Down syndrome, the risk of recurrence is probably less than 1%.[6] However, if the mother carries a 14;21 Robertsonian translocation, the risk of detecting translocation Down syndrome in a subsequent pregnancy at the time of amniocentesis is approximately 10% to 15%. If the father is the carrier, the risk is lower, at about 3% to 5%.[5] When a parent is a carrier of a homologous 21;21 Robertsonian translocation, the risk of having a fetus with Down syndrome in any future pregnancy is 100%. The other possible chromosome imbalance would result in monosomy 21 and an early spontaneous abortion.[6]

The risk associated with a Robertsonian translocation varies, then, depending on which acrocentric chromosomes are involved in the translocation. For example, a Robertsonian translocation involving chromosome 21 indicates a greater likelihood of a viable outcome than a Robertsonian translocation involving chromosomes 13, 14, or 15. The risk that the fetus will inherit an unbalanced rearrangement is also greater when the mother, rather than the father, is the translocation carrier. Robertsonian translocation carriers also have an increased risk for miscarriage.

QUESTION 4: WHAT ARE THE RISKS WHEN AN INVERSION IS DISCOVERED AT THE TIME OF AMNIOCENTESIS?

An inversion (inv) occurs when a single chromosome breaks in two places and the broken pieces reunite in such a way that the segment between the two breakpoints is inverted or reversed relative to its original position. When the inverted area includes the centromere, it is called a *pericentric inversion*. A *paracentric inversion* occurs when the centromere is not part of the inversion (Figure 5-3). The human genome contains common variant inversions that do not appear to be associated with an increased risk for abnormalities. For example, the

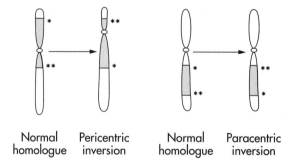

Normal   Pericentric   Normal   Paracentric
homologue   inversion   homologue   inversion

Fig. 5-3 Pericentric (left) and paracentric (right) inversions. The inverted segments are shaded. (From Gardner RJM, Sutherland GR: *Chromosome abnormalities and genetic counseling*, New York, 1989, Oxford University Press.)

common pericentric inversion of chromosome 9 [inv(9)(p11q12)] does not appear to increase the risk for abnormalities. Therefore, when a common variant inversion is prenatally diagnosed, karyotyping of the parents is rarely required.[6]

As with other types of chromosome rearrangements, parental karyotypes are needed for risk assessment when a less common inversion is diagnosed through amniocentesis. With a de novo inversion, the risk for birth defects or mental retardation or both is 9% to 10%.[13] A balanced familial pericentric inversion probably does not increase the risk for abnormalities in a carrier fetus. However, a recently published large review of paracentric inversions indicates that there may be a significant risk for birth defects or mental retardation or both in carrier fetuses, even for familial balanced paracentric inversions.[10]

A pericentric inversion carrier has an increased risk of having abnormal offspring as a result of crossover between the normal and the inverted chromosome. A pregnancy could result in a baby with partial trisomy or partial monosomy or both. If the inversion breakpoints are near the chromosome ends, there may be a significant risk for having a liveborn infant with a chromosome imbalance. If the breakpoints are proximal (closer to the centromere), the greatest risk may be for miscarriage.

Paracentric inversions are rarer than translocations, and pericentric inversions and their consequences are not as well understood. In general, the carriers of paracentric inversions appear to have a relatively low risk of having a child with an unbalanced karyotype secondary to the inversion. Such cases, however, have been reported in the literature. The actual magnitude of the risk probably depends on the location of the chromosomal breakpoints of the inversion and on the sex of the carrier parent.[6]

QUESTION 5: WHAT ARE THE RISKS WHEN A MARKER CHROMOSOME IS DISCOVERED AT THE TIME OF AMNIOCENTESIS?

A *marker chromosome* is a small extra chromosome of unknown cytogenetic origin. A marker chromosome can be inherited from a parent, can be de novo (sporadic), or can be the result of malsegregation in the gametes of a balanced translocation carrier. The latter two types are associated with an increased risk for abnormalities. Risks associated with inherited marker chromosomes vary, depending on the composition and mitotic stability of the marker and on the phenotype of the carrier parent.[11]

A de novo marker chromosome detected at amniocentesis poses an overall risk of about 13% of causing fetal abnormalities. Interestingly, this risk does not appear to be significantly different for mosaic versus nonmosaic cases.* The risk associated with nonsatellited markers appears to be higher than the risk associated with satellited markers.† To determine a specific risk, it is imperative to evaluate further the size and origin of the marker.[13]

---

*The term *mosaic* is used to describe an individual or a tissue that has at least two cell lines differing in genotype or karyotype but derived from a single zygote.

†*Satellites* are dark-staining regions attached to the ends of the short arms of the acrocentric chromosomes.

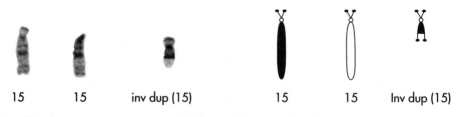

| 15 | 15 | inv dup (15) | 15 | 15 | Inv dup (15) |

Fig. 5-4 A submetacentric inverted duplication 15 (inv dup 15).

The most common marker chromosome is the inverted duplication 15 (inv dup 15), which comprises approximately half of all marker chromosomes.[2] As with other marker chromosomes, if this marker is familial, the risk to the pregnancy is variable. When a de novo inv dup 15 occurs, evaluation of the specific breakpoints is essential. A small metacentric inv dup 15, in which the breakpoint is close to the centromere, contains mostly heterochromatin (apparently inactive DNA) and can be associated with a normal phenotype. A larger submetacentric inv dup 15, in which the breakpoint is more distal, poses a high risk for mild to severe mental retardation, generally with no significant physical anomalies[9] (Figure 5-4).

QUESTION 6: WHEN A FAMILIAL CHROMOSOME REARRANGEMENT IS DISCOVERED, WHO SHOULD BE OFFERED TESTING?

When a familial chromosome rearrangement is diagnosed, additional family members should also be offered chromosome analysis. Some chromosome rearrangements can be inherited for many generations before being detected. Although certain family members may be past childbearing age, they should still consider being tested to determine whether their children are at risk for having reproductive problems. When a person of childbearing age is found to carry a balanced rearrangement, prenatal testing for future pregnancies is available to rule out unbalanced chromosome rearrangements in a fetus. For couples at risk, chorionic villus sampling (CVS) or amniocentesis is available. Other options include using a donor egg or sperm. In the case of a previous pregnancy with a de novo chromosome rearrangement, in which the recurrence risk is small, couples may still opt for prenatal diagnosis in future pregnancies because of the reassurance it can provide.

REFERENCES

1. Bogart MH, Bradshaw CL, Jones OW, Schanberger JE: Prenatal diagnosis and follow-up of a child with a complex chromosome rearrangement, *J Med Genet* 23:180, 1986.
2. Buckton KE, Spowart G, Newton MS, Evans HJ: Fourty-four probands with an additional "marker" chromosome, *Hum Genet* 69:353, 1985.
3. Burns JP, Kodru PRK, Alonso ML, Chaganti RSK: Analysis of meiotic segregation in a man heterozygous for two reciprocal translocations using the hamster in vitro penetration system, *Am J Med Genet* 38:954, 1986.
4. Daniel A, Boué A, Gallano P: Prospective risk in reciprocal translocation heterozygotes at amniocentesis as determined by potential chromosome imbalance sizes. Data of the European collaborative prenatal diagnosis centres, *Prenat Diagn* 6:315, 1986.

5. Ferguson-Smith MA: Prenatal chromosome analysis and its impact on the birth incidence of chromosome disorders, *Br Med Bull* 39:355, 1983.
6. Gardner RJM, Sutherland GR: *Chromosome abnormalities and genetic counseling*, New York, 1989, Oxford University Press.
7. Hook EB, Cross PK: Extra structurally abnormal chromosomes (ESAC) detected at amniocentesis: frequency in approximately 75,000 prenatal cytogenetic diagnoses and associations with maternal and paternal age, *Am J Hum Genet* 40:83, 1987.
8. Hook EB, Cross PK: Rates of mutant and inherited structural cytogenetic abnormalities detected at amniocentesis: results on about 63,000 fetuses, *Ann Hum Genet* 51:27, 1987.
9. Maraschio M, Cuoco C, Gimelli G et al: The cytogenetics of mammalian autosomal rearrangements. In Sandberg AA, editor: *Progress and topics in cytogenetics*, New York, 1988, Alan R. Liss.
10. Pettenati PN, Rao MC, Phelan MC et al: Paracentric inversions in humans: a review of 446 paracentric inversions with presentation of 120 new cases, *Am J Med Genet* 55:171, 1995.
11. Stamburg J, Thomas GH: Unusual supernumerary chromosomes: types encountered in a referred population, and high incidence of associated maternal chromosome abnormalities, *Hum Genet* 72:140, 1986.
12. Van Dyke DL, Weiss L, Roberson JR, Babu VR: The frequency and mutation rate of balanced autosomal rearrangements in man estimated from prenatal genetic studies for advanced maternal age, *Am J Hum Genet* 35:301, 1983.
13. Warburton D: De novo balanced chromosome rearrangements and extra marker chromosomes identified at prenatal diagnosis: clinical significance and distribution of breakpoints, *Am J Hum Genet* 49:995, 1991.
14. Weiss L, Van Dyke DL, Roberson J: The risk of mental retardation/multiple congenital anomalies (MR/MCA) related to de novo chromosome rearrangements: a first-order approximation, *Pediatr Res* 17:221A, 1983.

Evaluation of Fragile X Syndrome and Other Causes of Mental Retardation

NANCY P. CALLANAN
JEFFREY A. KULLER

The evaluation of a pregnant patient who has a family history of mental retardation requires careful pedigree analysis, medical record review to document the phenotype of each affected relative, and clinical evaluation or laboratory investigation of the patient and, when possible, each affected relative. The goals of this evaluation are the following: (1) to provide accurate risk assessment and genetic counseling; (2) to perform appropriate carrier testing when indicated; and (3) to identify genetic abnormalities for which prenatal diagnosis is available. This task can be complicated in that there are multiple causes of mental retardation. Genetic forms of mental retardation can be caused by chromosome disorders or can be inherited as autosomal dominant, autosomal recessive, X-linked, or multifactorial traits. Genetic conditions associated with mental retardation include inborn errors of metabolism, hereditary degenerative disorders, primary central nervous system defects, and some malformation syndromes. Mental retardation can also be caused by intrauterine infection or other teratogenic exposures or by postnatal illness or injury.[1] The most common nongenetic cause of mental retardation is the fetal alcohol syndrome.

When a patient's family history includes a mentally retarded relative with a specific diagnosis (e.g., Down syndrome or fragile X syndrome) that can be documented by medical records, including results of cytogenetic or molecular analysis, appropriate genetic counseling, carrier testing, or prenatal diagnosis can be initiated. Unfortunately, the more common situation is for a patient to report a family history that includes a relative or relatives with mental retardation of unknown cause. The following patient profiles illustrate essential components of the evaluation of this type of history and some of the factors that can enhance or limit the practitioner's ability to provide accurate risk assessment, counseling, and testing.

❧ Patient Profile: Evaluation of mentally retarded family members

A 22-year-old patient (gravida 1, para 0000) (IV:8) seeks obstetric care at 8 weeks' gestation. She mentions that she has two cousins with "Down syndrome" (IV:2 and IV:4) and wonders whether she has an increased risk for this condition in her offspring.

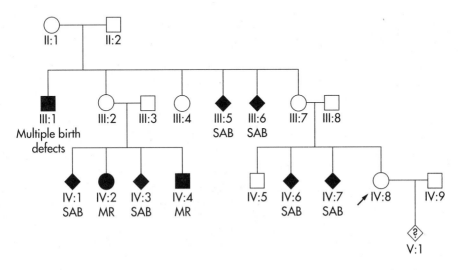

Fig. 6-1 Pedigree from *Patient Profile: Evaluation of mentally retarded family members. SAB*, spontaneous abortion; *MR*, mental retardation.

QUESTION 1: WHAT IS THE RISK FOR DOWN SYNDROME IN THE OFFSPRING OF RELATIVES OF AN AFFECTED PERSON?

Approximately 95% of all cases of Down syndrome are caused by nondisjunctional meiotic errors.[11] The empiric recurrence risk for trisomy 21 due to nondisjunction is 1% to 2%.[3] The risk for nondisjunctional Down syndrome in the offspring of other first- and second-degree relatives (siblings, aunts, and uncles) may be slightly increased.[9] There does not appear to be a significantly increased risk for Down syndrome in the offspring of more distant relatives.

Approximately 5% of cases of Down syndrome are caused by chromosome translocations, about a third of which are inherited from a carrier parent.[11] It is important, therefore, to differentiate between nondisjunctional trisomy 21 and Down syndrome caused by unbalanced chromosome translocations. Medical records, including results of chromosome analysis, should be requested for each affected relative. If it can be documented that the affected relatives of the patient in the case presented here had nondisjunctional trisomy 21, then she can be reassured that she does not have a significantly increased risk of having a child with Down syndrome.

QUESTION 2: WHAT IF MEDICAL RECORDS ARE NOT AVAILABLE OR THE AFFECTED RELATIVES WERE NOT KARYOTYPED?

The main issue here is the accuracy of the diagnosis of Down syndrome in the relatives. Patients frequently misuse the term "Down syndrome" to describe any form of mental retardation. Asking for descriptions of the affected relatives or having photographs reviewed by a medical geneticist experienced in dysmorphology can sometimes be helpful. It is inappropriate to provide risk assessment and genetic counseling without documentation of the relatives' diagnoses.

Careful review of the family history is essential in the evaluation of a family history of mental retardation. In this example, review of the family history (see Figure 6-1) revealed that the patient's mother (III:7) and maternal aunt (III:2) had histories of unexplained miscarriages. Furthermore, her maternal grandmother (II:1) had a history of miscarriages and a stillborn infant with multiple birth defects (III:1). The patient was able to provide photographs of her affected cousins. In fact, the clinical history and physical features of each cousin were not consistent with the diagnosis of Down syndrome. This family history suggested a possible familial chromosome translocation, and a blood karyotype revealed that the patient was a carrier of a balanced translocation. Genetic counseling and chromosome analysis were recommended for other at-risk relatives.

QUESTION 3: WHAT ARE THE REPRODUCTIVE RISKS AND OPTIONS FOR CARRIERS OF BALANCED CHROMOSOME TRANSLOCATIONS?

Balanced translocation carriers have an increased risk for early miscarriage and for having liveborn infants with unbalanced translocations and their associated birth defects and mental retardation. The specific risk depends on the nature of the translocation, the mode of ascertainment, and the family history, but it is generally in the range of 3% to 30%.[2] Translocation carriers should be offered prenatal diagnosis by chorionic villus sampling (CVS) or amniocentesis. Furthermore, genetic counseling and chromosome analysis should be recommended for relatives of translocation carriers. Patients who are found to be translocation carriers should be encouraged to share this information with their families so that they can seek medical attention.

In this patient profile, careful review of the family history resulted in appropriate laboratory testing, genetic counseling, and accurate risk assessment for the patient.

❧ Patient Profile: Testing for fragile X syndrome

A 30-year-old patient (gravida 2, para 1001) (III:3) seeks prenatal care at 12 weeks' gestation. The patient's 2-year-old son (IV:3) is demonstrating moderately delayed language develop-

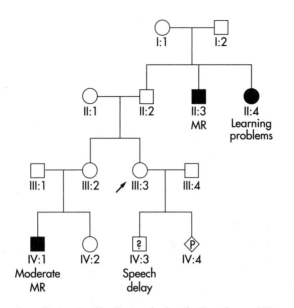

Fig. 6-2 Pedigree from *Patient Profile: Testing for fragile X syndrome. MR,* mental retardation.

ment, for which he receives speech therapy. The patient's sister (III:2) has a 7-year-old son (IV:1) with moderate mental retardation. A paternal uncle is mentally retarded (IV:1), and a paternal aunt (II:4) has a learning disability (see Figure 6-2). The speech therapist has suggested that the patient's son be evaluated for fragile X syndrome. The patient and her husband request information about fragile X syndrome and wonder whether prenatal diagnosis of this condition is possible.

QUESTION 1: WHAT IS FRAGILE X SYNDROME?

Fragile X syndrome is the most common inherited cause of mental retardation, with an estimated frequency of 1 in 1100 to 1 in 1500 males and 1 in 2000 to 1 in 3000 females.[11] Down syndrome is the single most common genetic cause of mental retardation but, as previously stated, is rarely inherited. Fragile X syndrome is inherited as an X-linked dominant trait with incomplete penetrance. Several unusual aspects of the inheritance of fragile X syndrome were described by Sherman and colleagues.[7,8] Approximately 30% of carrier females are clinically affected, and 20% of carrier males show no clinical expression of the disorder (called *normal-transmitting males [NTMs]*). These NTMs pass the gene to all of their daughters, who themselves are clinically unaffected but can have clinically affected sons. It was also observed that the risk for mental retardation in both males and females was greater in the offspring of clinically affected females and of females with clinically affected siblings.

Affected males have normal growth but relatively large heads, connective tissue abnormalities, and developmental and behavioral abnormalities. Characteristic physical features, such as a long face, prominent forehead, large ears, and macroorchidism, become more apparent after puberty. Many affected males are hyperactive and have speech characterized by perseveration. Autistic behavior may also be seen in some patients. Clinically affected females may have similar features, but the expression is generally milder than in affected males.

Fragile X syndrome is associated with a folate-sensitive, cytogenetically identifiable fragile site at band Xq27.3. Cytogenetic testing for fragile X can identify most clinically affected males, but NTMs and a significant proportion of carrier females cannot be identified by cytogenetic testing.[10]

The fragile X gene (*FMR-1*), isolated in 1991,[6,12,13] contains a region of unstable DNA with a $(CGG)_n$ repeat sequence. Amplifications of the CGG repeat sequence are associated with clinical expression of fragile X syndrome. Therefore, the preferred test for fragile X is now molecular rather than cytogenetic.

Two classes of mutations in the *FMR-1* gene have been identified. The normal variation in the number of CGG repeats ranges from 6 to 45 copies. Small amplifications (50 to 230 copies) represent premutations that are not usually associated with clinical expression of the fragile X phenotype and are found in NTMs and in many carrier females. Larger amplifications (>230 copies) represent full mutations and are found in clinically affected males and females and in some carrier females.[10] About 50% of carrier females with full mutations are clinically affected.[6] Premutations appear to remain stable during spermatogenesis, but amplification to the full mutation range can occur during oogenesis. In the carrier female, the risk of amplification from premutation to full mutation varies with the size of the premutation. A female premutation carrier can, therefore, have clinically affected sons or daughters, but can also transmit the premutation in a stable form.[10]

QUESTION 2: WHEN IS IT APPROPRIATE TO SCREEN FOR FRAGILE X SYNDROME?

Fragile X testing should be considered in males and females with developmental delay or mental retardation of unknown cause, especially if there is a family history of mental retardation or developmental delay. The fact that the physical abnormalities associated with fragile X syndrome are subtle, especially in young children, makes it difficult to diagnose fragile X clinically. Unless a family history of fragile X syndrome can be confirmed by laboratory studies, fragile X testing should be performed in combination with routine chromosome analysis to identify individuals whose mental retardation is caused by detectable chromosome abnormalities.[5,10]

QUESTION 3: IS ACCURATE PRENATAL DIAGNOSIS AVAILABLE FOR FRAGILE X SYNDROME?

Prenatal diagnosis of fragile X syndrome by amniocentesis is available. Chorionic villus sampling is a less ideal means of testing because of the possibility of obtaining inconclusive molecular results. Women who are identified as carriers of a premutation or a full mutation in the *FMR-1* gene are candidates for prenatal diagnosis. Because experience with prenatal diagnosis by DNA analysis is limited, the current recommendation is that testing be performed by both cytogenetic methods and DNA analysis.[10]

The couple described in this profile should be encouraged to have their son tested for fragile X syndrome and for other chromosome abnormalities. If the diagnosis of fragile X syndrome is confirmed in the child, prenatal diagnosis can be offered. In addition, genetic counseling and carrier testing should be offered to appropriate relatives when such a diagnosis is made.

❧ Patient Profile: Family history of mental retardation

A 22-year-old woman (gravida 1, para 0000) (III:4) seeks prenatal care at 16 weeks' gestation. As indicated in her pedigree (Figure 6-3), she has a maternal first cousin (III:2) with mental retardation. Her partner has a paternal first cousin (III:5), a maternal first cousin (III:8), and a maternal aunt (II:9) with mental retardation. All of the affected relatives live out of state. The couple is not able to provide specific details about the clinical status of their affected relatives, and they are not willing to request medical records because they do not wish their families to know about the pregnancy. They are concerned about the risk for mental retardation in their offspring and request amniocentesis for reassurance. Because of the advanced gestational age, the time available for evaluation is limited.

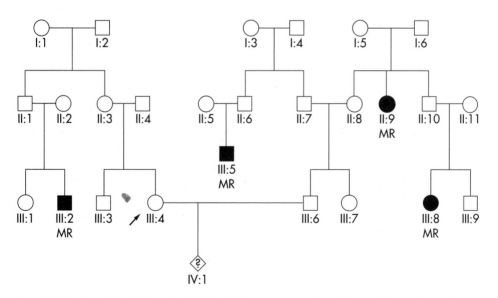

Fig. 6-3 Pedigree from *Patient Profile: Family history of mental retardation. MR*, mental retardation.

QUESTION 1: IN THE ABSENCE OF DEFINITIVE DIAGNOSES OF AFFECTED RELATIVES, SHOULD PRENATAL DIAGNOSIS BE OFFERED TO A PATIENT WITH A FAMILY HISTORY OF MENTAL RETARDATION?

A patient with a family history of mental retardation may request prenatal diagnosis by chorionic villus sampling or amniocentesis for reassurance. It is appropriate to offer this testing, provided that the patient and her partner understand the limitations of the test results. They should be encouraged to obtain as much information as possible about their affected relatives and should be informed that an accurate risk assessment is not possible without this information.

If the patient is unwilling or unable to provide additional information or if late gestational age prevents a more extensive evaluation, detailed ultrasound examination and amniocentesis for cytogenetic studies can be offered as mechanisms with which to rule out conditions that can be diagnosed by these procedures. The patient and her partner should be clearly informed that not all genetic conditions can be identified by these procedures and that there may still be a risk for genetic conditions that are not associated with chromosome abnormalities and for fetal abnormalities that cannot be detected by ultrasound.

QUESTION 2: WHAT LABORATORY TESTS SHOULD BE CONSIDERED IN EVALUATING A PATIENT WITH A FAMILY HISTORY OF MENTAL RETARDATION?

In some circumstances, it may be appropriate to recommend parental blood chromosome analysis or fragile X testing or both for a couple with a family history of mental retardation of unknown cause. Careful pedigree analysis may suggest the possibility of a familial chromosome rearrangement (translocation or inversion) or may be consistent with the possibility of X-linked mental retardation, as is found in fragile X syndrome.

For example, if the patient reports that affected relatives have birth defects, growth problems, or unusual facial features associated with mental retardation or if there is an extensive family history of unexplained miscarriage, intrauterine fetal demise, or neonatal death, a chromosome analysis of the patient and her partner might be indicated. Even if the patient is considering amniocentesis, parental karyotyping should still be offered, since subtle structural chromosome abnormalities might not be detected by routine karyotype analysis of amniotic fluid cells. This is because of the superior cytogenetic analysis that can be performed on blood versus amniotic fluid. Thus, if a structural rearrangement is found in the chromosomes of parental blood cells, the cytogeneticist can focus attention on the relevant fetal chromosomes cultured from amniocytes.

In some cases, the family history might strongly suggest X-linked mental retardation, and carrier testing for fragile X should be considered. Fragile X carrier testing is preferred to fragile X testing in the fetus by prenatal diagnosis because it will provide information not only for the current pregnancy but for future pregnancies as well. In addition, invasive fetal testing is not without risk of pregnancy loss. Furthermore, if a patient is identified as a fragile X premutation carrier, genetic counseling and carrier testing can be recommended for other relatives.

Routine screening by chromosome analysis and fragile X carrier testing of all patients with a family history of mental retardation is cost prohibitive. Currently, the cost of a chromosome analysis ranges from $400 to $500, and the cost of fragile X carrier testing ranges from $200 to $300. In the absence of a suggestive family history, it is not cost effective to screen all patients with a family history of mental retardation by these methods. Rather, it is preferable to arrange for cytogenetic testing or fragile X testing of the affected relative. The results, positive or negative, have important implications not only for the patient but also for other relatives.

QUESTION 3: WHAT ARE THE POTENTIAL LIMITATIONS IN THE EVALUATION OF A PATIENT WITH A FAMILY HISTORY OF MENTAL RETARDATION?

The evaluation of a patient with a family history of mental retardation can be limited by four factors: (1) lack of availability of medical records or other documentation of the diagnosis or clinical status of the affected relative or relatives; (2) lack of cooperation on the part of the patient or the relatives in performing necessary clinical or laboratory evaluation that might lead to a more specific diagnosis; (3) the wide variety of genetic and nongenetic causes of mental retardation and the limited capability of laboratory testing to identify carriers of genetic mental retardation syndromes caused by mutations in single genes; and (4) the high cost of chromosome analysis and fragile X testing.

•   •   •

Evaluation of a pregnant patient with a family history of mental retardation should include careful pedigree analysis, documentation of each affected relative's diagnosis by medical record review and, when possible, by clinical evaluation or laboratory investigation, and consideration of carrier screening by chromosome analysis or fragile X testing or both. In some cases, this evaluation may result in confirmation of a specific diagnosis, allowing for accurate risk assessment, genetic counseling, and prenatal diagnosis. If a specific diagnosis cannot be identified, the couple must be made aware of the limitations of the evaluation.

REFERENCES

1. Berini RY, Kahn E: *National Genetics Foundation, Inc. clinical genetics handbook*, Oradell, N.J., 1987, Medical Economics Company.
2. Gardner RJM, Sutherland GR: *Chromosome abnormalities and genetic counseling*, New York, 1989, Oxford University Press.
3. Harper PS: *Practical genetic counseling*, ed 4, Oxford, 1993, Butterworth Heinemann.

4. Oberle I, Rousseau F, Heitz D et al: Instability of a 550-base pair DNA segment and abnormal methylation in fragile X syndrome, *Science* 252:1097, 1991.
5. Oostra BA, Jacky PB, Brown WT, Rousseau F: Guidelines for the diagnosis of fragile X syndrome, *J Med Genet* 30:410, 1993.
6. Rousseau F, Heitz D, Biancalana V et al: Direct diagnosis by DNA analysis of the fragile X syndrome of mental retardation, *N Engl J Med* 325:1673, 1991.
7. Sherman SL, Jacobs PA, Morton NE et al: Further segregation analysis of the fragile X syndrome with special reference to transmitting males, *Hum Genet* 69:289, 1985.
8. Sherman SL, Morton NE, Jacobs PA, Turner G: The marker (X) syndrome: a cytogenetic and genetic analysis, *Ann Hum Genet* 48:21, 1984.
9. Tamaren J, Spuhler K, Sujanski E: Risk of Down syndrome among second- and third-degree relatives of a proband with trisomy 21, *Am J Hum Genet* 15:393, 1983.
10. Tarleton JC, Saul RA: Molecular genetic advances in fragile X syndrome, *J Pediatr* 122:169, 1993.
11. Thompson MW, McInnes RR, Willard HF: *Genetics in medicine*, ed 5, Philadelphia, 1991, WB Saunders.
12. Verkerk AJMH, Pieretti M, Sutcliffe JS et al: Identification of a gene (*FMR-1*) containing a CGG repeat coincident with a breakpoint cluster region exhibiting length variation in fragile X syndrome, *Cell* 65:905, 1991.
13. Yu S, Pritchard M, Kremer EJ et al: Fragile X genotype characterized by an unstable region of DNA, *Science* 252:1179, 1991.

CHAPTER 7

Hemoglobinopathies and Coagulation Disorders

BARBARA A. WEDEHASE
JEFFREY A. KULLER

Hemoglobinopathies

It is estimated that approximately 5% of the world's population are carriers of genes for hemoglobin disorders. Hemoglobin is a tetramer composed of two pairs of distinct globin chains. Hemoglobin A (HbA), the normal adult hemoglobin, comprises two alpha (α) and two beta (β) chains. Each person has four genes that encode for α-globin chains (located on chromosome 16) and two genes that encode for β-globin chains (located on chromosome 11). Abnormalities of hemoglobin can be caused by changes or mutations in any of these genes. Structural variants, such as sickle cell anemia, alter the hemoglobin molecule. Decreased production of one or more of the globin chains results in thalassemia.

❦ Patient Profile: Testing for thalassemia

A 25-year-old Asian woman (gravida 1, para 0000) and her 27-year-old African-American husband seek obstetric consultation at 11 weeks' gestation. She reports that her sister's child is anemic, but she does not know what treatment, if any, the child receives. They want to learn whether they could have a child with anemia and whether prenatal testing is available.

QUESTION 1: WHAT IS β-THALASSEMIA AND WHAT ARE ITS CLINICAL MANIFESTATIONS?

A mutation in the β-globin gene, located on chromosome 11, can cause a lack of or a decreased rate of synthesis of β-globin chains. Over 90 different mutations have been identified, all of which result in a similar clinical picture. A person with β-thalassemia trait has one normal β-globin gene and one altered β-globin gene. Patients with β-thalassemia trait are asymptomatic and only rarely have mild anemia. If both parents have β-thalassemia trait, they have a one in four (25%) chance of having a child with β-thalassemia major. This

45

disease is characterized by severe anemia and requires life-long medical management, but gradations of severity do exist. Frequent transfusions are necessary to maintain an adequate hemoglobin level. When patients are adequately transfused, development is usually normal until early puberty. By age 10 or 11, treated patients begin to show signs of progressive hepatic, cardiac, and endocrine disturbances. These changes are caused largely by accumulation of iron from transfusion and deposition in the tissues. Expansion of the bone marrow due to excessive extramedullary hematopoiesis in response to anemia leads to characteristic skeletal changes and a typical thalassemia facies caused by frontal bossing of the skull and protrusion of the jaws and cheekbones. Unless iron overload is controlled by chelation therapy, affected persons generally die in the second or third decade of life as a result of cardiac failure.

QUESTION 2: WHAT IS α-THALASSEMIA AND WHAT ARE ITS CLINICAL MANIFESTATIONS?

There are two α-globin gene loci on chromosome 16. A mutation of the α-globin gene can affect either one or both α genes, resulting in any one of four α-thalassemia states: (1) silent carrier (three functional α genes); (2) α-thalassemia trait (two functional α genes); (3) hemoglobin H (HbH) disease (one functional α gene); or (4) hemoglobin Bart's hydrops fetalis syndrome (no functional α genes). Silent carriers are asymptomatic, whereas patients with α-thalassemia trait may have mild anemia and microcytosis. Hemoglobin H disease is associated with mild to moderate hemolytic anemia and splenomegaly. Infants with Bart's hydrops are usually stillborn between 20 and 40 weeks' gestation.

QUESTION 3: HOW IS SICKLE CELL ANEMIA INHERITED AND WHAT ARE ITS CLINICAL MANIFESTATIONS?

Sickle cell hemoglobin (HbS) was the first abnormal hemoglobin to be detected and is currently the only genetic disorder identifiable by direct diagnostic testing. Every patient with sickle cell anemia has the same mutation, with a substitution of valine for glutamic acid at position 6 of the β-globin chain (Figure 7-1). A person with sickle cell trait has HbA and HbS and is clinically normal. Although a number of clinical abnormalities have been reported for individuals with sickle cell trait, most of them are anecdotal. However, patients with sickle cell trait are probably at risk for splenic infarction when flying at high altitude under conditions of inadequate cabin pressurization (not usually encountered in commercial flights) and for urinary tract infections during pregnancy. The risk of having a fetus with sickle cell disease is one in four (25%) if both parents have sickle cell trait. Sickle cell disease, homozygous HbS, is characterized by life-long hemolytic anemia, increased propensity to infection, and repeated vasooclusive episodes and acute exacerbations called *crises*.

Hemoglobin C (HbC) is a electrophoretic hemoglobin variant. Hemoglobin C trait is found in approximately 3% of African-Americans at birth. An individual heterozygous for

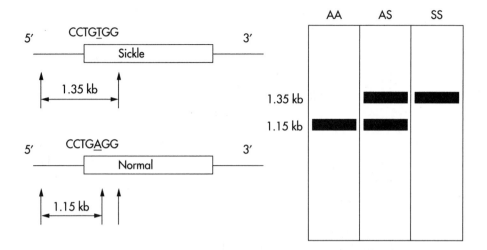

Fig. 7-1 Diagnosis of sickle cell disease by restriction endonuclease analysis. The *Mst*II restriction sites are indicated on the left. The resulting fragments are seen on the Southern blot analysis. (From Goldberg JD: Basic principles of recombinant DNA use for prenatal diagnosis, *Semin Perinatol* 14:439, 1990.)

HbC and HbS has sickle–HbC disease. This disease is generally milder than homozygous HbS, sickle cell disease, but the severity of the disease varies among patients. Patients with homozygous HbC disease have mild to moderate chronic anemia.

QUESTION 4: WHICH POPULATIONS ARE AT RISK FOR HEMOGLOBINOPATHIES?

Sickle cell disease occurs most frequently in equatorial Africa and is also common in the Mediterranean region, India, and countries to which people from these regions have migrated. Approximately 8% to 10% of African-Americans have sickle cell trait (HbA, HbS), with a disease incidence of 1 in 600. Approximately 1% of African-Americans are carriers of HbC.

People from the Mediterranean basin (Italy, Greece, and Sardinia), Southeast Asia, India, Africa, and Indonesia may have as high as a 1% chance of carrying the gene for β-thalassemia. α-Thalassemia is common in Southeast Asian, South Chinese, and Filipino populations. Approximately 30% of African-Americans are silent carriers, and 3% have α-thalassemia trait. The α-thalassemia trait in African-Americans is usually caused by the deletion of a single α gene on *both* number 16 chromosomes (*trans*). Therefore, Bart's hydrops is generally not seen in fetuses of African-American α-Thalassemia carriers. This is in contrast to the usual Asian genotype in which there is a deletion of both α genes on *one* chromosome (*cis*). Specific mutations have been identified for the various ethnic groups, most differing from normal by only one amino acid.

QUESTION 5: HOW IS CARRIER TESTING PERFORMED FOR HEMOGLOBINOPATHIES?

Hemoglobin electrophoresis to determine HbA, HbS, and HbC is the recommended test for persons at risk for sickle cell anemia. A sickle prep, although an excellent test for mass screening, cannot distinguish between the heterozygote and the homozygote nor determine the presence of HbC.

A complete blood count (CBC) with red blood cell (RBC) indices is recommended as a screening test for the thalassemias. In most thalassemic heterozygotes, the RBC indices are low, with a mean corpuscular hemoglobin (MCH) <27 pg and a mean corpuscular volume (MCV) <79 fl. If the RBC indices are lowered and the hematocrit is decreased, the patient should be evaluated for iron deficiency (also associated with low RBC indices) before screening for the thalassemias.

If the RBC indices are low and iron deficiency is ruled out, hemoglobin electrophoresis should be performed. Hemoglobin A_2 is elevated in most β-thalassemic heterozygotes to a level between 3.5% and 7%. On the other hand, patients who are heterozygous for α-thalassemia have a normal HbA_2 level.

Carrier testing should ideally be performed during the preconceptional period. If performed during pregnancy, the patient may not have the option of prenatal testing because of the time required to obtain complete results.

QUESTION 6: WHEN SHOULD PRENATAL TESTING BE OFFERED?

Couples who have α-thalassemia trait have a 1 in 4 (25%) risk of having a fetus with Bart's hydrops, in which there are no functional α genes. Populations at risk for Bart's hydrops include Southeast Asian, South Chinese, and Filipino. Bart's hydrops has not been seen in African-Americans. Prenatal diagnosis of α-thalassemia is performed by DNA analysis of cultured cells obtained by chorionic villus sampling (CVS) or amniocentesis to detect α-globin deletions.

Prenatal diagnosis of β-thalassemia is offered if both members of the couple are β-thalassemia carriers (giving them a 1 in 4 [25%] risk). Direct detection of the β-globin gene mutation in cultured cells from CVS or amniocentesis can indicate whether the couple has a fetus with β-thalassemia.

The risk of having a child with sickle cell disease is 1 in 4 (25%) for couples who have sickle cell trait. Prenatal diagnostic testing for sickle cell disease can be performed directly on chorionic villi or amniotic fluid to determine the presence or absence of the characteristic single-base mutation.

Coagulation Disorders

Coagulation disorders are characterized clinically by excessive bleeding after trauma or surgery, hemarthroses, and muscle hematomas. They are caused by the absence of a plasma protein that causes blood to clot. Approximately 1 to 2 in 10,000 males suffer from hemophilia, the majority from hemophilia A (classic hemophilia), which is caused by a deficiency of clotting factor VIII. The deficiency of factor IX causes hemophilia B (Christmas disease). Hemophilias A and B are clinically similar and can be distinguished only by specific assays for the deficient coagulation factor. The gene for hemophilias A and B is on the X chromosome, causing males to be affected and females to be carriers.

Von Willebrand disease (vWD) is the most common inherited bleeding disorder. It is generally thought to be an autosomal dominant disorder, but autosomal recessive forms have been described. The disease is characterized by a prolonged bleeding time because of a qualitative or quantitative defect in the von Willebrand factor. This factor, a plasma protein, is required for normal primary hemostasis because it mediates the adhesion and aggregation of platelets. The exact incidence of vWD is not known, since mild cases may not be diagnosed. The severity of symptoms may vary among individuals and even among affected members of the same family.

✤ Patient Profile: Prenatal testing for coagulation disorders

A 20-year-old woman (gravida 1, para 0000) seeks obstetric consultation because her brother has a bleeding disorder. She does not know his diagnosis and denies any additional family history of bleeding problems. She reports that her brother's medical problems have been numerous and that he has spent a significant proportion of his life in the hospital. This situation has been very stressful for the woman and her family, and she does not wish to have a child with similar problems. She wants to know what her risk is of having a child with this problem and whether prenatal testing is available.

QUESTION 1: WHAT IS HEMOPHILIA AND WHAT ARE ITS CLINICAL MANIFESTATIONS?

Hemophilia A, or classic hemophilia, is caused by a deficiency of clotting factor VIII. Affected males are easily bruised, have prolonged bleeding from wounds, and have joint and muscle hemorrhages resulting from defective fibrin formation. Hemophilia A is caused by changes in the factor VIII gene, located near the tip of the long arm of the X chromosome. The gene consists of 186,000 base pairs, representing approximately 0.1% of the X chromosome. Many different mutations in this gene have been described, a majority of which are specific for individual families. Mutations have been found for almost all mild and moderately affected patients, but for only half of severely affected patients. Inversions in the gene may account for 50% of severe disease, specifically in many patients without a family history of hemophilia.

About 20% of the total hemophiliac population is deficient in clotting factor IX, resulting in hemophilia B. Patients with severe hemophilia B have spontaneous bleeding in the joints and muscles. Mild hemophilia B may not be detected until a person has increased bleeding from trauma or surgery in adulthood. The gene for factor IX is located near the factor VIII gene on the X chromosome. The gene consists of 34,000 base pairs, and mutations in the gene have been identified by DNA sequencing.

Female carriers of hemophilia A or B usually do not have any bleeding manifestations. Occasionally, carriers may have unusually low levels of factors VIII or IX, presumably because a large proportion of the normal X chromosome undergoes inactivation. These women may have menorrhagia and, occasionally, hemarthroses. Pregnancy and delivery, however, are generally free of serious hemorrhagic complications.

QUESTION 2: WHAT IS VON WILLEBRAND DISEASE AND WHAT ARE ITS CLINICAL MANIFESTATIONS?

Von Willebrand disease is a heterogeneous autosomal dominant and sometimes autosomal recessive bleeding disorder. More than 20 variants of vWD have been reported, with type I vWD (classic vWD) accounting for over 70% of all cases. Type I vWD is characterized by a deficiency of the von Willebrand factor, resulting in a prolonged bleeding time. Bleeding usually occurs from mucocutaneous sites rather than from joints or muscles. Symptoms of the disorder vary both among individuals and within families. The gene is located on the short arm of chromosome 12, and no distinct molecular defect has yet been identified for type I. Type II vWD is the least common type and has several variants that are usually dominantly inherited.

Type III vWD is the severe form of the disease, similar to severe hemophilia A, but often with mucosal bleeding. Inheritance is usually autosomal recessive, and parents of these patients rarely show symptoms. Point mutations and large deletions spanning the entire von Willebrand gene are associated with type III vWD.

QUESTION 3: HOW ARE HEMOPHILIA CARRIERS IDENTIFIED?

Any woman whose father has hemophilia or who has had an affected son *and* another affected maternal relative is an obligate carrier of the gene; she therefore has a 50% chance with each pregnancy of having an affected son. A woman may or may not be a carrier if she has only one affected son or affected maternal relatives. Approximately 30% to 50% of the hemophilic population is composed of sporadic cases caused by new mutations. The mother of an isolated (the only known case in the family) hemophilic male has an empiric 85% probability of being a gene carrier. Carrier risk in these situations is determined by pedigree analysis and bayesian calculations,* clotting factor assays, and DNA studies.

Bayesian analysis is a mathematical method used to calculate risk for genetic disease. The method combines information that may come from several sources, including pedigree information, laboratory results, and genetic inheritance data and is used to determine the probability that a specific individual will develop or transmit a certain disorder.

Confirmation of the diagnosis in each affected individual is imperative for accurate risk determination and testing. Carriers of hemophilia A or B have, on average, approximately 50% of the normal levels of factor VIII or factor IX, respectively. Coagulant assays can establish an odds ratio for carrier status, but this status may still be uncertain because of the overlap of levels in carriers and noncarriers. The assay can be confounded if the woman is past 22 weeks' gestation or is taking oral contraceptives at the time of testing because of the resulting increase in factor VIII levels. Carrier assays for hemophilia A also depend on the woman's age and blood group status. For hemophilia B carrier assays, identification of cross-reactive material in affected males is necessary.

If DNA analysis of the affected male identifies a mutation or an inversion, the carrier status of female relatives can be accurately determined. Accurate carrier diagnosis is often not possible because of the high incidence of new mutations in the hemophilia gene. For many families, restriction fragment length polymorphism (RFLP)* analysis is used to track the affected factor VIII gene or factor IX gene within the family, using an intragenic polymorphism. This testing has an error rate of less than 1%. Restriction fragment length polymorphism analysis in families with an isolated affected male can never prove carrier status. Carrier status can, however, be excluded by DNA testing if the female relative can be shown to have inherited a different X chromosome than the proband.

QUESTION 4: HOW IS PRENATAL DIAGNOSIS OF COAGULATION ABNORMALITIES PERFORMED?

Women who are known hemophilia carriers by DNA analysis have the options of chorionic villus sampling or amniocentesis for accurate diagnosis. Fetal blood sampling to measure either factor VIII or factor IX is offered to women for whom DNA analysis is either not available or not informative. A detailed ultrasound examination is offered to all possible hemophilia carriers for fetal sex determination. If the fetus is found to be female, invasive prenatal testing can be avoided.

Prenatal diagnosis of type I vWD by RFLP analysis can be performed if there are several affected individuals in a family. Because of the heterogeneity of this disorder, accurate prognostic information regarding affected fetuses is not possible. Prenatal diagnosis of type III vWD by DNA analysis is offered to couples with an affected child because of the severe hemorrhagic manifestations associated with the disease.

*An RFLP is a difference in the DNA sequence between individuals that can be recognized by enzymes used to cut DNA in vitro.

REFERENCES

1. Brocker-Vriends AHJT, Bakker E, Kanhai HHH et al: The contribution of DNA analysis to carrier detection and prenatal diagnosis of hemophilia A and B, *Ann Hematol* 64:2, 1992.
2. Forget BG: The pathophysiology and molecular genetics of beta thalassemia, *Mt Sinai J Med* 60:95, 1993.

3. Ginsburg D: Biology of inherited coagulopathies: von Willebrand factor, *Hematol Oncol Clin North Am* 6:1011, 1992.

4. Hedner U, Davie EW: Introduction to hemostasis and the vitamin K-dependent coagulation factors. In Scriver CR, Beaudet AL, Sly WS et al, editors: *The metabolic basis of inherited disease*, ed 6, New York, 1989, McGraw-Hill.

5. Higgs DR: The molecular genetics of the alpha globin gene family, *Eur J Clin Invest* 20:340, 1990.

6. Kazazian HH: The thalassemia syndromes: molecular basis and prenatal diagnosis in 1990, *Semin Hematol* 27:209, 1990.

7. Kazazian HH: The molecular basis of hemophilia A and the present status of carrier and antenatal diagnosis of the disease, *Thromb Hæmost* 70:60, 1993.

8. Lakich D, Kazazian HH, Antonarakis SE et al: Inversions disrupting the factor VIII gene are a common cause of severe hæmophilia A, *Nature Genet* 5:236, 1993.

9. Old JM: Prenatal diagnosis of the hemoglobinopathies. In Milunsky A, editor: *Genetic disorders and the fetus: diagnosis, prevention and treatment*, ed 3, Baltimore 1992, The Johns Hopkins University Press.

10. Oldenburg J, Schwaab R, Grimm T et al: Direct and indirect estimation of the sex ratio of mutation frequencies in hemophilia A, *Am J Hum Gen* 53:1229, 1993

11. Peake IR, Lillicrap DP, Boulyjenkov V et al: Haemophilia: strategies for carrier detection and prenatal diagnosis, *Bull World Health Organ* 71:429, 1993.

12. Sadler JE: Von Willebrand disease. In Scriver CR, Beaudet AL, Sly WS et al, editors: *The metabolic basis of inherited disease*, ed 6, New York, 1989, McGraw-Hill.

13. Thompson MW, McInnes RR, Willard HF: The hemoglobinopathies: models of molecular disease. In *Genetics in medicine*, ed 5, Philadelphia, 1991, WB Saunders.

14. Vehar GA, Lawn RM, Tuddenham EGD et al: Factor VIII and factor V: biochemistry and pathophysiology. In Scriver CR, Beaudet AL, Sly WS et al, editors: *The metabolic basis of inherited disease*, ed 6, New York, 1989, McGraw-Hill.

15. Weatherall DJ, Clegg JB, Higgs DR, Wood WG: The hemoglobinopathies. In Scriver CR, Beaudet AL, Sly WS et al, editors: *The metabolic basis of inherited disease*, ed 6, New York, 1989, McGraw-Hill.

CHAPTER 8

Autosomal Disorders:

Cystic Fibrosis, Tay-Sachs Disease, and Huntington Disease

MYRA I. ROCHE
JEFFREY A. KULLER

Of all the recognized single-gene traits, more than half are inherited in an autosomal dominant pattern, one third are inherited in an autosomal recessive pattern, and the remainder are X linked.[27] For an increasing number of genetic conditions, carrier testing, either before conception or during pregnancy, can identify couples who are at increased risk of having an affected child. Reproductive options, including prenatal diagnosis, can then be offered. In this chapter, carrier testing and prenatal diagnosis will be discussed for three conditions: cystic fibrosis (CF), Tay-Sachs disease, and Huntington disease (HD). Cystic fibrosis and Tay-Sachs disease are inherited in an autosomal recessive pattern; HD is inherited in an autosomal dominant pattern.

In autosomal recessive conditions, both unaffected parents are carriers and each has one mutant copy and one normal copy of the gene. When both parents are carriers, they have a 25% chance with each pregnancy of having an affected child who inherits both copies of the mutant gene. When there is a known family history of a genetic disorder or the couple's ethnicity places them at an increased risk of carrying a mutant gene, carrier testing may be available. Cystic fibrosis carrier testing relies on DNA mutation analysis, while enzymatic screening has traditionally been used to identify Tay-Sachs gene carriers. There are problems inherent in offering carrier testing for an autosomal recessively inherited condition to persons in the general population when there is no family history of the disease. The magnitude of these problems is inversely proportional to the sensitivity of the screening test.

For autosomal dominantly expressed genes, a gene carrier has one copy of the mutant gene and, therefore, a 50% chance of passing on the gene with each pregnancy. Depending upon the disease, a gene carrier may or may not be symptomatic by the time of reproductive age. The adult-onset nature of HD raises several issues: Is it ethical to offer presymptomatic testing for an untreatable progressive disease? How can the confidentiality of test results be maintained? How can discrimination against asymptomatic gene carriers be minimized? The effect of the recent availability of a direct DNA test for HD on presymptomatic testing and prenatal diagnostic options is currently being debated.[22]

Cystic Fibrosis

Cystic fibrosis is the most common autosomal recessively inherited single-gene disease in the Caucasian population, with an incidence of approximately 1 in 2500 live births.[16] The clinical features of CF are obstructive lung disease, repeated respiratory infections and, often, pancreatic insufficiency. Neonatal meconium ileus occurs in 5% to 10% of cases and is considered pathognomonic.[2] Other organs, notably the reproductive tract, can also be affected, and males with CF are usually sterile. In 1989, several groups, led by Tsui and colleagues, identified the CF gene.[13,19] Because affected persons have abnormally high sweat sodium and chloride levels, it has long been suspected that the abnormal CF gene product interferes with the regulation of electrolyte transport. This product, called *cystic fibrosis transmembrane conductance regulator*, has two ATP-binding domains, one of which is disrupted by the most common mutation causing CF, the ΔF508 mutation. Approximately 70% of chromosomes carrying a mutant CF allele have this specific mutation. Screening for this mutation alone identifies almost half of the CF carrier couples in the general population.[14]

Unfortunately, the other 30% of CF chromosomes contain mutations that are much rarer. Only a few of the more than 400 mutations in the CF gene that have been identified to date are present in the population at a frequency of 1% or greater. According to the most recent Cystic Fibrosis Genetic Analysis Consortium data, the six most common mutations occur on about 75% of the CF chromosomes in the U.S. population.[25] Separate ethnic populations differ in their proportions of these known mutations. In the Ashkenazi Jewish population, for example, three mutations account for over 93% of the total CF mutations. Carrier screening in that population is, therefore, relatively sensitive.[21] Currently, no single DNA test detects all CF carriers in any population.

Controversy exists regarding whether individuals in the general Caucasian population should be offered screening because of the concomitant need for extensive education and counseling due to the low sensitivity of the current test. Regardless of this controversy, some laboratories have begun offering this screening to pregnant couples.[11] Pilot studies, sponsored by the Human Genome Project Working Group on Ethical, Legal, and Social Issues (ELSI), are currently under way to identify and begin to address the social effects of widespread screening. Meanwhile, advances in gene therapy for CF are continuing, with human trials already in progress. Effective treatment for CF may eventually lower the demand for carrier testing.

❧ Patient Profile: Carrier testing for cystic fibrosis

A 27-year-old Caucasian woman (gravida 1, para 0000) seeks genetic counseling because her sister has a child with CF. The woman is interested in determining whether she is a CF carrier. Her husband, who is also Caucasian, has no family history of CF.

QUESTION 1: WHAT IS THE PATIENT'S RISK OF BEING A CYSTIC FIBROSIS CARRIER, HOW IS CARRIER TESTING PERFORMED FOR A PATIENT WITH A POSITIVE FAMILY HISTORY, AND WHAT ARE THE LIMITATIONS OF THIS TESTING?

The patient's risk of being a CF carrier can be calculated using mendelian principles. The parents of the affected child are assumed to be obligate carriers. The affected child's mother (the patient's sister) inherited the mutant CF gene from one of her parents. Because the pregnant patient and her sister have the same parents, the pregnant patient had a 1 in 2 (50%) chance of also inheriting that mutant CF gene. This is her estimated risk before any carrier testing is performed. Her husband's risk of being a carrier is estimated using the general Caucasian population carrier incidence of about 1 in 25 (4%). Thus the chance of this couple's having an affected child is $1/2 \times 1/25 = 1/50$, or 2%.

It may be possible to identify the specific mutation or mutations in the niece's CF alleles. If this can be accomplished, accurate carrier testing of collateral relatives can be performed. As shown in Figure 8-1, if the woman's niece is homozygous for the ΔF508 mutation (both of her CF alleles have this mutation), other interested relatives can also be screened for that mutation. If the pregnant patient is positive for the mutation, she is definitely a

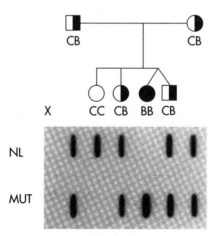

Fig. 8-1 Detection of the three-base deletion that causes cystic fibrosis, using DNA amplification and allele-specific oligonucleotides. Squares represent male family members, and circles represent female family members. Solid symbols denote affected members, half-solid symbols heterozygotes, and open symbols noncarriers. *NL* denotes the autoradiogram with the normal allele-specific oligonucleotide, and *MUT* denotes the autoradiogram with the mutant allele-specific oligonucleotide. The *X* denotes the black lane in which no genomic DNA was added to the polymerase chain reaction. Letters below the pedigree symbols indicate the *XV-2c* and *KM-19* haplotypes. (From Lemna W, Feldman G, Kerem B et al: Mutation analysis for heterozygote detection and the prenatal diagnosis of cystic fibrosis, *N Engl J Med* 322:293, 1990.)

carrier, and her husband should be offered carrier testing. If her husband also tests positive, their risk of having an affected child is 25% (1 in 4). If the pregnant patient does not have the ΔF508 mutation, she is not likely to be a carrier. However, a negative result does not mean that her risk of being a carrier is zero because of the presence of other CF mutations in the general population. Thus, performing mutation analysis can often yield more precise risk estimates for couples with positive family histories than simply using mendelian principles alone.

QUESTION 2: WHAT IF THE AFFECTED RELATIVE DIED WITHOUT HAVING HAD DNA TESTING FOR CYSTIC FIBROSIS OR IS UNWILLING TO BE TESTED?

In this case, the pregnant woman could be screened for a group of the most common mutations. Currently, six or more mutations are typically screened using the polymerase chain reaction (PCR). Detection of a mutation classifies the patient as a carrier. A negative result indicates that the patient has a significantly reduced risk of being a carrier. This risk approaches but does not reach zero because not all CF mutations have been identified. In addition, most CF mutations occur so infrequently that screening for all of them would be cumbersome, time consuming, expensive, and would not indicate a corresponding significant reduction in the patient's risk of being a carrier. If the pregnant woman is screened for the six most common mutations (accounting for 75% of all CF mutations), a negative result indicates that her risk of being a carrier is reduced from 1 in 2 (50%) to approximately 1 in 5 (20%). The patient's husband can also be tested. If he tests negative, his risk of being a carrier is reduced from 1 in 25 (4%) to less than 1 in 100 (1%). Thus, after factoring in these negative results, the couple's risk of having an affected child is estimated to be only 1 in 2000. This level of risk is comparable to that of couples in the general Caucasian population who have negative family histories and who have not had mutation screening (1 in 2500).

QUESTION 3: WHAT ARE THE PRENATAL DIAGNOSTIC OPTIONS WHEN BOTH PARENTS ARE CARRIERS OF THE CYSTIC FIBROSIS GENE?

Cystic fibrosis mutation analysis can be performed on the fetus by chorionic villus sampling (CVS), amniocentesis, or percutaneous umbilical blood sampling. Prenatal diagnosis is most accurate when both parental mutations are known. Successful preimplantation diagnosis of CF has been reported.[10] Ultrasound detection of fetal echogenic bowel is not definitively diagnostic of CF and should not be offered as such to couples at increased risk.

QUESTION 4: WHAT ARE THE LIMITATIONS OF FETAL CYSTIC FIBROSIS TESTING WHEN ONE PARENT HAS AN IDENTIFIABLE MUTATION AND THE OTHER TESTS NEGATIVE?

If 75% of mutations are detectable by carrier screening, the fetal risk for CF (before invasive fetal testing) is predicted to be approximately 1 in 400. Subsequent fetal testing will yield one of two scenarios. When the fetal testing is negative, the fetus did not inherit the known mutation from the parent who was identified as a carrier. It is unknown whether the fetus inherited an unidentifiable CF mutation from the other parent. In this situation, the fetus is predicted to be unaffected but, because there is still a chance that the fetus inherited an unidentifiable mutation, the carrier status is not definitively known. Of greater concern is the situation in which the mutation identified in the carrier parent is found in the fetus. The interpretation in this case is also ambiguous because the fetus carries at least one mutant CF allele. The possibility that the fetus may have inherited an unidentified mutant allele from the other parent and, consequently, is affected cannot be ruled out. The risk that the fetus is affected in this case is approximately 1 in 200.

QUESTION 5: ARE THERE OTHER PRENATAL INDICATORS THAT COULD CLARIFY THIS RISK?

Because of the high false-positive rate (2.5%) and false-negative rate (2% to 10%) of amniotic fluid microvillar enzyme studies, a positive enzyme result in this case is more likely to be a false positive rather than a true positive.[2] Thus, microvillar enzyme analysis of amniotic fluid is no longer performed.

Recently, fetuses with echogenic bowels have been detected during ultrasound examination. Some reports have indicated an associated increased risk of CF in these fetuses; other reports have found an increased risk of Down syndrome.[18] Cystic fibrosis carrier testing by mutation analysis may be offered to these parents, and amniotic fluid may be obtained for fetal CF testing (and fetal karyotyping). Even when echogenic bowel is noted, however, the chance of finding a CF mutation in both parents when neither has a family history is low. The resulting interpretation problems inherent in finding a mutation in only one parent are outlined in Question 4, above.

QUESTION 6: WHAT ARE THE LIMITATIONS OF SCREENING CAUCASIAN COUPLES TO DETERMINE THEIR CYSTIC FIBROSIS CARRIER STATUS WHEN BOTH HAVE NEGATIVE FAMILY HISTORIES?

The major problem lies in the interpretation of a negative result. If both members of a couple test negative, ruling out 75% of the total CF mutations, the couple's estimated risk of having an affected child is reduced from 1 in 2500 to approximately 1 in 40,000. However, in about 6% of these couples, one parent will have a detectable mutation and one will have a negative test result. Before prenatal testing, this couple's estimated risk of having an affected child is now increased from 1 in 2500 to about 1 in 400. Furthermore, prenatal diagnosis (as described in Question 4, above) is ambiguous under these circumstances. The determination of increased risk may heighten the couple's anxiety, yet no definitive prenatal testing can be offered. If the sensitivity of the CF carrier testing is increased, the proportion of couples with ambiguous results will decrease. However, for the near future, a dramatic improvement in sensitivity is probably not a realistic goal given currently available techniques.

Tay-Sachs Disease

Tay-Sachs disease is a neurodegenerative disorder involving the accumulation of GM_2 gangliosides and related glycolipids caused by a deficiency of the alpha subunit of the lysosomal enzyme hexosaminidase A. *Tay-Sachs disease* usually refers to (and in this discussion will be limited to) the classical infantile type in which there is virtually no detectable enzymatic activity. Symptoms, including hypotonia, a progressive loss of vision, and loss of interest in surroundings and previously attained motor milestones, usually begin in infancy. Death typically occurs at about 4 years of age. The macular cherry-red spot detected by ophthalmologic examination is found in virtually all affected patients.[20] The incidence of classical Tay-Sachs disease in two distinct populations, Ashkenazi Jews and French-Canadians, is approximately 1 in 3600. About 1 in 30 persons in these populations is a carrier. Carrier frequency in the general population is usually reported as 1 in 300 (when estimated using the incidence of the disease), but this frequency is much higher when enzymatic testing estimates are used, falling in the range of 1 in 167.[12] The discrepancy may be explained by the existence of one or more pseudodeficiency alleles, which produce false-positive results.[28] Active carrier screening in the Ashkenazi Jewish population has been in place since the 1980s and serves as an effective model of a population-based screening program because of its successful mobilization of community and religious groups.[17] The effect of carrier screening can be measured by the fact that in the U.S. and Canada in the late 1980s the incidence of classical Tay-Sachs disease in non-Jewish infants exceeded the incidence in Jewish infants.[20] The identification of DNA mutations within the hexosaminidase A gene has begun to play a role in carrier screening.

❧ Patient Profile: Carrier testing for Tay-Sachs disease

A 28-year-old Jewish woman (gravida 1, para 0000) visits her obstetrician, who obtains her family history. It is negative for birth defects, mental retardation, genetic diseases, and Tay-Sachs disease. Her husband is also of Ashkenazi Jewish ancestry and also has a negative family history.

QUESTION 1: SHOULD TESTING BE OFFERED TO THIS COUPLE EVEN THOUGH THEY HAVE NO FAMILY HISTORY OF TAY-SACHS DISEASE?

In autosomal recessively inherited conditions, the altered gene can be passed from one carrier to another for many generations before an affected child is born. Thus, the lack of a positive family history is not a sensitive indicator of this couple's risk of being carriers. The incidence of carriers in their ethnic group is high enough to justify offering testing.

QUESTION 2: HOW IS ENZYMATIC CARRIER TESTING PERFORMED?

Ideally, both members of the couple should be tested preconceptionally. If the woman is already pregnant, both members should be tested because of time constraints. A decreased level of serum hexosaminidase A activity in the presence of normal or elevated hexosaminidase B (an isoenzyme) is characteristic of carrier status. Pregnancy, the use of birth control pills, and disease states (e.g., diabetes) can confound enzymatic results. During pregnancy, hexosaminidase levels determined using leukocytes, in addition to serum, should be measured to confirm carrier status. The presence of one or more pseudodeficiency alleles, primarily in the non-Jewish population, can cause false-positive results, some of which can be clarified by DNA mutation analysis.

QUESTION 3: HOW ACCURATE IS DNA ANALYSIS IN TAY-SACHS CARRIER TESTING?

Three mutations in the hexosaminidase A gene account for over 90% of the mutations causing classical Tay-Sachs disease in the Ashkenazi Jewish population.[7] The range of mutations in most other ethnic groups is much larger. As a result, in most cases, enzyme testing is used for population-based screening programs and DNA testing is reserved for instances in which enzymatic results are inconclusive.

QUESTION 4: IF BOTH MEMBERS OF THE COUPLE ARE KNOWN TO BE CARRIERS OF THE TAY-SACHS DISEASE GENE, EITHER BY ENZYMATIC OR DNA ANALYSIS, WHAT ARE THE PRENATAL DIAGNOSTIC OPTIONS?

Prenatal diagnosis is typically performed using cultured amniocytes or direct or cultured material from CVS. Enzymatic testing is accurate in experienced hands, but DNA analysis can provide optimal accuracy when the parental mutations are known. Tay-Sachs disease is a likely candidate for preimplantation diagnosis in the future. This technique, discussed in greater detail in Chapter 30, relies on DNA analysis.

Huntington Disease

Huntington disease is a neurodegenerative disorder, with symptoms usually delayed until adulthood and typically occurring between ages 30 and 50. It is characterized by involuntary movements, intellectual deterioration, and behavioral changes. It is estimated that 5% of HD gene carriers have a juvenile-onset form, with rigidity rather than chorea and an onset in late childhood or early adolescence.[9]

One of the first clinically useful markers, discovered in 1983 by Gussella and colleagues,[8] localized the HD gene to the short arm of chromosome 4.[8] Using this and other, closer DNA markers, the HD gene could be tracked through a family and asymptomatic individuals could learn (with some chance of error) whether or not they carried the HD gene.

Identification of the HD gene proved elusive until the spring of 1993, when the molecular mechanism of mutation was discovered to be a polymorphic trinucleotide repeat (CAG) that occurs in tandem within the gene.[26] A similar mechanism has been identified in several other disorders.[24] The trinucleotide repeats in these genes are unstable and usually expand in size as they are passed from one generation to the next. Each of these genes has a specific "threshold"; if the number of repeats exceeds the threshold, that allele is associated with the disease. The number of repeats in non-HD alleles ranges from 11 to the mid-30s. In comparison, HD alleles typically have repeats of over 40.[26] However, a few exceptions have been reported in which clinically affected individuals have repeats within the "normal" range. These patients may have a different change in the HD gene (e.g., a point mutation) or may have been misdiagnosed. In addition, there appears to be a range between 30 and 40 repeats (called an *intermediate allele*) that may not cause the individual himself to have symptoms but when passed from father to child has the capacity to expand into the disease range. This phenomenon is associated with advanced paternal age.[15]

An inverse relationship exists between the number of repeats and the age of onset of symptoms: those with a juvenile onset have the largest number of repeats. However, this relationship does not allow and should not be used for prediction of a specific age of onset when an individual is presymptomatically or prenatally tested.[1] Although repeat expansions occur in both sexes, the largest expansions occur during sperm formation. This finding is consistent with the clinical observation that those with juvenile HD have inherited the gene from their fathers.[9]

The mechanism by which the trinucleotide repeats are involved in the pathogenesis of HD is unknown. Many articles have been written about the ethical and counseling implications of predictive testing for a late-onset disorder that has no cure.[29] These issues will remain and will perhaps be exacerbated by the availability of a simplified direct DNA test.

✤ Patient Profile: Carrier testing for Huntington disease

A 32-year-old pregnant woman (gravida 1, para 0000) has a family history of HD. Her mother has clinical features of HD and is currently institutionalized with severe neurologic symptoms. She also has other, similarly affected relatives.

QUESTION 1: WHAT IS THE RISK THAT THE PATIENT HAS INHERITED THE HUNTINGTON DISEASE GENE?

If her mother is, in fact, an HD gene carrier, the patient had a 50% chance at the time of her conception of inheriting the HD gene. Documentation of the diagnosis in other relatives by obtaining medical records is vital. The most definitive diagnosis of HD in a deceased relative is usually by autopsy of the brain. Information concerning the age of onset of symptoms as well as any unusual features in affected relatives is also important. Some families have chosen to obtain and store blood of affected relatives, which has allowed testing for some individuals that otherwise would not have been possible. Polymerase chain reaction-based DNA testing, like the direct test for HD, can potentially be performed on paraffin blocks (typically stored in a pathology laboratory) from a presumably affected relative.

QUESTION 2: HOW WILL THE AVAILABILITY OF A DIRECT DNA TEST FOR HUNTINGTON DISEASE AFFECT DIAGNOSTIC AND PRESYMPTOMATIC TESTING?

Before the HD gene was characterized, linkage studies, in which a series of DNA markers near the HD gene was used to "track" the gene through a family, were used for predictive and prenatal testing. Linkage studies impose an array of problems, most significantly the lack of available or cooperative affected relatives. The cloning of the gene will greatly simplify laboratory testing and will be more accurate. In principle, only the person who wants to know his or her status need be tested. In clinical practice, however, the presence of the expanded trinucleotide repeats in each affected relative should be confirmed. At the same time, the complex counseling and ethical issues remain regarding presymptomatic testing for a progressive disease that has no cure. For example, an asymptomatic person who is at 25% risk (who has an affected grandparent) may wish to have predictive testing, but the patient's parent (who is at 50% risk) may not want to learn whether he or she carries the gene. If the person at 25% risk is tested and has a repeat in the disease range, the parent will have simultaneously been tested but without consent.[22]

QUESTION 3: WHAT ARE THE CURRENT GUIDELINES FOR PRESYMPTOMATIC TESTING FOR HUNTINGTON DISEASE?

The general protocol for predictive testing for HD includes several components. A complete family and medical history is taken and the diagnosis is documented, including age of onset and type of symptoms present in affected relatives. A neurologic assessment is performed to determine whether clinical signs are already present in the presymptomatic individual. Psychologic and psychiatric testing and interviews are used to determine whether the individual is mentally ill or unstable and to assess his or her coping skills and support systems. The testing limitations and the potential effect of negative as well as positive results are discussed. Follow-up contacts and referral to a local professional for support are integral parts of the process.[3] These guidelines were proposed in part because the rate of suicide is substantially increased in newly diagnosed HD patients.[6] Other predictive testing issues include confidentiality of results, discrimination in employment, the ability to obtain health or life insurance, and the right not to be tested. These complex issues are reviewed in detail by Smarl and Weaver.[23]

QUESTION 4: IS IT POSSIBLE FOR A PREGNANT WOMAN TO HAVE FETAL TESTING WITHOUT LEARNING WHETHER SHE TOO IS A HUNTINGTON DISEASE GENE CARRIER?

Since predictive testing is not ideally undertaken during a pregnancy, fetal exclusion testing was designed with the specific purpose of allowing information about the fetus to be obtained without revealing whether the at-risk parent has inherited the HD gene. Linkage testing can assess whether the fetus has received the chromosome 4 that the at-risk woman described in the profile received from her (affected) mother or, alternatively, the one she inherited from her (unaffected) father. If the fetal markers match the woman's paternally inherited ones, the risk that the fetus is a gene carrier is low. If the maternal set of markers is inherited instead, the fetal risk is the same as that of the at-risk pregnant woman (approximately 50%).[5]

Fetal exclusion testing is controversial because if the results show that the fetus and the mother have the same risk and the mother later becomes symptomatic, the child will have been presymptomatically tested without his or her consent. However, pregnancy termination of a fetus at 50% risk is, to some, an unacceptable option. The discovery of the HD gene allows for more definitive fetal testing. At the same time, the main benefit of exclusion testing, allowing the fetal and predictive tests to be uncoupled, is not preserved when the fetus has a repeat in the disease range. Prenatal exclusion testing may become less desirable or may be challenged as unethical as more experience is gained with the direct test.

REFERENCES

1. Andrew S, Goldberg YP, Kremer B et al: The relationship between trinucleotide (CAG) repeat length and clinical features of Huntington's disease, *Nature Genetics* 4:398, 1993.
2. Boat T, Welsh M, Beaudet A: Cystic fibrosis. In Scriver C, Beaudet A, Sly W et al, editors: *The metabolic basis of inherited disease*, ed 6, New York, 1989, McGraw-Hill.
3. Brandt J, Quaid K, Folstein S et al: Presymptomatic diagnosis with delayed-onset disease with linked DNA markers, *JAMA* 261:3108, 1989.
4. Brock D, Clarke H, Barron L: Prenatal diagnosis of cystic fibrosis by microvillar enzymes assay on a sequence of 258 pregnancies, *Hum Genet* 78:271, 1988.
5. Brock D, Curtis A, Barron L et al: Predictive testing for Huntington's disease with linked DNA markers, *Lancet* 8661:463, 1989.
6. Farrer LA: Suicide and attempted suicide in Huntington disease: implications for preclinical testing of persons at risk, *Am J Med Genet* 24:305, 1986.
7. Fernandes M, Kaplan F, Clow C et al: Specificity and sensitivity of hexosaminidase assays and DNA analysis for the detection of Tay-Sachs disease gene carriers among Ashkenazi Jews, *Genet Epidemiol* 9:169, 1992.
8. Gusella J, Wexler N, Conneally P et al: A polymorphic marker genetically linked to Huntington's disease, *Nature* 306:234, 1983.
9. Harper PS: *Huntington's disease*, London, 1991, Saunders.
10. Handyside A, Lesko J, Tarin J et al: Birth of a normal girl after in vitro fertilization and preimplantation diagnostic testing for cystic fibrosis, *N Engl J Med* 327:905, 1992.
11. Harris H, Scotcher D, Hartlet N et al: Cystic fibrosis carrier testing in early pregnancy by general practitioners, *BMJ* 306:1580, 1993.
12. Kaback M, Hirsh P, Roy C et al: Gene frequencies for Tay-Sachs disease (TSD) and Sandhoff's disease (SD) in Jewish and non-Jewish populations, *Pediatr Res* 12:530A, 1978.
13. Kerem B, Rommens J, Buchanan J et al: Identification of the cystic fibrosis gene: genetic analysis, *Science* 245:1073, 1989.
14. Lemna W, Feldman G, Karem B et al: Mutation analysis for heterozygote detection and prenatal diagnosis of cystic fibrosis, *N Eng J Med* 322:291, 1990.
15. MacDonald M, Barnes G, Srinidhi J et al: Gametic but not somatic instability of CAG repeat length in Huntington's disease, *J Med Genet* 30:982, 1993.
16. McRae W, Williamson R: Cystic fibrosis. In Emery AE, Rimon DL, editors: *Principles and practices of medical genetics*, ed 2, Edinburg, 1990, Churchill Livingstone.
17. Natowicz M, Alper J: Genetic screening: triumphs, problems, and controversies, *J Pub Health Policy* 12:475, 1991.

18. Nyberg D, Dubinsky T, Resta R et al: Echogenic fetal bowel during the second trimester: clinical importance, *Radiology* 188:527, 1993.
19. Riordan JR, Rommens JM, Karem B et al: Identification of the cystic fibrosis gene: cloning and characterization of complementary DNA, *Science* 245:1066, 1989.
20. Sandhoff K, Conzelmann E, Neufeld E et al: The GM$_2$ gangliosides. In Scriver C, Beaudet A, Sly W et al, editors: *The metabolic basis of inheritance*, ed 6, New York, 1989, McGraw-Hill.
21. Shosani T, Augarten A, Gazit E et al: Association of a nonsense mutation (W1282X): the most common mutation in the Ashkenazi Jewish cystic fibrosis patients in Israel, with presentation of severe disease, *Am J Hum Genet* 50:222, 1992.
22. Simpson S, Harding A: Predictive testing for Huntington's disease: after the gene, *J Med Genet* 30:1036, 1993.
23. Smurl J, Weaver D: Presymptomatic testing for Huntington chorea: guidelines for moral and social accountability, *Am J Med Genet* 26:247, 1987.
24. Sutherland G, Richards R: Dynamic mutations: a new class of mutations causing human disease, *Cell* 70:709, 1992.
25. The Cystic Fibrosis Genetic Analysis Consortium: Population variation of common cystic fibrosis mutations, *Hum Mutat* 4:167, 1994.
26. The Huntington Disease Collaborative Research Group: a novel gene containing a trinucleotide repeat that is expanded and unstable on Huntington disease chromosomes, *Cell* 72:971, 1993.
27. Thompson M, McInnes R, Willard H: *Thompson and Thompson genetics in medicine*, ed 5, Philadelphia, 1991, WB Saunders.
28. Triggs-Raine B, Mules E, Kaback M et al: A pseudodeficiency allele common in non-Jewish Tay-Sachs carriers: implications for carrier screening, *Am J Hum Genet* 51:793, 1992.
29. Wiggins S, Whyte P, Huggins M et al: The psychological consequences of predictive testing for Huntington's disease, *N Engl J Med* 327:1401, 1992.

CHAPTER 9

Recurrent Pregnancy Loss

JEFFREY A. KULLER
VERN L. KATZ

Recurrent miscarriage, which affects approximately 1% of couples, is commonly defined as three consecutive spontaneous abortions of less than 20 menstrual weeks' duration. This is a devastating problem for most couples and has significant psychosocial ramifications.[5] After evaluation, a definite cause for recurrent miscarriage is identified 50% to 60% of the time. The etiology of recurrent miscarriage is diverse, and for purposes of classification it can be divided into three categories: (1) genetic causes, such as chromosome anomalies; (2) maternal reproductive anatomic disease, both developmental and acquired, such as septate uterus or cervical incompetence; and (3) systemic maternal disease, such as antiphospholipid antibody syndrome or maternal diabetes. Importantly, with no treatment, couples still have a 60% to 70% chance of subsequently delivering a viable infant.

❦ Patient Profile: Evaluation of a couple with recurrent spontaneous miscarriage

A 34-year-old woman (gravida 5, para 0040) is referred for consultation to evaluate her history of four spontaneous miscarriages. The patient and her husband have had two early spontaneous abortions at 7 weeks, one early fetal demise at 14 weeks, and an 8-week loss after fetal heart motion had been noted at 6 weeks' gestation. An evaluation is performed, including parental karyotypes, a hysterosalpingogram, an endometrial biopsy, cervical cultures for Ureaplasma and Chlamydia, and testing for antiphospholipid antibodies. All studies have normal results except for positive anticardiolipin antibodies (IgG and IgM). The lupus anticoagulant evaluation is negative. The patient is started on 80 mg/day of aspirin after a missed menses. She is currently 25 weeks' pregnant.

QUESTION 1: IF THE COUPLE IS OF NORMAL INTELLECTUAL FUNCTION, HOW COULD A GENETIC CAUSE EXPLAIN RECURRENT PREGNANCY LOSS?

Chromosome abnormalities cause at least 50% of spontaneous abortions. Autosomal trisomies form the largest group of cytogenetic abnormalities in spontaneous abortions, and monosomy X (45,X) is the single most common chromosome abnormality in spontaneous abortions. Though chromosome anomalies are the most common cause of spontaneous abortion, for such anomalies to be the cause of recurrent loss, the parents must have a chromosome rearrangement themselves. The most common parental structural chromosome rearrangement is a translocation. While parents with balanced translocations are phenotypically normal, offspring may demonstrate unbalanced rearrangements, such as chromosome duplications or deletions (Figures 9-1 and 9-2). Parental chromosome inversions are another cause of recurrent pregnancy loss.

A summary of reports of recurrent pregnancy loss published before 1985 concluded that 3% of parents had balanced chromosome rearrangements (six times the rate in the general population).[11] It is debatable whether to perform parental karyotypes after two

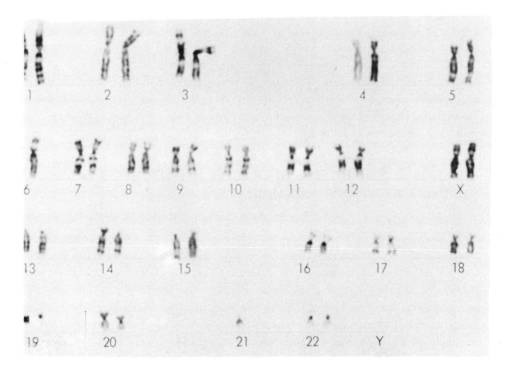

Fig. 9-1 Karyotype showing a balanced Robertsonian 14:21 translocation.

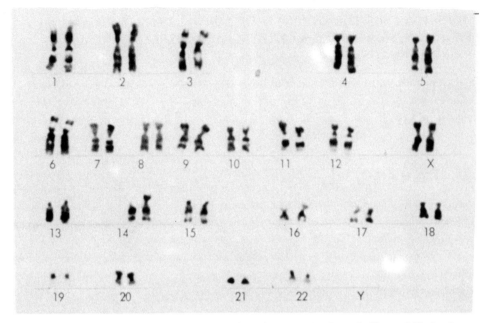

Fig. 9-2 Karyotype (of a fetus of the mother whose karyotype is shown in Figure 9-1) showing an unbalanced rearrangement resulting in an extra 21st chromosome (trisomy 21).

versus three consecutive losses. Therefore, we recommend performing parental karyotypes after three consecutive miscarriages. However, this evaluation may be performed after two miscarriages when the couple is particularly anxious or when the woman is 35 years of age or older at the time of evaluation.[3]

QUESTION 2: WHICH TYPES OF UTERINE MALFORMATION CAN CAUSE RECURRENT MISCARRIAGE?

Anatomic defects that lead to recurrent loss can be subdivided into three categories: (1) müllerian abnormalities; (2) uterine myomas; and (3) congenital or acquired cervical factors. Many women with uterine abnormalities have completely normal pregnancies. However, when they are associated with recurrent miscarriage, the treatment is surgical. Evaluation of the endometrial cavity with hysterosalpingogram or hysteroscopy should be part of the evaluation of all patients with recurrent loss. Müllerian anomalies, including septae, bicornate uterus, and uterus didelphis, when associated with recurrent pregnancy loss can be corrected hysteroscopically. Elective cervical cerclages are of questionable benefit for these anomalies. Occasionally a hysteroscopic examination will reveal uterine synechiae during an investigation for recurrent pregnancy loss. Hysteroscopic removal of the synechiae with subsequent estrogen treatment is extremely successful. Uterine myomas may be a cause of pregnancy loss when they are large, multiple, or occur in the submucosal area.[3,4] Because myomas only rarely cause recurrent miscarriage, a thorough evaluation for other causes must also be undertaken.[8]

Cervical factors in recurrent pregnancy loss, both congenital and acquired, have been referred to as *cervical incompetence*. The clinical presentation of premature cervical dilation ranges from silent dilation to bulging amniotic membranes, ruptured membranes, or sudden painless loss. Losses generally occur during the second trimester and are treated by cervical cerclage to prevent recurrent loss.

QUESTION 3: CAN GENITAL TRACT INFECTIONS CAUSE RECURRENT MISCARRIAGE?

To cause repeated miscarriage, an organism would have to persist for a prolonged period of time, be relatively asymptomatic, in order to escape diagnosis and treatment, be benign enough not to cause infertility, and also have access to the fetal compartment. The two organisms that fulfill these criteria are *Ureaplasma urealyticum* and *Chlamydia trachomatis*. Higher rates of cervical and endometrial colonization of *U. urealyticum* may be found in women with recurrent spontaneous abortion when compared with controls.[10] Erythromycin and doxycycline are the antibiotics of choice for genital T-strain mycoplasma. In addition, one study found a significantly higher incidence of high-titer IgG to *C. trachomatis* in women with recurrent abortion than in those without spontaneous losses.[12] Because many women who have had successful pregnancies may be carriers of *Ureaplasma*, it is still unclear whether these organisms are definite causes of recurrent loss. Although a debatable issue, the authors' policy is to recommend cervical cultures for *Ureaplasma* and *Chlamydia* in women with recurrent loss because the risk-benefit ratio favors treatment if these organisms are found in this clinical setting.[3]

QUESTION 4: CAN ENDOCRINE ABNORMALITIES CAUSE RECURRENT MISCARRIAGE?

The relationship of diabetes mellitus and spontaneous abortion has been studied extensively. Diabetic women with elevated blood glucose and glycosylated hemoglobin levels do have an increased rate of spontaneous abortion. However, most women with hyperglycemia significant enough to cause recurrent miscarriage are already known to be diabetic at the time of their evaluation.[7] Thus, a random glucose assay may be all that is needed to evaluate a patient with recurrent loss.

Luteal phase defect as a cause of recurrent pregnancy loss is extremely controversial.[2] The diagnosis of luteal phase defect is suggested by an elevation of basal body temperature lasting 10 days or less (short luteal phase) or an endometrial biopsy histologically more than 2 days out of phase in more than one menstrual cycle, or decreased serum progesterone concentration in the luteal phase. The most widely prescribed treatment is progesterone. A recent review of this subject concluded that there is insufficient evidence at this time to make recommendations concerning treatment of luteal phase defect.[2] If luteal phase abnormalities are a cause of recurrent miscarriage, the diagnosis would be suggested by losses very early in gestation, at 4 to 7 weeks. When no other cause can be found to explain recurrent miscarriage, it is certainly reasonable to measure serum progesterone levels or to perform an endometrial biopsy in the late luteal phase or both.

QUESTION 5: CAN IMMUNE MECHANISMS CONTRIBUTE TO RECURRENT MISCARRIAGE?

Antiphospholipid antibody syndrome causes between 5% and 40% of recurrent pregnancy loss. Though this family of antibodies reacts in vitro against several negatively charged phospholipids, assay for anticardiolipin antibody is the only test widely used at this time. There are several proposed and verified mechanisms by which the antiphospholipid antibodies induce pregnancy loss, including inhibition of the thrombolytic system, placental thrombosis, placental infarction, abnormal prostacyclin metabolism, direct cytotoxic effects, and fetal demise.[1,6] Serum from patients with lupus anticoagulant will demonstrate prolonged clotting time in vitro even after mixing with serum from normal controls. A dilute Russell viper venom test or kaolin clotting time should be used to test for the lupus anticoagulant. When affected patients are identified, as in the patient profile, treatment should be instituted as soon as an intrauterine pregnancy is verified. Low-dose aspirin (60-80 mg/day) should be prescribed for women with positive anticardiolipin antibodies. For women with a positive lupus anticoagulant test, the preferred treatment is low-dose aspirin and subcutaneous low-dose heparin. Even after miscarriage is prevented, antiphospholipid antibodies are associated with adverse pregnancy outcomes, including stillbirth, abruption, preeclampsia, and fetal growth retardation. Thus, treatment should be continued throughout pregnancy.

Finally, considerable research has been conducted during the past two decades regarding allogenic-immunologic causes of recurrent loss. Alloimmune causes may theoretically be related to an abnormal maternal immune response directed toward placental or fetal antigens. Therapeutic approaches for correction of an abnormal immune response have been aimed at inducing normal maternal immune responses to paternal antigens. However, information is still incomplete regarding the proper method of diagnosis and the nature of the immunologic cause of recurrent miscarriage.[9] Since the long-term consequences of immunotherapy are uncertain, therapy should be conducted only in research centers with carefully designed study protocols.

This chapter is based on and derived from the authors' review article on recurrent miscarriage.[3]

REFERENCES

1. Infante-Rivard AC, David M, Gauthier R, Rivard GE: Lupus anticoagulants, anticardiolipin antibodies, and fetal loss: a case-control study, *N Engl J Med* 325:1063, 1991.
2. Karamardian LM, Grimes DA: Luteal phase deficiency: effect of treatment on pregnancy rates, *Am J Obstet Gynecol* 167:1391, 1992.

3. Katz VL, Kuller JA: Recurrent miscarriage, *Am J Perinatol* 11:386, 1994.

4. Katz VL, Dotters DJ, Droegemueller W: Complications of uterine leiomyomas in pregnancy, *Obstet Gynecol* 73:593, 1989.

5. Kuller JA, Katz VL: A historical perspective on miscarriage, *Birth* 21:227, 1994.

6. Landy HJ, Kessler C, Kelly WK, Weingold AB: Obstetric performance in patients with lupus anticoagulant and/or anticardiolipin antibodies, *Am J Perinatol* 9:146, 1992.

7. Miodovnik M, Skillman C, Holroyde JC et al: Elevated maternal glycohemoglobin in early pregnancy and spontaneous abortion among insulin-dependent diabetic women, *Am J Obstet Gynecol* 153:439, 1985.

8. Rosenfeld DL: Abdominal myomectomy for otherwise unexplained infertility, *Fertil Steril* 46:328, 1986.

9. Scott JR, Rote NS, Branch DW: Immunologic aspects of recurrent abortion and fetal death, *Obstet Gynecol* 70:645, 1987.

10. Stray-Pedersen B, Eng J, Reikvan TM: Uterine T-mycoplasma colonization in reproductive failure, *Am J Obstet Gynecol* 130:307, 1978.

11. Tharapel AT, Tharapel SA, Bannerman RM: Recurrent pregnancy losses and parental chromosome abnormalities: a review, *Br J Obstet Gynæcol* 92:899, 1985.

12. Witkin SS, Ledger WJ: Antibodies to *Chlamydia trachomatis* in sera of women with recurrent spontaneous abortions, *Am J Obstet Gynecol* 167:135, 1992.

CHAPTER 10

Grief Counseling

DONNA JEANE HITCHCOCK PAPPAS
M. CATHLEEN McCOY

The vast majority of pregnancies have a positive outcome: a healthy child. However, in 3% of newborns a birth defect is detected, ranging from a minor anomaly of minimal concern to a lethal abnormality. When a fetal anomaly is detected, it is vital to explore the emotional responses of the patient and her partner in conjunction with a discussion of the perinatal management. The counseling the patient and her partner receive and the interaction they have with the physician and other health care professionals can positively influence how a woman and her family cope with and recover from a poor pregnancy outcome.

❧ Patient Profile: Discovery of a fetal anomaly

A 33-year-old married woman (gravida 2, para 1001) has a history of secondary infertility since the delivery of her first child, who is now 5 years old. The current pregnancy was achieved with ovulation induction and had been uncomplicated until 17 weeks' gestation, when an office ultrasound examination was performed to rule out anomalies. The fetal ultrasound examination revealed a large cystic hygroma, fetal ascites, and pleural effusions. The physician is concerned that the findings might indicate a karyotypic abnormality, probably Turner syndrome. He must inform the patient of the ultrasound findings, differential diagnosis, options for further evaluation, and overall prognosis.

QUESTION 1: HOW SHOULD THIS INFORMATION BE CONVEYED TO THE PATIENT?

Patients often regard ultrasound as a way to view their baby, without ever considering the possibility and the effect of the sonologist finding an anomaly. If a problem is detected, the patient does not necessarily need to be given a specific explanation of the defect while the ultrasound examination is being performed. However, the sonologist can make a statement such as, "I'm seeing some things that concern me. I need to focus on looking at the baby, but afterward we will sit down and talk about what I'm seeing and what it means." This statement gives the sonologist the opportunity to evaluate further what he or she is seeing, while acknowledging the patient who is undergoing the scan.

Reporting bad news to a patient is never easy. In a single moment a patient's hopes and dreams about the pregnancy are shattered. Giving an absolute prognosis at this point is often not possible. Although a patient may press for such information, it is preferable to describe what was seen during the ultrasound examination without quoting exact numbers, unless one is very certain of the diagnosis.

As the news of a problem is presented to the patient and her partner, they may be shocked and can quickly become overwhelmed. For this reason, the information given should be limited to what the patient and her partner need to know at that time. If the patient is alone, it is important to give her the opportunity to contact a support person, who also may help her process the information.

In this patient profile, one recommendation is to refer the patient to a prenatal diagnosis center, where further noninvasive and invasive testing could be performed. Before a definite prognosis can be given, more information is needed. Since it may be a threatening experience for a patient to leave the comfort of her primary care practice to go to an unknown setting, patients often find it helpful for their provider to tell them what to expect at this appointment. In addition, the referring physician should send medical records to the center at which the patient will be evaluated, thus providing better continuity of care. The referring physician may remain in touch with the patient via phone calls and visits to ease her anxiety while she awaits her consultation. Even if it becomes necessary to transfer care to a medical center for more specific pediatric or obstetric care, continued communication from the referring physician helps the patient to feel supported.

QUESTION 2: WHAT FEELINGS DO PATIENTS HAVE AFTER AN ABNORMALITY IS DIAGNOSED PRENATALLY?

Most women begin pregnancy with the knowledge that complications, such as a miscarriage, can occur, but they frequently believe that these happen only to other people. When news is relayed of a problem, the very foundation of their belief system, including their trust in God, is often shaken. This event is often the first tragedy that has affected the patient or couple so personally.

The most frequently asked question is, "Why did this happen?" This question reflects both the patient's search for a concrete explanation of why the problem occurred and, in particular, why it happened to her. The patient's first response may be to internalize the problem; she may think that she caused the abnormality in some way. Common examples include drinking an alcoholic beverage before she knew she was pregnant or using over-the-counter cold medications. It is reasonable to anticipate these ruminations and to clarify associations between an anomaly and teratogenic exposure. Most patients will continue to need reassurance regarding these concerns and to be told that they did not cause the anomaly. It may be helpful at different points during the pregnancy to ask the patient whether she continues to have any feelings of guilt.

Along with guilt, the patient and her partner often have a lingering feeling of hope. Some couples take a measure of comfort in thinking that the referring doctor may be incorrect. Many patients hope that the consulting physician at the prenatal diagnostic center will be able to tell them that everything is normal or that the anomaly is minor. Coming to terms with the problem is a process, and hope is a legitimate part of that evolution, allowing the couple to continue to cope. There is, however, a definite difference between hope and denial. With hope, the patient is still hearing about and responding to the problems in the pregnancy. Denial is problematic in that the patient refuses to respond to or act on the information. This can occasionally be harmful to the baby's prognosis.

The couple described in this profile was referred to a prenatal diagnostic center. At that visit, the couple had genetic counseling and ultrasound evaluation by a perinatologist. When the diagnosis of Turner syndrome was eventually confirmed, the couple was presented with the options of either continuing or interrupting the pregnancy. This is not a choice many couples ever imagine themselves having to make. Even for the couple who thought they had certain feelings regarding pregnancy termination, the circumstances of reality may not match what they had imagined. They may feel that they must make a decision even though there are no good options. Several issues enter into decision making: (1) concerns about the baby's suffering if the long-term prognosis is poor; (2) the effects on their other children of having a sibling with special needs; (3) the effect of the decision on the couple as a unit; (4) financial and employment considerations; (5) family influence; and (6) religious or spiritual beliefs.

The process of hearing the diagnosis, absorbing all the medical information, and then working toward a decision is extremely draining and traumatic for couples. When they eventually make a decision regarding whether or not to continue the pregnancy, they may have a sense of calm because they feel that the worst is over for them. However, this is just the first phase of grief. The practitioner can acknowledge this sense of resolution, but he or she must still prepare the couple for the next phase of treatment. A couple who elects to terminate their pregnancy needs to be prepared for the hospitalization, which will involve physically parting with their baby. In addition, they must be prepared for the sadness that they will face after the hospitalization.

QUESTION 3: WHAT TYPES OF SUPPORT SHOULD BE PROVIDED TO THE PATIENT DURING HOSPITALIZATION?

Whether a couple chooses to continue or to interrupt the pregnancy, the patient and her family will require a great deal of support. Communication is vital among physicians and nursing staff who will be caring for the patient during her stay. Along with the necessary medical information, it is helpful for hospital staff to provide psychosocial support and information. The more information the staff has about a patient, the better prepared they are to meet her needs.

Patients often look to the medical staff for guidance. In a situation that appears to be out of the patient's control, practitioners can give some control back to the patient and her family by discussing the choices that can be made during and after the pregnancy termination or delivery.

Years ago, anomalous babies were often whisked away from their mothers. Today, couples are encouraged to see and hold their baby. In addition, a variety of other options are offered to the parents. Tiny outfits may be provided for the patient to dress the baby or for the baby to be dressed by the nursing staff. A certificate of delivery with the baby's footprints is provided. This can be done even after a dilation and evacuation. In many hospitals, photographs are taken for the family. Naming the baby is discussed, and baptism or a visit with the hospital chaplain is offered. The number of family members allowed with the patient is usually flexible. If the couple has other children, they may want the children to see the baby after the delivery, depending on the children's ages. Decisions must also be made regarding autopsy and whether a funeral or cremation is preferred.

Ideally, the physician should initiate discussion of these options before hospitalization. Frequently, the patient or couple is disturbed by the idea of seeing the baby. The patient should not be made to feel that she has to make an immediate decision about any of the options. Many times a patient will be uncertain about whether she wishes to see the baby until the baby is actually delivered. The physician and nurse can help tremendously in facilitating this process by holding the baby themselves and describing to the patient what they are seeing. The patient's fears are frequently far worse than the reality of the situation. Parents often have a remarkable ability to see the beauty in their own baby even when he or she has multiple defects. Research indicates that parents usually do not regret the decision to hold and see their baby. In fact, those who elect not to do so may later wish that they had. Ultimately, the patient must be responsible for making this decision.

Since the patient sometimes declines to see the baby or even to have pictures taken, it should be standard protocol for the nursing staff to take photographs. In too many cases the patient comes back after a few weeks or months or sometimes even longer than a year and wants to know whether photographs are available. It is important to have a system for keeping the photographs on file, where they can be retrieved for the interested patient.

While much attention is directed toward the patient's medical care, if the father of the baby is present, he too will require support. Some men will not show a great deal of emotion but do appreciate being included in the process. Sometimes the patient and her partner will have disparate feelings about seeing and holding the baby. As long as each member of the couple is comfortable with his or her own decision, the staff should make the arrangements that best fulfill each person's wishes.

Frequently the patient will have other people present for support, including family members or friends. The staff should first ensure that the patient's needs are being met. For example, she may prefer to be alone with her husband at the time of delivery and for a short time afterward. The preferred time to discuss these arrangements is before delivery.

The amount of time a family chooses to be with their baby can vary greatly, ranging from several minutes to a number of hours. Because this is the only time they will have, every allowance should be made to give the family the time they need. Some families may have difficulty letting go. At some point the staff may have to suggest separation, while acknowledging that no time would ever be enough and that it is always difficult to say goodbye to someone you love, especially one's child. If the patient was sedated at the time of delivery, a later visit with the baby's body can be offered. Family members who were not present at the time of delivery may wish to see the baby. Admittedly, the logistics of this are not always easy; however, every effort should be made to fulfill the patient's wishes.

If after the delivery the patient continues her stay on the postpartum ward, all the medical and ancillary staff must be made aware of the baby's death. In many hospitals, a special sign is hung on the door of the room of any mother whose baby has died. Those who are caring for the mother can acknowledge the difficulty of the parents' situation and allow them to focus on their feelings. This is also the time to prepare a patient for some of the well-meaning but misguided statements that friends and family might make. Finally, it is critical that support from the medical staff not end with the hospital discharge.

QUESTION 4: HOW CAN FOLLOW-UP AFTER DELIVERY HELP THE PATIENT COPE WITH HER GRIEF?

When asked what aided the healing process after the death of a baby, parents frequently say that communication from their physician was critical. Conversely, when a patient has no contact with her physician, she often feels abandoned and hurt. Her relationship with the physician may be one of the deepest connections a patient has with her baby. Although it may be sad and emotional for the patient to speak with her physician, the caring and concern he or she expresses is appreciated. Even a call from a nurse or other staff member to the patient may not substitute for hearing from her physician.

The first visit back to the physician's office can be traumatic for the patient; the last time she visited the office, she was pregnant. It helps to schedule the appointment at a time when the patient will not have to wait to be seen. Sitting and talking with her in an office before the physical examination is often very helpful. When the patient does not feel emotionally ready for an examination, it may be preferable to reschedule it. The staff should be alerted to the patient's appointment so that they will be sure not to ask her questions such as, "How is your new baby?" When talking to the patient, the physician should ask whether she named the baby and, if so, he or she should use the baby's name in conversation. It is probably best not to use the term *abortion*, since it has both political and emotional implications. For the patient who interrupted her pregnancy, this may become an issue that needs to be addressed.

During the time of the diagnosis and the decision-making process, the patient receives a great deal of information that is often incompletely retained. Therefore, a follow-up meeting, included as part of the postpartum examination or as a separate meeting, should take place to review the information regarding the pregnancy and diagnosis. If an autopsy or karyotype was performed, a review of the findings may take place at that time. Other items to be discussed include the risk for recurrence and the management of a subsequent pregnancy. In some instances, referral to a perinatologist or geneticist for this information is warranted.

Both medical and emotional issues need to be considered in determining the timing of a subsequent pregnancy. From an emotional perspective, there is no perfect interval between pregnancies. The couple must decide for themselves when they are ready to face the complexity of another pregnancy.

Defining a normal time frame for recovery is difficult because patients have unique responses. The couple's families and friends may have unrealistic expectations of how long it will take to recover. During the first few weeks after the baby's death, the patient may find that she cries often. Approximately a month after the death, the reality of the situation often manifests itself, representing another acute phase of grief. The next difficult period is often the baby's original due date. For some patients, just as they were beginning to feel in control they find themselves feeling distressed several weeks or days before the original due date. A good gauge of how well the patient is coping is to ask whether she has been less distressed (crying less during the day, sleeping better, and eating more consistently) and whether she and her husband have begun to return to regular activities.

The grief responses of the mother and the father might be different because their experiences with the pregnancy were not the same. In some instances, the patient may express frustration with her partner for what she perceives as his lack of emotion. Alternatively, the father may wonder why she is not getting over the experience more quickly. Mentioning that men and women may differ in their responses to the loss prepares the couple and acknowledges that each partner's response is normal.

QUESTION 5: WHAT MANAGEMENT AND COUNSELING STRATEGIES FACILITATE A SUCCESSFUL SUBSEQUENT PREGNANCY?

Many couples talk of losing their innocence regarding pregnancy after the experience of the death of a baby. No longer do they assume that pregnancy is uncomplicated. Even when the risk of recurrence is low, some couples note that their risk was low for the problem to occur the first time. In addition, some couples begin to worry about all the other complications that can occur in a pregnancy.

For these couples, preconceptional counseling and planning of the pregnancy offers an element of control. It also gives the couple the opportunity to discuss with their physician their anxieties about a subsequent pregnancy and to develop strategies that will help them cope with their fears. The patient may need extra reassurance during her pregnancy. Telling her that she may come to the office at any time to listen to the baby's heartbeat will often help to alleviate some of the stress. Supportive office staff also help to ease the patient's anxiety.

Prenatal diagnostic choices must also be discussed. Each couple approaches prenatal diagnosis differently. Some couples choose to have every available test, whereas others decide that they would rather not have any prenatal testing. Despite all the preparation for a subsequent pregnancy and the implementation of strategies to cope with the anxiety, it cannot be totally eliminated. For many couples, it is not until they finally hold their new baby that the anxiety begins to ease. The parent and child relationship has been forever changed by the death of the couple's previous child. The emotional investment a physician makes and the time he or she spends caring for these patients and their families are paramount to the healing process.

REFERENCES

1. Blumberg BD, Golbus MS, Hanson KH: The psychological sequelae of abortion performed for a genetic indication, *Am J Obstet Gynecol* 122:799, 1975.
2. Brost L, Kenney J: Pregnancy after perinatal loss: parental reactions and nursing intervention, *J Obstet Gynecol Neonatal Nurs* 21:457, 1992.
3. Defain L: Learning about grief from normal families: SIDS, stillbirth and miscarriage, *J Marital Fam Ther* 17:215, 1991.
4. Elder S, Laurence K: The impact of supportive intervention after second trimester termination of pregnancy for fetal abnormality, *Prenat Diagn* 11:47, 1991.
5. Hunfeld JA, Wladimiroff JW, Passchier J et al: Emotional reactions in women in late pregnancy following the ultrasound diagnosis of a severe or lethal fetal malformation, *Prenat Diagn* 13:603, 1993.
6. Leon I: Perinatal loss: a critique of current hospital practices, *Clin Pediatr* 31:366, 1992.
7. Seller M, Barnes C, Ross S et al: Grief and mid-trimester fetal loss, *Prenat Diagn* 13:341, 1993.
8. Van Putte A: Perinatal bereavement crisis: coping with negative outcomes from prenatal diagnosis, *J Perinat Neonatal Nurs* 2:12, 1988.
9. White-Van Mourick M, Conner JM, Ferguson-Smith MA: The psychological sequelae of a second-trimester termination of pregnancy for fetal abnormality, *Prenat Diagn* 12:189, 1992.

PART THREE

MATERNAL SERUM
SCREENING

CHAPTER 11

Evaluation of Elevated Maternal Serum α-Fetoprotein

WILLIAM J. SWEENEY
NANCY C. CHESCHEIR

During the last several years, important advances have been made in the implementation of maternal serum α-fetoprotein (MSAFP) screening programs in the United States. It has become a standard part of obstetric care to offer this screening test to all pregnant women between 15 and 20 weeks' gestation. Advances in ultrasound technology have improved the ability to diagnose open neural tube and other defects. Maternal serum α-fetoprotein screening makes it possible to determine who is at increased risk of having a fetus with an open neural tube defect, allowing further testing to be performed to diagnose these defects. This chapter will focus on α-fetoprotein and on the proper evaluation of elevated MSAFP.

❧ Patient Profile: Diagnostic options for a patient with an elevated maternal serum α-fetoprotein value

The patient is a 22-year-old Caucasian woman (gravida 1, para 0000) determined to be at 17 weeks' gestation based on menstrual history. As part of her routine obstetric care, she was counseled about MSAFP screening, and she consented to undergo this test. Her MSAFP was 3.5 multiples of the median (MoM) for 17 weeks, and she was referred for evaluation.

Targeted ultrasound at 17.5 weeks showed a singleton live fetus with an anterior, normal-appearing placenta and a normal amount of amniotic fluid. The biparietal diameter (BPD), femur length, and abdominal circumference were consistent with her dates. The shapes of the cranium and cerebellum were normal, with a normal-appearing cisterna magna. The posterior horns of the lateral ventricles were measured at 0.5 cm, with a normal-appearing choroid plexus bilaterally. Transverse and longitudinal views of the spine showed nondiverging spinal echo centers and intact skin covering from the level of the skull through the sacrum. The abdominal wall appeared to be intact, with a normal umbilical cord insertion. Based on the normal ultrasound findings, her estimated risk for an open neural tube defect (ONTD) was lowered by 90%. Amniocentesis for α-fetoprotein (AFP) and acetylcholinesterase (AChE) was offered and declined. The patient was counseled that an unexplained elevation in MSAFP is associated with an increased risk for stillbirth, low birthweight, preeclampsia, and preterm labor.

QUESTION 1: WHAT IS α-FETOPROTEIN?

α-Fetoprotein is a glycoprotein with a molecular weight of approximately 70,000 daltons. It is produced by the yolk sac and liver equally at 4 to 8 weeks' gestation. When the yolk sac involutes, the liver becomes the dominant source of AFP production for the remainder of pregnancy.[5] Normally, most MSAFP is derived from the fetal circulation via its continuity with the maternal circulation, a process that seems to occur by diffusion.[2] Transmembranous transport of AFP from the amniotic cavity contributes approximately 6% of MSAFP.[2] Any condition of the fetus that leads to increased production of AFP (twins), increased passage of AFP from fetal compartment to maternal compartment (abnormal placentation), or an increased level of AFP in the amniotic fluid (open spina bifida) can lead to an increase in MSAFP.

QUESTION 2: HOW ARE THE NORMAL AND ABNORMAL RANGES OF MATERNAL SERUM α-FETOPROTEIN VALUES ESTABLISHED?

The MSAFP value is expressed as multiples of the median (MoM) value for normal pregnancies at a given gestational age. Each laboratory should establish its own range of normal values based on the population sampled. Laboratories should provide interpretation of results and risk assessment that takes into account variables such as maternal race and weight, multiple pregnancies, insulin-dependent diabetes mellitus, and multiple gestation. For example, black women are known to have higher MSAFP levels at any given gestational age than white women; therefore, the level of MSAFP required for a pregnancy to be considered at risk is higher for black women (see Table 11-1). Extremes of maternal weight require adjustment as well, since the MSAFP can be either concentrated or diluted in very thin or obese women, respectively. In general, multiple fetuses produce more AFP, and diabetics have been shown to have less MSAFP; both conditions require adjustment. In

Table 11-1 Sample limits for MSAFP values by race, diabetic status, and gestational age*†

	Gestational age (weeks)	
	15-18	**19-21**
Race		
White	2.25	2.00
Black	2.50	2.25
Other	2.25	2.00
Unknown	2.25	2.00
Diabetic‡	1.50	1.50

*These limits are used by the University of North Carolina Prenatal Diagnosis Program.
†All limits are expressed as multiples of the median (MoM) value for normal pregnancies.
‡Singleton pregnancy, any race.

Table 11-2   Sample limits for MSAFP values in the patient with a positive family history of neural tube defects[7]

Affected family member	Recurrence risk	MSAFP limit*
Previous child, or either parent of fetus	2.0%	1.0 MoM
Patient's sister's child	1.0%	1.0 MoM
Patient's brother, sister, aunt, uncle, niece, or nephew	0.3%	1.5 MoM
Patient's cousin or more distant relative	General population	Unchanged

*An MSAFP level below the various limits indicates that the patient's risk for ONTDs is the same as or less than that of the general population.

addition, diabetic patients have an overall increased risk for congenital malformation, which is also considered in making the adjustment. Recent data suggest that the differences in MSAFP seen with diabetic women may be more closely related to the efficacy of diabetic control than to diabetic status.1 Maternal serum AFP MoM limits are also adjusted for patients who have positive family histories of neural tube defects (see Table 11-2).

QUESTION 3: WHAT IS THE ROLE OF SONOGRAPHY IN THE EVALUATION OF ELEVATED MATERNAL SERUM α-FETOPROTEIN?

Until recently, it was recommended that all women with elevated MSAFP or increased *a priori* risk undergo amniocentesis for evaluation of amniotic fluid AFP and acetyl-cholinesterase levels for the detection of ONTDs. This recommendation has become controversial since the discovery of certain cranial features detectable by high-level ultrasound that are almost always present in cases of spina bifida.

When a woman is referred for an evaluation of MSAFP, a detailed ultrasound examination is performed. Miscalculation of gestational age, multiple gestation, fetal demise, and anencephaly are readily detectable. A detailed anatomic survey is performed, with careful attention given to the cranium, spine, and abdominal wall. The placenta and amniotic fluid are also evaluated. Normal findings on high-resolution ultrasound allow a 90% reduction in the MSAFP-based estimated risk of an ONTD. For example, if a woman presents with a risk of 1 in 100 for an ONTD based on MSAFP, a normal ultrasound with adequate views of *all* relevant anatomic features lowers her estimated risk to less than 1 in 1000.[4] Inability to visualize relevant features or the discovery of any abnormality prohibits risk reduction. Amniocentesis is offered to all patients with elevated MSAFP; however, many decline invasive testing when the fetal anatomy is found by the ultrasound to be apparently normal.

For a second-trimester ultrasound examination to be considered satisfactory, the following views of the fetus should be clearly seen: (1) serial sections of the fetal spine showing nondivergent spinal echo centers and intact skin covering from the level of the skull through the sacrum; (2) normal ventricles (posterior horns <1 cm); (3) BPD appropriate for gestational age; (4) normal cisterna magna; (5) absence of frontal notching (lemon sign); and (6) normal cerebellar anatomy, without distortion or caudal displacement (banana sign). If the scan is inadequate for technical reasons, the patient is informed that the ultrasound examination was suboptimal, and the estimated MSAFP-related risk for spina bifida is not reduced. This protocol has significantly lowered the frequency of amniocentesis, with no decrease in detection rates for ONTDs.[4]

QUESTION 4: WHAT ARE THE TYPICAL SONOGRAPHIC FINDINGS ASSOCIATED WITH OPEN SPINA BIFIDA?

The prenatal diagnosis of open spina bifida has been facilitated by the almost universal presence during the second trimester of certain cranial abnormalities, which include the Arnold-Chiari malformation (banana sign) and frontal notching (lemon sign). Microcephaly and ventriculomegaly may also be present but are not as predictive in the early diagnosis of spina bifida. The Arnold-Chiari malformation is a congenital downward displacement of the hind brain into the cervical portion of the spinal canal. It is thought to be caused by either traction on the brainstem resulting from fixation of the spinal cord at the meningocele site[3] or by decreased spinal pressure.[9] Hydrocephalus eventually develops in 80% to 90% of cases as part of the Arnold-Chiari type II malformation; however, during the midtrimester, ventriculomegaly may be associated with a BPD that is actually small for dates. Frontal notching is seen as a concave frontal contour of the fetal calvaria, rather than a normal convex frontal contour. It is postulated that this may be caused by leakage of cerebrospinal fluid from an open spina bifida, resulting in a partial collapse of the soft fetal calvaria.

Nicolaides and colleagues[6] were the first to report the usefulness of these cranial findings in diagnosing open spina bifida. Others have confirmed that these features are almost always detectable in cases of open spina bifida if the ultrasound examination is performed between 16 and 24 weeks' gestation. Demonstration of a rachischisis is also diagnostic of spina bifida. This defect can usually be seen in transverse and longitudinal views. Disruption of the overlying integument is another important clue to the diagnosis of spina bifida. A myelomeningocele sac may be found, as it is present in most fetuses with spina bifida. These sacs are most commonly located in the lumbosacral region.

QUESTION 5: HOW DOES AMNIOCENTESIS AID IN THE DIAGNOSIS OF OPEN NEURAL TUBE DEFECTS?

Amniotic fluid can be evaluated for AFP and acetylcholinesterase. As with MSAFP, the level of amniotic fluid AFP (AFAFP) is expressed as MoM for normal pregnancies of the same gestational age. Using a cut-off level of 2.5 MoM, 93% to 96% of fetuses with open spina bifida and virtually all anencephalic fetuses can be detected. False-positive results still occur frequently, however, as a result of contamination of the amniotic fluid by fetal blood. This is especially true if the needle traverses the placenta during the amniocentesis.

Acetylcholinesterase is an enzyme found in large quantities in cerebrospinal fluid, accounting for its presence in the amniotic fluid of pregnancies affected by ONTDs. Its molecular weight is so large that it is not normally secreted in the urine, making it useful as a marker for ONTDs. Contamination of the amniotic fluid by fetal blood can also lead to a small number of false-positive results (1%). The measurement of amniotic fluid acetylcholinesterase has proved to be a slightly better diagnostic test than the measurement of amniotic fluid AFP, with a detection rate for open spina bifida of up to 99%.

QUESTION 6: SHOULD CHROMOSOME ANALYSIS BE PERFORMED WHEN EVALUATING AMNIOTIC FLUID FOR α-FETOPROTEIN?

Watson and colleagues[8] suggested that there may be an increased incidence of chromosome abnormalities in patients with elevated levels of MSAFP. They found that the rate of detection of significant cytogenetic abnormalities in patients whose sole indication for amniocentesis was elevated MSAFP was 1 in 157. One fourth of these were sex chromosome abnormalities, which present different counseling problems than those of the autosomal aneuploidies. In the presence of fetal or placental abnormalities or both, the risk of chromosome abnormalities increases to approximately 15%. These issues should be presented to the patient who is considering amniocentesis for evaluation of elevated MSAFP.

QUESTION 7: WHY IS GESTATIONAL AGE SO IMPORTANT IN EVALUATING MATERNAL SERUM α-FETOPROTEIN?

Maternal serum AFP screening is best performed between 16 and 18 weeks' gestation because it is at this time that there is the widest disparity between levels of MSAFP for affected and unaffected pregnancies. The most common reason for a false-positive result is incorrect gestational age when the sample is drawn. Ultrasound examination logically becomes the next step in the evaluation to ensure that the sample was drawn at the appropriate time. The BPD is the only measurement used, since it actually will help increase the detection rate of ONTDs. This is because in affected pregnancies the biparietal diameter is usually smaller, which in turn leads to a lower gestational age estimate so that the level of MSAFP expressed in MoM would be higher.

QUESTION 8: WHAT OTHER FETAL ANOMALIES CAUSE AN ELEVATION IN MATERNAL SERUM α-FETOPROTEIN?

Many conditions are associated with an elevation of MSAFP. Some of the more common abnormalities include abdominal wall defects, renal agenesis, fetal demise or impending fetal demise, teratoma, congenital nephrosis, congenital diaphragmatic hernia, and some tumors. Other conditions are fetomaternal hemorrhage, abnormal placental morphology, oligohydramnios, Rh isoimmunization, and low birthweight. Unexplained elevations in MSAFP have been associated with suboptimal pregnancy outcomes. These concerns will be addressed in Chapter 13.

QUESTION 9: HOW SHOULD AN OBSTETRIC PATIENT BE COUNSELED ABOUT MATERNAL SERUM α-FETOPROTEIN? SHOULD EVERY PATIENT BE OFFERED THIS TESTING?

Maternal serum AFP screening is designed for a low-risk population because 90% of neural tube defects occur in the absence of a positive history, making identification of neural tube defects by history alone impractical. A careful history should be taken either as part of a preconceptional counseling session or at the initial prenatal appointment. The history should include diabetic status, medication and drug exposures, and a detailed family history of birth defects, especially neural tube defects. Exposure to anticonvulsant medication is especially important because valproic acid and carbamazepine use have been associated with an increased incidence of neural tube defects. Any patient who is noted to be at risk for having a fetus with an ONTD should be referred for counseling and possible diagnostic testing.

Patients who have no risk factors should be offered MSAFP screening. Because of the nature of screening tests, it is important to remember that, regardless of what limits are used to define an abnormal result, false-negative and false-positive results will occur.

REFERENCES

1. Baumgarten A, Reece EA, Davis N, Mahoney MJ: A reassessment of maternal serum alpha-fetoprotein in diabetic pregnancy, *Eur J Obstet Gynecol Reprod Biol* 28:289, 1988.
2. Gitlin D: Normal biology of alpha-fetoprotein, *Ann NY Acad Sci* 259:7, 1975.
3. Ingraham FD, Scott HW Jr: Spina bifida and cranium bifidum v. the Arnold-Chiari malformation: a study of 20 cases, *N Engl J Med* 229:108, 1943.
4. Katz VL, Seeds JW, Albright SG, Lingley LH, Lincoln-Boyea B: Role of ultrasound and informed consent in the evaluation of elevated maternal serum alpha-fetoprotein, *Am J Perinatol* 8:73, 1991.
5. Lau HL, Linkins SE: Alpha-fetoprotein, *Am J Obstet Gynecol* 124:533, 1976.
6. Nicolaides KH, Campbell S, Gabbe SG, Guidetti R: Ultrasound screening for spina bifida: cranial and cerebellar signs, *Lancet* 2:71, 1986.
7. Wald NJ, Cuckle HS: Nomogram for estimating an individual's risk of having a fetus with open spina bifida, *Br J Obstet Gynæcol* 89:598, 1982.
8. Watson WJ, Chescheir NC, Katz VL, Seeds JW: The role of ultrasound in evaluation of patients with an elevated maternal serum alpha-fetoprotein: a review, *Obstet Gynecol* 78:123, 1991.
9. Williams B: Cerebral spinal fluid pressure gradients in spina bifida cystica with special reference to the Arnold-Chiari malformation and aqueductal stenosis, *Dev Med Child Neurol* 17(suppl 35):138, 1975.

CHAPTER 12

Triple-Marker Screening for Aneuploidy

CAROL C. COULSON
VERN L. KATZ
JEFFREY A. KULLER

Triple-marker screening refers to the use of three maternal serum markers to define or modify an individual patient's risk for fetal aneuploidy. The three markers are α-fetoprotein (AFP), human chorionic gonadotropin (hCG), and unconjugated estriol (uE$_3$). These markers are measured to estimate a patient's risk of having a fetus with trisomy 21 (Down syndrome) and trisomy 18. Results are reported as multiples of the median (MoM) value for each gestational age. Low levels of AFP, hCG, and uE$_3$ are associated with pregnancies affected by trisomy 18, while low levels of AFP and uE$_3$ accompanied by high levels of hCG are associated with pregnancies affected by Down syndrome. An abnormal screening result is followed by ultrasound assessment, which may detect misdated pregnancies, multifetal pregnancies, unsuspected midtrimester losses, and other anomalies. The biologic basis of these altered protein concentrations is unknown but may be related to immaturity of the placenta or of the fetal liver or adrenal glands.

Accurate dating of a pregnancy is critical to the correct interpretation of maternal serum markers. Results of each of the serum markers vary by gestational age; thus, screening may be falsely positive if the pregnancy is not as advanced at the time of screening as estimated by the patient's menstrual dating. Testing should be performed at 15 to 20 weeks' gestation. Ideally, the test should be conducted at approximately 16 weeks because the results are more accurate at this gestational age and because the patient will have enough time to pursue diagnostic testing if results are abnormal. In several large prospective series, 30% to 40% of women initially classified as being at high risk for having a child with Down syndrome were reassigned to a low-risk category after correction of gestational age by ultrasound evaluation.[20,33] It is recommended, however, that positive screening results for trisomy 18 not be corrected by sonographic measurements because trisomy 18 fetuses may demonstrate early-onset growth retardation.

Three specific adjustments are necessary to increase the accuracy of screening when low maternal serum AFP (MSAFP) values are found. The first correction is for maternal weight. Obese women generally have lower MSAFP values, presumably because of dilution of fetal

AFP in a larger maternal blood volume. The second adjustment is for diabetes mellitus. Insulin-dependent diabetic women generally have MSAFP levels equal to two-thirds those found in nondiabetic women. In the absence of medians from this subgroup, the lower limit cut-off requires reduction by one third. The effect of diabetes on hCG and uE_3 levels appears to be less significant. The third adjustment is for race. Racial differences in MSAFP levels are well documented. For reasons that are uncertain, black women have levels 9% to 15% higher than those of white women. A 10% correction is recommended when screening women from the African-American population. The effect of racial differences on hCG and uE_3 levels is not well defined at this time. Although maternal smoking is known to increase AFP and reduce hCG and uE_3 levels, generally no correction is applied. Interestingly, smokers appear to have a lower incidence of children with Down syndrome. Twin gestation raises AFP, hCG, and uE_3 levels; however, there are no published series on biochemical markers in twin pregnancies with one or both fetuses affected by Down syndrome.[14]

It has been suggested that the risk for Down syndrome can be approximated in a twin pregnancy by dividing the AFP, hCG, and uE_3 MOMs by the average analyte level in twin pregnancies and then calculating the risk as if it were a singleton pregnancy. Although not as reliable an estimate as in a singleton pregnancy, this risk can be used to determine whether the result is screen positive or negative. Preliminary data from Lockwood and colleagues[25] suggest that fetal sex affects the prediction of Down syndrome by MSAFP. They found that women carrying female fetuses with Down syndrome had significantly lower MSAFP values than their male counterparts, resulting in a disproportionate identification of affected female fetuses.

Before 1984, prenatal screening for fetal aneuploidy was restricted to second-trimester amniocentesis for women who would be 35 years of age or older at the time of delivery. This approach was based on Penrose's identification[7] in 1933 of the association between increasing maternal age and the birth of children with autosomal trisomies. Twenty percent to thirty percent of Down syndrome cases occur in fetuses of women age 35 or older. Although this group of older mothers is at higher risk for fetal aneuploidy, they constitute the minority of pregnant women in this country. Therefore, the majority of Down syndrome babies are born to women less than 35 years of age.

With the advent of widespread MSAFP screening for open neural tube defects (ONTDs) in the early 1980s, the relationship between low MSAFP values and autosomal trisomies was discovered. Merkatz and colleagues[30] reported the index case of "undetectable" MSAFP at 16 weeks' gestation in a 28-year-old primigravida whose infant was postnatally found to have trisomy 18. Further retrospective analysis of their data demonstrated that MSAFP concentrations at 14 to 20 weeks' gestation were approximately 25% lower in pregnancies affected with Down syndrome than in unaffected pregnancies.

Age and MSAFP levels are independent risk measures, as shown by Cuckle and associates.[13] The use of age and MSAFP values in combination yields a better risk estimate for Down syndrome than either one alone. Using this information, DiMaio and colleagues[16] investigated prospectively the utility of measuring MSAFP during the second trimester in over 34,000 pregnant women of less than 35 years of age. When the combined use of MSAFP and maternal age produced an estimated risk of Down syndrome of 1 in 270 (i.e., the *a priori* risk of a 35-year-old woman), 20% to 33% of Down syndrome pregnancies could be selected for amniocentesis, with a false-positive rate of 5%.

The discovery of the inverse relationship between Down syndrome and MSAFP stimulated the search for other biochemical markers of the abnormal fetus. In 1987, Bogart and colleagues[7] observed that both high and low extremes of hCG were found in pregnancies with chromosomally aberrant fetuses. Maternal serum hCG concentrations were significantly elevated in pregnancies affected with Down syndrome and decreased in those with trisomy 18. They found that 6 of 17 women (35%) with Down syndrome fetuses had elevated maternal serum levels of hCG, whereas less than 2% of pregnancies with normal outcomes had elevated hCG levels. Subsequent studies confirmed that hCG measurements alone can be used to detect Down syndrome at a rate equal to or better than that of MSAFP.[40,41] Maternal serum hCG appears to be an independent marker. Thus the combination of MSAFP, maternal serum hCG, and maternal age can be used to identify 55% to 60% of fetuses with Down syndrome, with a false-positive rate of 5%. Confirmatory studies have strengthened the association between low maternal serum concentrations of hCG and trisomy 18.[10] Most studies measure either intact hCG or intact hCG plus the small fraction of free β-hCG found in midtrimester. Some authors claim that the free β-hCG subunit is more specific for Down syndrome.[28,37,39] More data are needed before the relative predictive value of intact hCG versus free β-hCG can be assessed.

The precise mechanism by which AFP and hCG levels are altered in a chromosomally abnormal fetus is unclear. Many authors have suggested that either decreased synthesis or decreased secretion by the fetal liver may be responsible. Based on this supposition, Canick and associates[8] investigated the use of uE_3, another protein product of the fetoplacental unit, as a biochemical marker of the anomalous fetus. Second-trimester uE_3 levels were measured in 22 pregnancies affected with Down syndrome and in 110 unaffected control pregnancies. The uE_3 levels were significantly lower in the affected pregnancies. Wald and colleagues[42] showed a similar decrease of approximately 25% in midtrimester uE_3 values in pregnancies affected with Down syndrome when compared with unaffected pregnancies. In addition, at a cut-off value selected to indicate at least 35% of affected pregnancies, the uE_3 level was a stronger predictor of Down syndrome risk than the AFP level, although each provided statistically significant information. The level of uE_3 was independent of maternal age and largely independent of AFP value. A subsequent publication concluded that each marker (AFP, hCG, uE_3) provided an independent measure of risk and that all three biochemical tests could be combined with maternal age to calculate a patient-specific risk for having a fetus with Down syndrome.[41] Although other investigators have disputed the additional value of including uE_3 measurements in multiscreen testing for fetal chromosome abnormalities, triple-marker screening has become a commonly used technique for aneuploidy screening in this country.[27]

The new screening method can be used to detect over 60% of all Down syndrome pregnancies, more than double the percentage detected by prenatal screening based on historical age only. Unique patterns of maternal serum markers associated with fetal defects can be evaluated by judicious selection of analyses and algorithms to optimize the accuracy of individual risk assessment. The American College of Medical Genetics (ACMG) states that data are currently insufficient to recommend testing with any one specific combination of markers.[11]

✤ Patient Profile: Noninvasive testing for aneuploidy

A 33-year-old woman (gravida 1, para 0000) seeks obstetric consultation at 10 weeks' gestation. She will be 34 years old at the time of delivery. She and her husband have a long history of primary infertility and are elated that they have conceived after 8 years of using artificial reproductive techniques. They are also somewhat distressed by the recent birth of a child with Down syndrome to their closest friends. They wish to do everything possible to ensure a normal outcome for their pregnancy, and they ask about triple-marker screening. Assuming that their pregnancy goes well, they are planning to pursue another pregnancy almost immediately after this delivery. The couple also inquires about noninvasive prenatal diagnosis in women over age 35.

QUESTION 1: CAN TRIPLE-MARKER SCREENING BE USED TO DETECT DISORDERS OTHER THAN DOWN SYNDROME?

Second-trimester maternal serum AFP, hCG, and uE_3, when assessed in combination with maternal age, have been shown to define the risk of fetal Down syndrome more accurately than any other method previously described. The evaluation of these levels in pregnancies with other defects is of continued interest. Trisomy 18 is the second most common autosomal trisomy compatible with live birth, although the birth prevalence is significantly lower than that of trisomy 21. Risk estimates for trisomy 18 can be determined by triple-marker screening. The typical profile is one of low levels of maternal serum AFP, hCG, and uE_3. Prevalence of trisomy 18 at birth or amniocentesis is positively correlated with maternal age.

Lindenbaum and associates[24] retrospectively studied 58 pregnancies affected with trisomy 18. Midtrimester MSAFP levels were markedly reduced in those affected pregnancies uncomplicated by either fetal omphalocele or neural tube defect. The presence of either or both of these defects raised the MSAFP value to normal or elevated levels, respectively. Greenberg and colleagues[19] described 14 patients whose pregnancies were affected with trisomy 18. Most had decreased levels of hCG and uE_3 as well as AFP; however, as previously noted, some AFP values were elevated. This series, in addition, showed markedly elevated levels of hCG in three cases. They concluded that maternal serum AFP and hCG may be bimodally distributed in pregnancies affected with trisomy 18, irrespective of neural tube or ventral wall defects.

Some authors feel that ultrasound examination may be a more reliable modality than maternal serum screening for the detection of trisomy 18. In a small series of 15 patients with trisomy 18 fetuses, Benacerraf and colleagues[5] reported ultrasound detection of 12 affected fetuses. Ultrasound examination frequently shows limb abnormalities consistent with those typically seen at birth in affected fetuses: limb reductions, clubbed or rockerbottom feet, and clenched fists with overlapping index fingers. Major congenital anomalies, such as diaphragmatic hernias, cardiac abnormalities, omphaloceles, neural tube defects, and single umbilical arteries, are also common. In addition, there is an association with choroid plexus cysts, although these can be found in 1% of normal fetuses. The sonographic detection of trisomy 18 is likely to improve with increasing awareness of the sonographic appearance of facial and limb abnormalities.

Nyberg and colleagues[34] reviewed the prenatal sonographic findings in 47 consecutive fetuses with trisomy 18. Thirty-nine fetuses (83%) were noted to have one or more abnormalities, excluding choroid plexus cysts. All of the fetuses with trisomy 18 were noted to have anomalies detectable by ultrasound when examined initially after 24 weeks, while 72% of the fetuses were found to have anomalies detectable by ultrasound when the examination was performed between 14 and 24 weeks. The most frequent abnormalities seen before 24 weeks included cystic hygromas, nuchal thickening, and meningomyelocele. Although the single most common abnormality, intrauterine growth retardation, was detected in 51% of all fetuses with trisomy 18, it was more pronounced after 24 weeks, when 89% of fetuses demonstrated growth delay. Cardiac defects and enlargement of the cisterna magna were also noted more often after 24 weeks. Awareness of the pathologic features that are associated with trisomy 18, particularly early-onset intrauterine growth retardation, will help to identify the patients who are at greatest risk.

Although trisomy 21 and trisomy 18 are the conditions most often discussed, counseling and prenatal diagnosis should emphasize the risk for all chromosomal anomalies, not just these two aneuploidies. In a series of 1154 patients who had amniocentesis for low MSAFP values, Drugan and colleagues[17] identified 13 chromosome abnormalities. Only half of these were autosomal trisomies. The remainder were sex chromosome aberrations, deletions, or triploidies. Additionally, Wenstrom and colleagues[44] reported the detection of eight fetuses with Turner syndrome using multiple-marker screening. Many of these abnormalities may not be detectable antenatally by ultrasound examination alone and may require invasive testing via amniocentesis, placental biopsy, or cordocentesis when indicated. Triple-marker screening can detect approximately 60% of fetuses with trisomy 18, but the detection rate for most other chromosome abnormalities is unknown.[9]

QUESTION 2: CAN DOWN SYNDROME BE DETECTED BY ANTENATAL ULTRASOUND EVALUATION?

Ultrasound confirmation of menstrual dating should be the first step in the evaluation of the patient with an abnormal triple-marker screening result that indicates an increased fetal risk of Down syndrome. In contrast to patients with elevated MSAFP values, positive serum screening results for Down syndrome should not be repeated. Of the biometric measurements used in the ultrasound examination, the biparietal diameter (BPD) is generally the most reliable midtrimester biometric measurement of dating because some fetuses with Down syndrome may have lagging femur lengths. After the gestational age and accurate interpretation of the serum multiscreen results have been confirmed, the patient should be offered karyotype analysis, the definitive diagnostic test for chromosome abnormalities. Amniocentesis is usually performed, although in some cases of advanced gestations placental biopsy or percutaneous umbilical blood sampling may be warranted for more rapid results. A detailed anatomic survey of the fetus at the time of counseling for abnormal results is recommended.

The increased use of prenatal ultrasound evaluation allows the detection of visible patterns of malformation in patients at risk for fetal aneuploidy. Fifty percent to sixty percent of Down syndrome fetuses can be identified by performing a sophisticated ultrasound examination.[43] Several different anthropomorphic features that may help identify the fetus with Down syndrome have been suggested based on findings in affected infants (see the box below). For instance, infants with Down syndrome are generally brachycephalic (with normal BPDs and short occipitofrontal diameters, leading to an increased cephalic index). However, second-trimester evaluation of fetuses known to have Down syndrome, when compared with normal controls, shows no difference in the cephalic indices, making this an unreliable screening criterion for Down syndrome.[38] Fetuses with Down syndrome may have shortened femur lengths (FLs), leading to increased BPD-FL ratios. Dicke and others[15,22,38] reported conflicting BPD-FL results, perhaps related to the great regional variation in norms and the need for institution-specific normative data. Sixty percent of infants with Down syndrome have hypoplasia of the middle phalanx of the fifth digit. This feature can often be confirmed in the second-trimester fetus with Down syndrome and may be a useful adjunct to other sonographic signs in the fetus at risk for chromosome abnormalities.[3]

SONOGRAPHIC FEATURES ASSOCIATED WITH DOWN SYNDROME

Nuchal thickness >5 mm
Short femur or humerus or both
Pyelectasis
Hyperechogenic bowel
Hypoplasia of the middle phalanx
    of the fifth digit
Duodenal atresia

Endocardial cushion defect
Cystic hygroma
Nonimmune hydrops
Mild cerebral ventriculomegaly
Possible increased biparietal
    diameter-femur length ratio

Similarly, excess soft-tissue thickening at the occiput and neck is well recognized in the neonate with Down syndrome. In 1985, Benacerraf and associates[2] reported 11 cases of Down syndrome in a series of 1704 consecutive genetic amniocenteses. Four of the 11 fetuses demonstrated soft-tissue thickening at the fetal occiput.[2] The nuchal thickening was flat and symmetric, unlike that of a cystic hygroma, and may represent resolution of a cystic hygroma present earlier in gestation. A nuchal measurement >5 mm (taken from the surface of the occiput to the skin surface on a transverse plane of the head through the thalami and angled through the posterior fossa and cisterna magna) was considered to be abnormal at 15 to 20 weeks' gestation (Figure 12-1). Additional prospective investigations have confirmed the potential usefulness of nuchal thickening as a screening criterion for Down syndrome.[12,25,43]

Renal and gastrointestinal abnormalities have also been reported with Down syndrome. In Nyberg and colleagues' series,[35] hyperechogenic bowel was an unexpected abnormality previously seen primarily in fetuses with cystic fibrosis or in association with periplacental

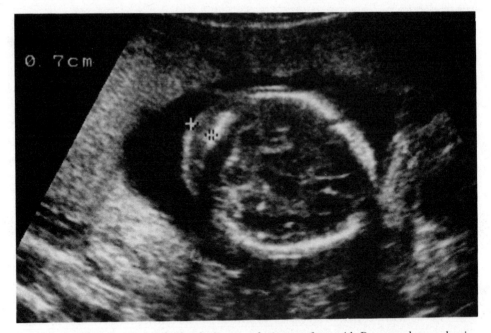

Fig. 12-1 Transverse view of the head of a second-trimester fetus with Down syndrome, showing nuchal skin thickening.

hemorrhage and elevated AFP levels. Benacerraf and associates[4] suggested an association of fetal pyelectasis with Down syndrome. A retrospective review of 210 consecutive fetuses with renal pyelectasis (anteroposterior diameter of the renal pelvis ≥4 mm between 15 and 20 weeks' gestation; ≥5 mm between 20 and 30 weeks' gestation; ≥7 mm between 30 and 40 weeks' gestation) among 7400 patients scanned over a 1-year period demonstrated seven fetuses with Down syndrome. Conversely, a review of 44 fetuses with Down syndrome, compiled over a 5-year period, showed 11 with pyelectasis. The overall incidence of Down syndrome was approximately 3% when fetal pyelectasis was present.

Occasionally a major anomaly associated with Down syndrome is detected sonographically, but these anomalies are rare. For example, although the classic prenatal ultrasound finding (generally found late in gestation) of duodenal atresia, the "double bubble" sign, represents a 30% risk of Down syndrome, only 3% of fetuses with Down syndrome have duodenal atresia. Another characteristic anomaly associated with trisomy 21 is an endocardial cushion defect. Nyberg and colleagues[35] published the results of a series of 94 fetuses with Down syndrome, most of which were between 14 and 24 weeks' gestation.[35] Thirty-seven abnormalities were detected among 31 fetuses. Sonographic findings included those previously mentioned, as well as cystic hygroma, nonimmune hydrops, omphalocele, and mild cerebral ventriculomegaly. An increased sonographic detection of abnormalities in fetuses with Down syndrome was found with advancing gestational age.

Similar to the use of a combination of maternal serum markers to improve Down syndrome detection, a sonographic scoring index for prenatal detection of chromosome abnormalities has been proposed by Benacerraf and associates.[6] The weighted system allots 2 points each for thickened nuchal fold or a major structural defect and 1 point each for short femur, short humerus, or pyelectasis. The sonographic features of 43 trisomic fetuses and 588 normal controls were examined and scored between 14 and 20 weeks' gestation. Selecting fetuses with a score ≥2 would have identified 26 of 32 Down syndrome fetuses and 9 of 9 trisomy 18 fetuses, with a false-positive rate of 4.4%. This scoring system can be used to increase presumed risk; however, its accuracy has not been validated for risk reduction. Preliminary data compiled by Lockwood and colleagues[25] suggest that the assessment of a combination of biometric parameters, adjusted specifically for fetal sex, may improve the sonographic detection of Down syndrome fetuses. The future of noninvasive identification of fetuses at risk for aneuploidy may lie in combining ultrasound evaluation and assessment of biochemical markers.

QUESTION 3: WHAT ARE THE EMOTIONAL RAMIFICATIONS OF TRIPLE-MARKER SCREENING?

"Screening" is the operative word in the phrase *triple-marker screening*. All patients should be made aware that triple-marker screening is not a diagnostic test, but rather a way to identify pregnancies at increased, *not absolute*, risk of fetal abnormalities, including both neural tube defects and chromosome abnormalities. In fact, most women with abnormal multiscreen results will have normal fetuses. Approximately 5% to 10% of patients who undergo triple-marker screening will have abnormal serum results. Although only 3% to 5% of these patients will ultimately be found to have fetuses with structural or chromosome defects, the initial report of an abnormal result inevitably creates anxiety for the patient.

Several authors have addressed this topic with specific reference to low levels of MSAFP. Unlike high levels, for which the principal risks of neural tube and ventral wall defects can be assessed with reasonable accuracy by ultrasound examination, the woman at risk for having a fetus with Down syndrome is faced with the prospect of undergoing an invasive procedure such as amniocentesis. Evans and associates[18] demonstrated that this knowledge creates significantly more anxiety in younger women with low MSAFP values than in women 35 years of age or older. Keenan and associates[23] confirmed that there is generally an exaggerated anxiety reaction when the patient is informed of her increased risk of having an infant with Down syndrome. Assessing anxiety by using an established scoring method before and after a counseling intervention, they demonstrated that, although heightened anxiety may persist at least until definitive chromosome diagnosis is made, the high level of initial anxiety can be reduced through comprehensive genetic counseling. Interestingly, among the 52 couples studied, the partners of the women with low levels of MSAFP did not have as dramatic an increase in anxiety when informed of the abnormal results, nor did they have a significant reduction in anxiety after the counseling intervention.

QUESTION 4: IS MATERNAL SERUM SCREENING APPLICABLE TO WOMEN AGE 35 OR OLDER?

The historically accepted screening indication for Down syndrome is advanced maternal age. Women are selected for antenatal genetic testing based on an age of 35 years or older at the time of delivery. This is because the quantitative risks for fetal aneuploidy and for amniocentesis-related fetal loss are roughly equal at this age cut-off. In the United States, triple-marker assessment of Down syndrome risk has traditionally been limited to women younger than age 35. The ACMG and the American College of Obstetricians and Gynecologists recommend that serum screening be offered to all pregnant women who are less than 35 years of age unless their history suggests that amniocentesis or chorionic villus sampling (CVS) is indicated.[11]

The applicability of using triple-marker screening to reduce the estimated risk of fetal aneuploidy in pregnancies of women age 35 years or older is a topic of much investigation. In an initial study by Zeitune and colleagues,[45] MSAFP results were evaluated in 517 women undergoing amniocentesis because of advanced maternal age. Six fetuses with autosomal trisomy were identified by chromosome analysis: five with Down syndrome and one with trisomy 18. All six affected pregnancies diagnosed prenatally would have been predicted by screening in which MSAFP levels were assessed in combination with maternal age. In addition, 39% to 45% of the amniocenteses in this study would have been avoided if patients had been reclassified as "low risk" after MSAFP testing. The serum marker appeared to perform best in patients less than 38 years of age. A subsequent study of over 5000 women age 35 or older found that measuring maternal serum AFP, hCG, and uE_3 at 15 to 20 weeks' gestation could detect 89% of Down syndrome fetuses, with a 1 in 200 risk cut-off for Down syndrome and a false-positive rate of 25%.[21] In addition, approximately 45% of sex chromosome aneuploidies and other trisomies would also be revealed. Although these detection rates are significant and, in fact, superior to those of the triple-marker screenings performed in younger women, they must be contrasted with the detection of virtually all chromosome abnormalities if every woman over 35 chose to have amniocentesis or CVS. Amniocentesis and CVS, with their associated loss rates, could be avoided in 70% to 75% of older women at the expense of missing 10% to 15% of Down syndrome cases and more than 50% of other chromosome abnormalities.

The ACMG's position statement on multiple-marker screening in women 35 and older advises against replacing CVS or amniocentesis with multiple-marker screening in this age group.[11] Women over 35 should continue to be offered genetic counseling for advanced maternal age. Some patients will prefer to proceed directly with CVS or amniocentesis. However, for the select group of women who choose to avoid invasive procedures, triple-marker screening may be an option. All patients, regardless of whether they choose to undergo evaluation of any type for chromosome abnormalities, should be offered MSAFP screening for neural tube defects. Patients who have midtrimester amniocentesis should have concomitant amniotic fluid assessment of AFP, while those who undergo CVS may elect to have MSAFP screening at 15 to 20 weeks' gestation.

QUESTION 5: ARE THERE ANY SERUM MARKERS THAT CAN BE USED TO DETECT CHROMOSOME ABNORMALITIES DURING THE FIRST TRIMESTER?

Early reports suggesting an association between low first-trimester MSAFP and Down syndrome appeared in 1986. Milunsky and colleagues[31] described a group of 540 women whose blood samples were drawn for MSAFP screening before CVS.[31] Twenty-seven fetal chromosome defects were discovered by karyotype analysis. Twenty-two of these were autosomal trisomies. Seven of the 22 fetal trisomies (31.8%) had a decreased AFP value of 0.6 MoM. The false-positive rate of 11%, however, was more than double that accepted in second-trimester analysis.

It has been suggested that the patterns of serum markers for Down syndrome established during the second trimester (low AFP, low uE_3, high hCG) and trisomy 18 (low AFP, low uE_3, low hCG) may also be exhibited during the first trimester. Aitken and associates[1] described the measurement of AFP, uE_3, hCG, and free β-hCG in 21 chromosomally abnormal fetuses at 6 to 14 weeks' gestation. Significant reductions in AFP and uE_3 levels as well as a significant increase in free β-hCG were found in all 16 fetuses with Down syndrome. Intact hCG levels, the most widely used test in midtrimester, were within the normal range. Similarly, levels of all four biochemical markers were shown to be reduced in the five pregnancies affected with trisomy 18. Macri and colleagues[29] have presented similar data showing altered levels of the free β analyte in Down syndrome and trisomy 18.[29] Thus, it appears that measurement of free β-hCG in combination with AFP and maternal age may have utility in the first-trimester assessment of fetal aneuploidy.

Preliminary data by Ozturk and associates[36] have demonstrated that measurement of free α and β subunits of hCG between 8 and 12 weeks' gestation may be a useful adjunct to the early prenatal diagnosis of trisomy 18. In a select group of 704 women at increased risk for fetal trisomies because of advanced maternal age or previous birth of a child with a chromosome abnormality, serum levels of free α- and β-hCG were determined. This testing was followed by karyotype analysis from CVS. Of eight fetuses with trisomy 18, six had a calculated ratio of free β-hCG to free α-hCG of less than 0.25 MoM. Only 3.2% of mothers carrying a normal fetus had a ratio in this range. This ratio in mothers carrying fetuses with trisomy 21 was not significantly different from the ratio in those carrying normal fetuses.

Schwangerschafts protein 1 (SP1), also known as *pregnancy-specific β-1 glycoprotein*, is a product of placental syncytiotrophoblast. The first-trimester relationship between maternal serum SP1 and fetal karyotype was explored in a series by MacIntosh and associates.[26] A cohort of 692 women underwent CVS at 6 to 12 weeks' gestation. Thirty pregnancies with abnormal karyotypes included fourteen with Down syndrome and eight with trisomy 18. The median SP1 of the abnormal group was half that of the normal group. This relationship was maintained in the subanalysis of Down syndrome pregnancies but not in those with trisomy 18. At a false-positive rate of 5%, the combination of age and SP1 could be used to detect 43% of fetal chromosome abnormalities and 50% of Down syndrome cases. Similarly, measurement of pregnancy-associated plasma protein A (PAPP-A) in early pregnancy showed a statistically significant reduction in the PAPP-A levels among Down syndrome cases, compared with controls.[32] Data are currently insufficient to draw firm conclusions about prospective screening with first-trimester markers.

REFERENCES

1. Aitken DA, McCaw G, Crossley JA et al: First-trimester biochemical screening for fetal chromosome abnormalities and neural tube defects, *Prenat Diagn* 13:681, 1993.
2. Benacerraf BR, Frigoletto FD, Laboda LA: Sonographic diagnosis of Down syndrome in the second trimester, *Am J Obstet Gynecol* 153:49, 1985.
3. Benacerraf BR, Harlow BL, Frigoletto FD: Hypoplasia of the middle phalanx of the fifth digit: a feature of the second-trimester fetus with Down syndrome, *J Ultrasound Med* 9:389, 1990.
4. Benacerraf BR, Mandell J, Estroff JA et al: Fetal pyelectasis: a possible association with Down syndrome, *Obstet Gynecol* 76:58, 1990.
5. Benacerraf BR, Miller WA, Frigoletto FD: Sonographic detection of fetuses with trisomies 13 and 18: accuracy and limitations, *Am J Obstet Gynecol* 158:404, 1988.
6. Benacerraf BR, Neuberg D, Bromley B, Frigoletto FD: Sonographic scoring index for prenatal detection of chromosomal abnormalities, *J Ultrasound Med* 11:449, 1992.
7. Bogart MH, Pandiant MR, Jones OW: Abnormal maternal serum chorionic gonadotropin levels in pregnancies with fetal chromosome abnormalities, *Prenat Diagn* 7:623, 1987.
8. Canick JA, Knight GJ, Palomaki GE et al: Low second-trimester maternal serum unconjugated oestriol in pregnancies with Down syndrome, *Br J Obstet Gynæcol* 95:330, 1988.
9. Canick JA, Palomaki GE, Osathanonah R: Prenatal screening for trisomy 18 in the second trimester, *Prenat Diagn* 10:546, 1990.
10. Canick JA, Stevens LD, Abell KB et al: Second-trimester maternal serum unconjugated estriol and human chorionic gonadotropin in pregnancies affected with fetal trisomy 18, anencephaly, and open spina bifida, *Am J Hum Genet* 45:A255, 1989.
11. Crandall BF, Corson VL, Goldberg JD et al: ACMG position statement on multiple marker screening in women 35 and older, *American College of Medical Genetics College Newsletter* 2:11, 1994.
12. Crane JP, Gray DL: Sonographically measured nuchal skinfold thickness as a screening tool for Down syndrome: results of a prospective clinical trial, *Obstet Gynecol* 77:533, 1991.
13. Cuckle HS, Wald NJ, Lindenbaum RH: Maternal serum alpha-fetoprotein measurement: a screening test for Down syndrome, *Lancet* 28:926, 1984.
14. Cuckle HS, Wald NJ: HCG, estriol, and other maternal blood markers of fetal aneuploidy. In Elias S, Simpson JL, editors: *Maternal serum screening for fetal genetic disorders,* New York, 1992, Churchill Livingstone.
15. Dicke JM, Gray DL, Songster GS, Crane JP: Fetal biometry as a screening tool for the detection of chromosomally abnormal pregnancies, *Obstet Gynecol* 74:726, 1989.
16. DiMaio MS, Baumgarten A, Greenstein RM et al: Screening for fetal Down syndrome in pregnancy by measuring alpha-fetoprotein levels, *N Engl J Med* 317:342, 1987.
17. Drugan A, Dvorin E, Koppitch FC et al: Counseling for low maternal serum alpha-fetoprotein should emphasize all chromosome anomalies, not just Down syndrome, *Obstet Gynecol* 73:271, 1989.
18. Evans M, Bottoms S, Carlucci T et al: Determinants of altered anxiety after abnormal maternal serum alpha fetoprotein screening, *Am J Obstet Gynecol* 159:1501, 1988.
19. Greenberg F, Schmidt D, Darnule AT et al: Maternal serum alpha-fetoprotein, beta-human chorionic gonadotropin, and unconjugated estriol levels in midtrimester trisomy 18 pregnancies, *Am J Obstet Gynecol* 166:1388, 1992.
20. Haddow JE, Palomaki BS, Knight GJ et al: Prenatal screening for Down syndrome with use of maternal serum markers, *N Engl J Med* 327:588, 1992.
21. Haddow JE, Palomaki GE, Knight GJ et al: Reducing the need for amniocentesis in women 35 years of age or older with serum markers for screening, *N Engl J Med* 330:1114, 1994.
22. Hill LM, Guzick D, Belfar HL et al: The current role of sonography in the detection of Down syndrome, *Obstet Gynecol* 74:620, 1989.

23. Keenan KL, Basso D, Goldkrand J, Butler W: Low level of maternal serum alpha-fetoprotein: its associated anxiety and the effects of genetic counseling, *Am J Obstet Gynecol* 164:54, 1991.

24. Lindenbaum RH, Ryynänen M, Holmes-Siedle M et al: Trisomy 18 and maternal serum and amniotic fluid alpha-fetoprotein, *Prenat Diagn* 7:511, 1987.

25. Lockwood CJ, Lynch L, Ghidini A et al: The effect of fetal gender on the prediction of Down syndrome by means of maternal serum alpha-fetoprotein and ultrasonographic parameters, *Am J Obstet Gynecol* 169:1190, 1993.

26. MacIntosh MCM, Brambati B, Chard T, Grudzinskas JG: First-trimester maternal serum Schwangerschafts protein 1 (SP1) in pregnancies associated with chromosomal anomalies, *Prenat Diagn* 13:563, 1993.

27. Macri JN, Kasturi RV, Krantz DA et al: Maternal serum Down syndrome screening: unconjugated estriol is not useful, *Am J Obstet Gynecol* 162:672, 1990.

28. Macri JN, Kasturi RV, Krantz DA et al: Maternal serum Down syndrome screening: free ß-protein is a more effective marker than human chorionic gonadotropin, *Am J Obstet Gynecol* 163:1248, 1990.

29. Macri JN, Spencer K, Aitken D et al: First-trimester free beta (hCG) screening for Down syndrome, *Prenat Diag* 13:557, 1993.

30. Merkatz IR, Nitowsky HM, Macri JN, Johnson WE: An association between low maternal serum alpha-fetoprotein and fetal chromosomal abnormalities, *Am J Obstet Gynecol* 148:886, 1984.

31. Milunsky A, Wands J, Brambati et al: First-trimester maternal serum alpha-fetoprotein screening for chromosome defects, *Am J Obstet Gynecol* 158:1209, 1988.

32. Muller F, Cuckle H, Teisner B, Grudzinskas JG: Serum PAPP-A levels are depressed in women with fetal Down syndrome in early pregnancy, *Prenat Diagn* 13:633, 1993.

33. New England Regional Genetics Group Prenatal Collaborative Study of Down Syndrome Screening: Combining maternal serum alpha-fetoprotein measurements and age to screen for Down syndrome in pregnant women under age 35, *Am J Obstet Gynecol* 160:575, 1989.

34. Nyberg DA, Kramer D, Resta RG et al: Prenatal sonographic findings of trisomy 18: review of 47 cases, *J Ultrasound Med* 2:103, 1993.

35. Nyberg DA, Resta RG, Luthy DA et al: Prenatal sonographic findings of Down syndrome: review of 94 cases, *Obstet Gynecol* 76:370, 1990.

36. Ozturk M, Milunsky A, Brambati B et al: Abnormal maternal serum levels of human chorionic gonadotropin free subunits in trisomy 18, *Am J Med Genet* 36:480, 1990.

37. Ryall RG, Staples AJ, Robertson EF, Pollard AC: Improved performance in a prenatal screening programme for Down syndrome incorporating serum-free hCG subunit analyses, *Prenat Diagn* 12:251, 1992.

38. Shah YG, Eckl CJ, Stinson SK, Woods JR: Biparietal diameter/femur length ratio, cephalic indices, and femur length measurements: not reliable screening techniques for Down syndrome, *Obstet Gynecol* 75:186, 1990.

39. Spencer K, Coombes EJ, Mallard AS, Ward AM: Free beta human choriogonadotropin in Down syndrome screening: a multicentre study of its role compared with other biochemical markers, *Ann Clin Biochem* 29:506, 1992.

40. Suchy SF, Yeager MT: Down syndrome screening in women under 35 with maternal serum hCG, *Obstet Gynecol* 76:20, 1990.

41. Wald NJ, Cuckle HS, Densem JW et al: Maternal serum screening for Down syndrome in early pregnancy, *Br Med J* 297:883, 1988.

42. Wald NJ, Cuckle HS, Densem JW et al: Maternal serum unconjugated œstriol as an antenatal screening test for Down's syndrome, *Br J Obstet Gynæcol* 95:334, 1988.

43. Watson WJ, Miller RC, Menard MK et al: Ultrasonographic measurement of fetal nuchal skin to screen for chromosomal abnormalities, *Am J Obstet Gynecol* 170:583, 1994.

44. Wenstrom KD, Williamson RA, Grant SS: Detection of fetal Turner syndrome with multiple-marker screening, *Am J Obstet Gynecol* 170:570, 1994.

45. Zeitune M, Ben-Tovim T, Fejgin M et al: Screening for Down syndrome in older women based on maternal serum alpha-fetoprotein levels and age: preliminary results, *Prenat Diagn* 11:393, 1991.

CHAPTER 13

Unexplained Elevations of
Maternal Serum α-Fetoprotein

STEVEN R. WELLS
ROBERT C. CEFALO

First identified in 1956 by Bergstrand and Czar,[1] α-fetoprotein (AFP) is the major serum protein of the embryo and early fetus. In 1972, Brock and colleagues[2] reported the association of elevated levels of maternal serum AFP (MSAFP) with open neural tube defects in the fetus. The large U.K. Collaborative Study on AFP in 1977 confirmed the efficacy of detection of open neural tube defects by MSAFP screening.[8] Since that time, MSAFP screening programs have been widely used to detect anomalies such as anencephaly, encephalocele, open spina bifida, and ventral wall defects (gastroschisis and omphalocele). It has recently become known also that low levels of MSAFP are associated with chromosomal trisomies. During the last 10 to 15 years, it has become apparent that unexplained elevations of MSAFP are also associated with adverse pregnancy outcomes, including low birthweight (both intrauterine growth retardation [IUGR] and preterm delivery), oligohydramnios, abruptio placentae, preeclampsia, and fetal death.[11] This growing body of evidence suggests that an unexplained elevation of MSAFP should categorize a pregnancy as "high risk." The current controversy centers on exactly how to manage such a pregnancy.

❧ Patient Profile: Negative diagnostic evaluation of an elevated maternal serum α-fetoprotein screen

A 24-year-old patient (gravida 1, para 0000) thought to be at 16 weeks' gestation based on last menstrual period and a first-trimester ultrasound examination elected to have AFP screening at 15 weeks' gestation; her MSAFP level was 4.7 multiples of the median (MoM). A level II ultrasound examination performed at 16 weeks' gestation confirmed a viable single intrauterine pregnancy consistent with dates, with a normal-appearing placenta and no fetal anomalies. Amniocentesis revealed a normal amniotic fluid AFP level, negative amniotic fluid acetylcholinesterase, and a normal karyotype.

QUESTION 1: WHAT ARE THE USUAL EXPLANATIONS FOR ELEVATED LEVELS OF MATERNAL SERUM α-FETOPROTEIN?

The most common reasons for elevated levels of MSAFP are incorrect dates (a more advanced pregnancy), multifetal pregnancy, and fetal death. The association with open neural tube defects, such as open spina bifida, anencephaly, and encephalocele, was first reported by Brock and colleagues[2] in 1972. Since then, abdominal wall defects, sacrococcygeal teratomas, cystic hygromas, renal anomalies, congenital nephrosis, oseteogenesis imperfecta, and a host of other fetal anomalies have been associated with elevated MSAFP levels. Most of these conditions can be detected by ultrasound examination with or without amniocentesis. By exclusion, if no abnormalities can be detected by these modalities, there is an unexplained elevation of MSAFP.

QUESTION 2: WHAT ARE THE POTENTIAL PROBLEMS ASSOCIATED WITH UNEXPLAINED ELEVATIONS OF MATERNAL SERUM α-FETOPROTEIN?

Brock and colleagues[2] were the first to report an increased incidence of low birthweight related to unexplained MSAFP elevations.[3] This association was confirmed by Wald and colleagues,[10] who also reported an increase in the incidence of preterm birth and perinatal loss. During the last 15 years, many investigators have reported similar findings. In 1990, Katz and colleagues[6] presented a review of more than 20 such studies that included over 225,000 screened pregnancies; an elevated MSAFP level was associated with up to a 38% incidence of adverse pregnancy outcome when anomalies were excluded by ultrasound or amniocentesis.[6] There was a twofold to fourfold increase in the incidence of low birthweight from preterm birth or IUGR or both, a tenfold increase in the frequency of placental abruption, and a tenfold increase in the rate of perinatal mortality.

QUESTION 3: IS THERE A POSITIVE CORRELATION BETWEEN THE LEVEL OF MATERNAL SERUM α-FETOPROTEIN AND THE LIKELIHOOD OF AN ADVERSE PREGNANCY OUTCOME?

The higher the level of MSAFP, the more likely an adverse pregnancy outcome appears to be. In 1991, Waller and colleagues[11] reported a case-control study that classified pregnancies according to the level of MSAFP. They found even small elevations of MSAFP (2.0 to 2.9 MoM) to be associated with risk of fetal death (odds ratio, 2.4; confidence interval, 1.7 to 3.4). But when MSAFP levels were elevated to three or more times the MoM value, the risk was very high (odds ratio, 10.4; 95% confidence interval, 4.9 to 22.0). In 1991, Crandall and associates[5] reported an increased fetal risk associated with higher values of MSAFP. They stratified elevated MSAFP values into three groups: group 1, 2.5 to 2.9 MoM; group 2, 3.0 to 5.0 MoM; group 3, ≥5.0 MoM. Among women whose sonographic and amniocentesis studies were normal, the risk of adverse pregnancy outcome was 19%, 29%, and 70% in groups 1,

2, and 3, respectively. These and other studies support the idea that the higher the level of MSAFP, the more likely an adverse pregnancy outcome.

QUESTION 4: WHAT IS THE ETIOLOGY OF THE ASSOCIATION BETWEEN UNEXPLAINED ELEVATIONS OF MATERNAL SERUM α-FETOPROTEIN AND ADVERSE PREGNANCY OUTCOMES?

The link between unexplained elevations of MSAFP and adverse pregnancy outcomes is probably attributable to some type of placental pathology. Abnormalities of the placenta increase the chance of a fetal-maternal hemorrhage, which would increase the amount of AFP transferred from the fetus to the mother. Therefore, the elevated MSAFP may actually be a marker for abnormal placentation. This etiology could help to explain the increased incidence of low birthweight, placental abruption, and perinatal mortality. Khalil and colleagues[7] documented a marked increase in AFP levels in the placentas of women with preeclampsia, compared with controls. Salafia and colleagues[9] in 1988 reported the occurrence of chronic villitis in 38% of placentas from pregnancies with unexplained MSAFP elevations, compared with 15% of those with normal MSAFP levels. Other placental abnormalities included vascular lesions, infarcts, and intervillous thromboses. These and many other studies point to placental pathology as the cause of increased MSAFP levels and subsequent poor pregnancy outcomes. Any pregnancy in which an unexplained elevation of MSAFP is noted warrants a detailed gross and histologic examination of the placenta.

QUESTION 5: ARE THERE OTHER PROBLEMS IN INFANTS BORN TO MOTHERS WITH UNEXPLAINED ELEVATIONS OF MATERNAL SERUM α-FETOPROTEIN?

In addition to the problem of decreased birthweight, other abnormalities have been noted. In 1984, Burton and Dillard[4] reported an increase in the incidence of a variety of abnormal physical findings, such as ventricular septal defects, pyloric stenosis, cleft lip and palate, hemangioma of the tongue, duodenal atresia, preauricular appendage, and multiple minor anomalies, in infants born to women with unexplained MSAFP elevations, compared with controls. However, there was no increased incidence of long-term developmental disability in infants born to mothers with elevated MSAFP levels. Also, interestingly, at 12 months of age, size differences between the two groups of infants were no longer evident when weight, length, and head circumference were measured.

QUESTION 6: HOW SHOULD PREGNANCIES OF WOMEN WHO HAVE UNEXPLAINED ELEVATIONS OF MATERNAL SERUM α-FETOPROTEIN BE MANAGED?

No prospective study has specifically addressed how to manage pregnancies with unexplained elevations of MSAFP (as described in the patient profile). Consequently, optimal management has not been defined. One of the most common findings is low birthweight. Therefore, it would seem reasonable, especially if a lagging fundal height is noted, to repeat the ultrasound examination later in pregnancy to document adequate growth and check amniotic fluid levels. Third-trimester fetal surveillance, such as non-stress tests and biophysical profiles, might be indicated, especially if there is a documented growth delay. Patients should be counseled about fetal kick counts and instructed regarding preterm labor symptoms. However, until prospective studies address the issue of optimal management, none of these approaches should be accepted as standard of care. Treatment modalities such as the use of low-dose aspirin to prevent IUGR and preeclampsia are intriguing but as yet untested and unproved.

REFERENCES

1. Bergstrand CG, Czar B: Demonstration of a new protein fraction in serum from the human fetus, *Scand J Clin Lab Invest* 8:174, 1956.
2. Brock DJH, Sutcliffe RG: Alpha-fetoprotein in the antenatal diagnosis of anencephaly and spina bifida, *Lancet* 2:197, 1972.
3. Brock DJH, Barron L, Jelen P et al: Maternal serum alpha-fetoprotein measurements as an early indicator of low birthweight, *Lancet* 2:267, 1977.
4. Burton BK, Dillard RG: Outcome in infants born to mothers with unexplained elevations of maternal serum alpha-fetoprotein, *Pediatrics* 77:582, 1986.
5. Crandall BF, Robinson L, Grau P: Risks associated with an elevated maternal serum alpha-fetoprotein level, *Am J Obstet Gynecol* 165:581, 1991.
6. Katz VL, Chescheir NC, Cefalo RC: Unexplained elevations of maternal serum alpha-fetoprotein, *Obstet Gynecol Surv* 45:719, 1990.
7. Khalil FK, Bonnet M, Guiboud S et al: Alpha-fetoprotein levels in placenta, maternal, and cord blood in normal and pathologic pregnancy, *Obstet Gynecol* 54:117, 1979.
8. Report of U.K. collaborative study: Maternal serum alpha-fetoprotein measurement in antenatal screening for anencephaly and spina bifida in early pregnancy, *Lancet* 1:1323, 1977.
9. Salafia CM, Silberman C, Herrerra NE, Mahoney MJ: Placental pathology at term associated with elevated midtrimester maternal serum AFP concentration, *Am J Obstet Gynecol* 158:1064, 1988.
10. Wald N, Cuckle H, Stirrat GM et al: Maternal serum alpha-fetoprotein and low birthweight, *Lancet* 2:268, 1977.
11. Waller DK, Lustig LS, Cunningham GC et al: Second-trimester maternal serum alpha-fetoprotein levels and the risk of subsequent fetal death, *N Engl J Med* 325:6, 1991.

PART FOUR

SONOGRAPHIC EVALUATION

CHAPTER 14

Overview of
Obstetric Sonography

NANCY C. CHESCHEIR

Fetal sonography is an integral part of obstetric care. With rapid technologic advances, the diagnostic potential of fetal sonography continues to broaden and the demands on the practitioner become more difficult to meet. Most patients expect any defect to be diagnosable, with little regard for the limitations imposed by gestational age, fetal positioning, maternal body habitus, the sonologist's skills, and the technologic limitations of the ultrasound equipment, which must be purchased within a budget. Most practitioners, for example, have been faced with the obese woman at 14 weeks' gestation who is irate because the sex of her breech fetus cannot be determined!

Yet none of these limitations, however real, should be used as an excuse for performing an inadequate fetal assessment. It is imperative to communicate to patients the purpose and findings of the study, including what was not seen. The "level 1" and "level 2" scan terminology is gradually eroding as it becomes clear that if someone "takes a peek" with the ultrasound unit, he or she is responsible for examining all of the accessible fetal anatomy to the best of his or her ability. As Benacerraf[4] discussed in an editorial, this distinction between level 1 and level 2 is artificial—there is no such thing as a level 1 or level 2 chest x-ray, for instance. A distinction arises, however, when a fetus is considered to be at significant risk for a birth defect or developmental problem. In such cases, it is important to refer the patient for more specialized scanning, whatever the terminology. To counter Benacerraf's x-ray argument, this referral is similar to requesting a CT scan of the thorax after an abnormality is suggested but not defined on a chest x-ray. While fetal sonography is a powerful tool in obstetrics, it can also be a dangerous tool if not used responsibly and carefully.

❧ Patient Profile: Missed diagnosis of a severe fetal anomaly

The patient is 27 years old (gravida 2, para 1001) and has had two prior ultrasound examinations: the first to confirm gestational age, at 18 weeks, and the second before she was transferred to a tertiary center because of a low platelet count, discovered at 32 weeks. Both scans were interpreted as normal. Upon arrival at the tertiary center, her platelet count was 15,000, she was normotensive, and her examination was otherwise within normal limits. Fundal height was 36 cm, and fetal heart tones were audible. Physical and laboratory evaluation led to a presumptive diagnosis of idiopathic thrombocytopenic purpura (ITP), and she was started on steroid therapy. On the second day of her hospitalization, a third ultrasound examination showed a fetus with mild polyhydramnios, femur and abdomen measurements of 32 weeks, and classic findings of anencephaly. The patient's platelet count rose in response to the steroids, and after a normal bleeding time was confirmed, labor was induced, with delivery of an anencephalic male fetus who expired within minutes of birth. The patient's postpartum course was uncomplicated.

QUESTION 1: DURING A SECOND- OR THIRD-TRIMESTER ULTRASOUND EXAMINATION PERFORMED FOR PROPER DATING OF A PREGNANCY (THE CLASSIC "LEVEL 1" SCAN), WHAT IS THE PRACTITIONER RESPONSIBLE FOR EXAMINING?

Both the American College of Obstetrics and Gynecology (ACOG) and the American Institute of Ultrasound in Medicine (AIUM) have published guidelines for the appropriate content of a basic second-trimester ultrasound.[1,3] In essence, a thorough confirmation of gestational age, with measurements of multiple fetal body parts, examination of the uterus and adnexa, placenta, and fluid, as well as a review of the fetal anatomy, is to be included. The AIUM, for instance, states that the study "should include, but not necessarily be limited to, the following fetal anatomy: cerebral ventricles, four-chamber view of the heart (including its position within the thorax), spine, stomach, urinary bladder, umbilical cord insertion site on the anterior abdominal wall, and renal region."[3] Had such basic features been included on either of the two prior scans in the patient described above, this lethal abnormality could have been detected at a much earlier gestational age, when induction of labor would have been safer. In addition, the patient would not have been so strongly reassured by "normal" scans.

The argument that women who are at high risk for having a fetus with a birth defect are routinely transferred to a qualified diagnostic center does not release the practitioner from responsibility. While many defects do occur in high-risk families, most fetal anomalies occur in families with no identifiable risk factors. Careful scrutiny of each fetus being scanned thus is essential.

QUESTION 2: IS THERE A ROLE FOR "ROUTINE" ULTRASOUND EXAMINATION IN OBSTETRICS? IF SO, WHEN SHOULD IT BE PERFORMED?

Cogent arguments have been made on each side of this question, and the answer remains elusive. From a health policy perspective, different countries have adopted a variety of recommendations. In European countries, the number of "routine" scans varies from one to three, while in the United States the official recommendation of the National Institutes of Health is that there is no strong evidence supporting the use of routine sonography.[10] Indeed, a large randomized study of routine obstetric ultrasound, known as the RADIUS study and sponsored by the National Institute of Child Health and Human Development, failed to support the idea of routine sonography.[7] Critics of this study point out that the outcomes chosen may not be relevant in the cost-benefit analysis of routine sonography. For example, it is difficult to imagine that routine ultrasound would cause a decrease in the rate of fetal and neonatal death or alter the frequency of neonatal morbidity, such as intraventricular hemorrhage. Moreover, the prenatal detection rate of congenital malformations was low, and there was significant variation in the detection rates among practitioners in the study. Another criticism is that 45% of the group randomized to undergo selective sonography actually underwent ultrasound evaluation, perhaps negating any potential benefit of routine scanning.[8]

A practical response to the question is that the value of routine sonography depends in part on the nature of one's practice. If the practice is largely composed of women with indications for ultrasound, the cost is not exorbitant, it is convenient for the patient, and the sonographer performing the scans is appropriately trained, then routine sonography may be cost effective. The most important advantage of routine scanning is that the information obtained may allow for better obstetric care by identification of multifetal pregnancies, proper dating of the pregnancy to ensure appropriate timing of age-specific tests and delivery plans, and identification of major structural abnormalities.

If a physician routinely performs sonography on all patients, a difficult question is when the scan should be done. Gestational age assessment is most accurate during the first trimester, when the variation in individual fetal growth is minimal. At present, however, identification of fetal anatomic defects is limited during the early period of pregnancy. There is some value in delaying such scans until by best estimate the patient is at approximately 15 to 18 weeks' gestation. This time period affords a reasonably good view of fetal anatomy, limited variation in fetal growth, and the opportunity to decrease the likelihood of false-positive results of maternal serum screening studies by accurately dating the gestational age, using biparietal diameter measurement. Thus, if a practitioner routinely performs only one examination, more information is obtained when the scan is undertaken at 15 to 18 weeks' gestation.

QUESTION 3: WHICH PATIENTS SHOULD BE REFERRED FOR ULTRASOUND EXAMINATION?

In most medical disciplines, screening tests are relied on to allow diagnostic tests to be focused on the highest-risk groups. Determining which patients to refer for diagnostic ultrasound during pregnancy is no different. Most birth defects occur in families with no significant risk factors. The inclusion of a thorough anatomic fetal survey allows these otherwise "low-risk" women to be referred for a diagnostic scan any time the fetal anatomy or uterine contents do not look completely normal to the office practitioner. Overall, about 50% of the fetuses of women referred for ultrasound evaluation because the outside scan "did not look quite right" will end up actually having an abnormality. This figure will vary widely, depending on the skills of the referring physician and the abnormality suspected. For instance, it is unusual for the screening study to suggest anencephaly only to result in the diagnostic study's demonstrating normal cranial anatomy, whereas suspicion of congenital heart disease is not confirmed approximately 50% of the time.

Other indications for referral include the patient whose fetus is considered to be at increased risk for karyotypic abnormalities. Many of these fetuses will have findings on ultrasound that are more compelling indications for karyotype analysis than age-related risk alone. On the other hand, most birth defects are not chromosomal, but rather structural, and amniocentesis would probably not detect them. If a woman is willing to accept the physical discomfort, financial cost, and potential risk to her pregnancy to rule out aneuploidy by submitting to amniocentesis or chorionic villus sampling, it is only reasonable to include a thorough search for the other abnormalities, for which she is at even higher risk. The box on p. 106 lists the other indications for ultrasound determined by the NIH task force.

QUESTION 4: WHAT ARE THE RISKS OF DIAGNOSTIC SONOGRAPHY?

The jury is still out on the biologic risks associated with ultrasound. While no study has ever confirmed a biologic risk associated with exposure of the human fetus to diagnostic levels of ultrasound, caution is still warranted. Although obstetric sonography has been performed since 1958, the expected lifespan of the first fetus so exposed is another 40 years.[6] No guarantee can be given that over the more than 70 years of the average lifespan of the exposed fetus there will be no adverse health effects.

The Bioeffects Committee of the AIUM issued in 1988 a thorough review of the data regarding the bioeffects of ultrasound. The committee concluded that "no confirmed biologic effects on patients or instrument operators caused by exposure to intensities typical of present diagnostic ultrasound instruments have ever been reported. Although the possibility exists that such biologic effects may be identified in the future, current data indicate that the benefits to patients of prudent use of diagnostic ultrasound outweigh the risks, if any, that may be present."[2]

Some researchers, however, are beginning to raise questions about other possible adverse effects of ultrasound. Salvesen and colleagues[9] studied over 2000 Norwegian children, ages 8 to 9 years, who had been part of randomized trials of fetal sonography as either scanned or unscanned fetuses. They reported no association between exposure to ultrasound and teacher-reported school problems. A related question was posed by Campbell.[5] This study suggested an increased rate of fetal ultrasound exposure among children with diagnosed speech delay. These developmental questions must continue to be examined with emphasis on the reasons that the scan was performed in the first place. Nonetheless, these concerns warrant continued study and conservatism in ultrasound use.

GUIDELINES FOR FETAL ULTRASOUND EXAMINATION*

The Consensus Development Conference, sponsored by the National Institute of Child Health and Human Development, has supported ultrasound examinations in the following clinical situations:

1. Estimation of gestational age for patients with uncertain clinical dates, or verification of dates for patients who are to undergo scheduled elective repeat cesarean delivery, indicated induction of labor, or other elective termination of pregnancy
2. Evaluation of fetal growth
3. Vaginal bleeding of undetermined cause in pregnancy
4. Determination of fetal presentation
5. Suspected multiple gestation
6. Adjunct to amniocentesis
7. Significant discrepancy between uterine size and clinical dates
8. Pelvic mass
9. Suspected hydatidiform mole
10. Adjunct to cervical cerclage placement
11. Suspected ectopic pregnancy
12. Adjunct to special procedures, such as fetoscopy, intrauterine transfusion, shunt placement, in vitro fertilization, embryo transfer, or chorionic villus sampling
13. Suspected fetal death
14. Suspected uterine abnormality
15. Intrauterine contraceptive device localization
16. Ovarian follicle development surveillance
17. Biophysical evaluation of fetal well-being
18. Observation of intrapartum events
19. Suspected polyhydramnios or oligohydramnios
20. Suspected abruptio placentae
21. Adjunct to external version from breech to vertex presentation
22. Estimation of fetal weight or presentation in premature rupture of membranes or vertex presentation
23. Abnormal serum α-fetoprotein value
24. Follow-up observation of identified fetal anomaly
25. Follow-up evaluation of placenta localization for identified placenta previa
26. History of previous congenital anomaly
27. Serial evaluation of fetal growth in multiple gestation
28. Evaluation of fetal condition in late registrants for prenatal care

*Reference 10.

The most significant risk of ultrasound is not a biologic one, however. Instead, it is the risk of a false diagnosis. Incorrect assessment of gestational age of a fetus, for instance, may alter clinical management regarding induction of labor or the use of tocolytic therapy. Failure to diagnose a fetal abnormality may falsely reassure a family about the health of the fetus, precluding the opportunity to make plans to optimize neonatal outcome by arranging delivery where pediatric subspecialists are available, or precluding the opportunity for the family to terminate the pregnancy if a severe abnormality is detected. A grave concern, of course, is the diagnosis of a fetal abnormality when none is present, which results in marked anxiety and grief for the family and potentially the induced abortion of a normal fetus. This last risk forms the crux of the reason for a close relationship with a tertiary perinatal center to confirm suspected malformations before an irrevocable decision is made regarding pregnancy continuation.

Performing prenatal sonography entails a weighty responsibility. Patients and their families deserve to receive an appropriate degree of fetal scrutiny by ultrasound examination and to be clearly informed of the sonologist's abilities and limitations.

REFERENCES

1. American College of Obstetricians and Gynecologists: *Ultrasonography in pregnancy,* Technical bulletin #187, Washington DC, Dec 1993, ACOG.
2. American Institute of Ultrasound in Medicine: Bioeffects considerations for the safety of diagnostic ultrasound, *J Ultrasound Med* 7(suppl 9):S1, 1988.
3. American Institute of Ultrasound in Medicine: *Guidelines for performance of the antepartum obstetrical ultrasound examination,* Rockville, Md, 1991, AIUM.
4. Benacerraf BR: Who should be performing fetal ultrasound? *Ultrasound Obstet Gynecol* 3:1, 1993.
5. Campbell JD, Elford RW, Brant RF: Case control study of prenatal ultrasonography exposure in children with delayed speech, *Canadian Med Assoc J* 149:1435, 1993.
6. Donald I, MacVicar J, Brown TG: Investigation of abdominal masses by pulsed ultrasound, *Lancet* 1:1188, 1958.
7. Ewigman BG, Crane JP, Frigoletto FD et al: Effect of prenatal ultrasound screening on perinatal outcome, *N Engl J Med* 329:821, 1993.
8. Romero R: Routine obstetric ultrasound, *Ultrasound Obstet Gynecol* (suppl 3):303, 1993.
9. Salvesen KA, Bakketeig LS, Eik-Nes SH et al: Routine ultrasonography in utero and school performance at ages 8-9 years, *Lancet* 339:85, 1992.
10. U.S. Department of Health and Human Services, Public Health Service, National Institutes of Health: *Diagnostic ultrasound imaging in pregnancy,* NIH publication no. 84-667, Washington, DC, 1984, U.S. Government Printing Office.

CHAPTER 15

Sonographic Identification of Fetal Aneuploidy

NANCY C. CHESCHEIR

Early prenatal diagnostic research focused primarily on cytogenetic abnormalities. This focus developed for a variety of reasons, including that amniocentesis and karyotype analysis predated clinical ultrasound in terms of accuracy and availability. In addition, the burden of life-long handicaps was greater for nonlethal trisomies than for most isolated structural abnormalities because the outcomes of neonatal surgery were relatively poor until recently. This increased burden prompted the greater effort to make possible the prenatal diagnosis of aneuploidy rather than the diagnosis of structural abnormalities.

Contemporary obstetric sonography is increasingly able to detect not only major malformations but also some of the more subtle phenotypic changes that characterize many of the trisomies. This expanding role for ultrasound augments the potential use of karyotype analysis for the standard indications: maternal age 35 or older at the time of delivery, abnormal maternal serum screening studies, and a previous child or fetus with a chromosome abnormality. The risk of second-trimester detection of trisomy for women who will be age 35 at delivery is about 1 in 190.[15] The presence of any factor that raises the risk of aneuploidy to 1 in 190 or greater should prompt the practitioner to offer karyotype analysis. It is important to individualize patient counseling regarding the risk of having a fetus with a trisomy based on the patient's age, results of maternal serum screening studies, family history, and results of the ultrasound examination.

Accurate assessment of each patient's risk and appropriate patient counseling are especially important because most babies with trisomy 21 are born to women under the age of 35. Although the incidence of autosomal trisomies increases to 1 in 190 at a maternal age of 35, 80% of mothers of Down syndrome babies are actually under age 35, since the birth rate is higher in these women. In fact, less than 3% of aneuploid fetuses occur in pregnancies with any known preconceptional risk factors.[17] The following patient profile illustrates the interaction of maternal age, maternal serum screening results, and ultrasound results in guiding genetic counseling and decision making regarding invasive prenatal diagnostic testing.

108

✤ Patient Profile: Ultrasound diagnosis of trisomy 21

The patient is a 23-year-old woman (gravida 1, para 0000) who presents for prenatal care and is uncertain about the date of her last menstrual period. The physical examination suggests a gestational age of about 15 to 17 weeks. An ultrasound performed to determine gestational age shows the following:

> *Biparietal diameter (BPD) consistent with 16 weeks*
> *Femur length consistent with 15 weeks*
> *Humerus length consistent with 14.5 weeks*
> *Abdominal circumference consistent with 16 weeks*

No gross structural disorders are seen. Amniotic fluid volume and placenta appear normal. The composite gestational age is determined to be 15 weeks, and a maternal serum screening study is ordered at the patient's request after she is counseled about the test. The gestational age recorded on the serum screening test is 16 weeks (because of the BPD measurement).

Two days later, the results show a positive screen for Down syndrome, with an MSAFP of 0.58 MoM, MS hCG of 2.06 MoM, and MS uE$_3$ of 0.72. The patient is then referred for genetic counseling and targeted ultrasound. Her age-related risk for second-trimester Down syndrome was 1 in 1100[15]; based on the maternal serum screening study the estimated risk has risen to 1 in 190. The targeted ultrasound examination reveals an increased nuchal skin

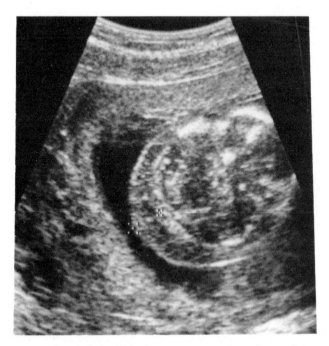

Fig. 15-1 Increased nuchal skinfold measurement (7 mm) in a fetus with Down syndrome.

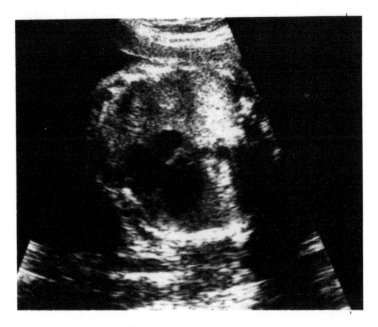

Fig. 15-2 Four-chamber view of the heart, showing a large ventricular septal defect.

thickness (measured from the skin edge to the outer edge of the occipital bone at the level of the cerebellum) of 7 mm (normal is <6 mm) (Figure 15-1). Fetal echocardiographic examination shows a normally positioned heart with four chambers, but a ventricular septal defect is present (Figure 15-2). The remainder of the examination is normal.

The patient is counseled that the findings of the ultrasound examination in conjunction with the results of the maternal serum screening studies indicate a high risk that the fetus has trisomy 21. Amniocentesis is performed at her request, and the results indeed show a 47,XY + 21 karyotype.

QUESTION 1: HOW SHOULD GESTATIONAL AGE BE DETERMINED IN THE PATIENT WITH AN ABNORMAL MATERNAL SERUM SCREENING RESULT?

The BPD data alone should be used to report ultrasound-derived gestational age assessment on maternal serum screening requests, since Down syndrome fetuses characteristically have foreshortened femurs and humeruses. Using measurements of the long bones to determine gestational age would cause the true gestational age to be underestimated, making a false-negative screening result more likely. (Similarly, the use of BPD alone is important in screening for open neural tube and abdominal wall defects, since the heads of second-trimester fetuses with open spina bifida are typically smaller than average for gestational age.)

QUESTION 2: WHAT ULTRASOUND FINDINGS ARE COMMON IN ANEUPLOID FETUSES?

Autosomal trisomies can cause a wide spectrum of phenotypic abnormalities. To identify aneuploid fetuses, the sonologist must be able to recognize these phenotypes. Growth disturbances, which may be evident as early as the late first or early second trimester,[11] are common in both trisomy 13 and trisomy 18, particularly in association with polyhydramnios, if the scan is performed during the third trimester. On the other hand, most fetuses and newborns with trisomy 21 are above the tenth percentile in weight, despite disproportionately short long bones. Among all fetuses identified as being growth retarded, 19% are aneuploid.[16,20] This incidence increases if polyhydramnios or dysmorphology is present. In a series by Gagnon and colleagues,[13] 21.4% of aneuploid fetuses showed symmetric intrauterine growth retardation (IUGR).

The features that are visible by ultrasound vary with gestational age. The boxes that follow list abnormalities that have been noted on ultrasound in cytogenetically proved cases of trisomies 21, 18, and 13, the three most common autosomal trisomies in liveborn infants. Not every fetus affected with a trisomy will display each of these phenotypic findings.

Monosomy X, or 45,X, is also often diagnosed prenatally. It is the most common cytogenetic abnormality in conceptuses, but 99% die in utero. Most second-trimester fetuses with serous effusions and cystic hygroma, hydrops, and monosomy X die in utero, and this condition is considered uniformly lethal.

Aneuploidies involving three copies of the sex chromosomes (gonosomal aneuploidy), such as 47,XXY or 47,XYY, are relatively common in series of abnormal amniocenteses performed because of increased maternal age; however, they do not often result in phenotypic abnormalities in either the newborn or the fetus and therefore are not commonly found in amniocenteses performed for ultrasound dysmorphology.

_____ **TRISOMY 21** _____

Normal growth
Short humerus and femur[9,19,21] (0.91 of expected length; femur length-abdominal circumference
    ratio lower than expected)[9]
Congenital heart defects (ventricular septal defects and atrioventricular septal defects most
    common)
Duodenal obstruction ("double bubble" sign in third trimester)
Polyhydramnios
Nuchal skin thickening (>0.5 cm in the second trimester)[8,14]
Pyelectasis[4,7]
Midphalangeal hypoplasia of the fifth digit[3]
Encephalocele[23]
Omphalocele[23]

_____ **TRISOMY 18** _____

IUGR with polyhydramnios   Omphalocele
IUGR with normal fluid   Urinary abnormalities
Congenital heart disease   Talipes (clubfoot)
Nuchal skin thickening   Clenched hands
Enlarged cisterna magna   Diaphragmatic hernia
    (seen in third trimester)[18]   Facial clefting
Open spina bifida   Encephalocele
Single umbilical artery

_____ **TRISOMY 13*** _____

IUGR   Urinary abnormalities
Congenital heart disease   Holoprosencephaly
Abnormal hands and feet   Single umbilical artery
    (polydactyly common)   Polyhydramnios
Omphalocele

---

*Reference 24.

Abnormalities of chromosome structures, such as ring chromosomes, deletions, or partial duplications, as well as mosaicism, can result in a variety of phenotypic abnormalities, depending on which chromosomes are affected and on what percentage of cells is abnormal.

QUESTION 3: WHAT IS THE INCIDENCE OF FETAL TRISOMY IN PATIENTS WITH ABNORMAL SCANS?

If dysmorphology is noted on ultrasound, the chance that the fetus is aneuploid increases. Certain malformations are thought to carry a relatively low risk of karyotypic abnormalities, especially if they occur in isolation. For instance, if open spina bifida occurs without other malformations, the risk is low that there is an associated karyotypic abnormality. In general, however, in the presence of any dysmorphology it is prudent to offer karyotype assessment: the standard of care is to offer amniocentesis when the risk of aneuploidy is greater than 1 in 190 (the risk associated with a maternal age of 35). Therefore, karyotyping should be offered whenever the risk exceeds 1 in 190.

The box on the next page lists the risk of aneuploidy associated with identified malformations of particular organs and systems. It is again important to remember that other factors that increase the prevalence of aneuploidy in a given population will increase the predictive value of these findings. For instance, in the patient profile above, although the patient's age would decrease the estimated risk of trisomy 21, the abnormal maternal serum screening study increases it. Even so, an abnormality in any of these organs or systems increases the risk above 1 in 190.

In a group of 74 fetuses with trisomy 21, 13, or 18, 63% (38 fetuses) were found on post-natal examination to have at least one malformation. Of these, 68% (26 of 38) were identified prenatally.[10] Most abnormalities associated with sex chromosome trisomies will not be noted on the scan and are usually detected only at the time of amniocentesis or CVS performed for increased maternal age.

The presence of more than one abnormality on ultrasound examination increases the risk of karyotypic abnormalities. Even so, in large series of prenatally diagnosed structural defects, the presence of any dysmorphology is associated with a risk of aneuploidy of 14% to 34%.[17,20] Van Zalen-Sprock and colleagues[23] showed that 17% of 288 fetuses with a single-organ abnormality identified on ultrasound had an abnormal karyotype, while 26% of those with multiple malformations were chromosomally abnormal. Brumfield and associates[6] showed that single malformations were associated with a 14% aneuploid rate, two separate anomalies with a 75% rate, and more than two malformations with a 100% aneuploid rate.

THE RISK OF ANEUPLOIDY ASSOCIATED WITH IDENTIFIED MALFORMATIONS OF SELECTED ORGANS AND SYSTEMS

Gastrointestinal[12]: 21%
Central nervous system[6,12]: 19%
Skeletal[12]: <1% if isolated, 37% if other systems involved
Cardiac[5,12]: 34%-36%
Diaphragmatic hernia[12]: 10% if associated with polyhydramnios or IUGR; <1% if isolated
Renal[12]: 11% if other systems involved, 2% if isolated
Bilateral hydronephrosis[6]: 40%
Omphalocele[6,12]: 6%-26%
Polyhydramnios[12]: 5% if isolated
Facial[12]: <1% if isolated, 27% if other systems involved
Cystic hygroma with hydrops[6]: 100%
Cystic hygroma without hydrops[6]: 25%

QUESTION 4: WHAT SHOULD BE INCLUDED IN A ROUTINE ULTRASOUND EXAMINATION?

The American College of Obstetrics and Gynecology[1] and the American Institute of Ultrasound in Medicine[2] have each published guidelines regarding the content of obstetric scans. It is important to remember that fetal ultrasound examination is a complex diagnostic test and that the practitioner's ability to recognize abnormalities increases over time and with repeated observation of abnormal fetuses. Neither of these professional groups condones the performance of a scan that does not assess fetal anatomy, however. The sonologist is potentially legally liable for failing to recognize major malformations at the time of a routine ultrasound examination. This legal risk and standards of good medical care demand that an attempt be made to evaluate fetal anatomy as thoroughly as possible.

The primary purposes of performing a routine screening, or so-called "level 1" scan, are to establish an accurate estimated gestational age, to diagnose multifetal pregnancies, and to confirm fetal presentation and placental positioning. Because most instances of fetal malformation occur in families with no significant family history of congenital defects or other *a priori* risk factors, however, the sonologist must carefully look for malformations by performing a systematic evaluation of fetal anatomy. After the early first trimester, in addition to the above information, an assessment of amniotic fluid volume, placental morphology, and fetal anatomy is essential. Multiple biometric parameters, including limb and head measurements, should be included.

A clear explanation of all findings should be given in a written report. In addition, a verbal report to the patient of what was seen and what was not seen is critical. Any special limitations of the examination should also be explained and documented.

QUESTION 5: CAN THE RESULTS OF A SCAN BE USED TO DIMINISH OR TO INCREASE THE ESTIMATED RISK OF FETAL ANEUPLOIDY?

Just as some centers use optimal ultrasound results to lower the estimated risk of open fetal defects for women with elevated MSAFP,[22] a normal ultrasound result determined by a sonologist skilled at evaluating fetal growth and anatomy may reasonably be used to decrease the estimated risk of aneuploidy. However, the percentage of fetuses with Down syndrome who have normal scans will be higher than the percentage of fetuses with open spina bifida who have normal scans. Thus, careful counseling will be required to give women enough information to make an informed decision about whether to undergo amniocentesis. In addition, first-trimester phenotypic abnormalities that suggest an increased risk of aneuploidy are poorly delineated, decreasing the ability of ultrasound to be useful for risk adjustment during the first trimester. Sonologists are currently less able to confidently exclude the diagnosis of a fetal trisomy during the second trimester than to exclude the presence of an open spina bifida. Further research should allow investigators to refine the combined data of maternal age, maternal serum screening studies, and targeted ultrasound to individualize genetic counseling in women over 35. As with risk adjustment for elevated MSAFP, such counseling must also include an offer to perform amniocentesis even when maternal serum screening studies and ultrasound results are normal.

REFERENCES

1. American College of Obstetricians and Gynecologists: *Ultrasonography in pregnancy*, Technical bulletin #187, Washington, D.C., Dec 1993, ACOG.
2. American Institute of Ultrasound in Medicine: *Guidelines for performance of the antepartum obstetrical ultrasound examination*, Rockville, Md, 1991, AIUM.
3. Benacerraf BR, Harlow BL, Frigoletto FD: Hypoplasia of the middle phalanx of the fifth digit, *J Ultrasound Med* 9:389, 1990.
4. Benacerraf BR, Mandell J, Estroff JA et al: Fetal pyelectasis: a possible association with Down syndrome, *Obstet Gynecol* 76:58, 1990.
5. Brown DL, Emerson DS, Shulman LP et al: Predicting aneuploidy in fetuses with cardiac anomalies: significance of visceral situs and noncardiac anomalies, *J Ultrasound Med* 3:153, 1993.

6. Brumfield CG, Davis RO, Hauth JC et al: Management of prenatally detected nonlethal fetal anomalies: is a karyotype of benefit? *Am J Perinatol* 8:255, 1991.

7. Corteville JE, Dicke JM, Crane JP: Fetal pyelectasis and Down syndrome: is genetic amniocentesis warranted? *Obstet Gynecol* 79:770, 1992.

8. Crane JP, Gray DL: Sonographically measured nuchal skinfold thickness as a screening tool for Down syndrome: results of a prospective clinical trial, *Obstet Gynecol* 77:533, 1991.

9. Dicke JM, Gray DL, Songster GS, Crane JP: Fetal biometry as a screening tool for the detection of chromosomally abnormal pregnancies, *Obstet Gynecol* 74:726, 1989.

10. Dicke JM, Crane JP: Sonographic recognition of major malformations and aberrant fetal growth in trisomic fetuses, *J Ultrasound Med* 10:433, 1991.

11. Drugan A, Johnson MP, Isada NB et al: The smaller than expected first-trimester fetus is at increased risk for chromosome anomalies, *Am J Obstet Gynecol* 167:1525, 1992.

12. Eydoux P, Choiset A, LePorrier N et al: Chromosomal prenatal diagnosis: study of 936 cases of intrauterine abnormalities after ultrasound assessment, *Prenat Diagn* 9:255, 1989.

13. Gagnon S, Fraser W, Fouquette B et al: Nature and frequency of chromosomal abnormalities in pregnancies with abnormal ultrasound findings: an analysis of 117 cases with review of the literature, *Prenat Diagn* 12:9, 1992.

14. Hill LM, Guzick D, Belfar HL et al: The current role of sonography in the detection of Down syndrome, *Obstet Gynecol* 74:620, 1989.

15. Hook EB, Cross PK, Schreinemachers DM: Rates of chromosomal abnormality at amniocentesis and in liveborn infants, *JAMA* 249:2034, 1983.

16. Khoury MJ, Erickson JD, Cordero JF, McCarthy BJ: Congenital malformations and intrauterine growth retardation: a population study, *Pediatrics* 82:83, 1988.

17. Nicolaides KH, Snijders RJM, Gosden CM et al: Ultrasonographically detectable markers of fetal chromosomal abnormalities, *Lancet* 340:704, 1992.

18. Nyberg DA, Kramer D, Resta RG et al: Prenatal sonographic findings of trisomy 18: review of 47 cases, *J Ultrasound Med* 2:103, 1993.

19. Nyberg DA, Resta RG, Luthy DA et al: Humerus and femur length shortening in the detection of Down's syndrome, *Am J Obstet Gynecol* 168:534, 1993.

20. Snijders RJ, Sherrod C, Gosden CM, Nicolaides KH: Fetal growth retardation: associated malformations and chromosomal abnormalities, *Am J Obstet Gynecol* 168:547, 1993.

21. Platt LD, Medearis AL, Carlson DE et al: Screening for Down syndrome with the femur length/biparietal diameter ratio: a new twist of the data, *Am J Obstet Gynecol* 167:124, 1992.

22. Richards DS, Seeds JN, Katz VW, Lingley SH, Cefalo RC: Elevated maternal serum alpha-fetoprotein with normal ultrasound: is amniocentesis always appropriate? A review of 26,069 screened patients, *Obstet Gynecol* 71:203, 1988.

23. Van Zalen-Sprock MM, Van Vugt JMG, Karsdorp VHM et al: Ultrasound diagnosis of fetal abnormalities and cytogenetic evaluation, *Prenat Diagn* 11:655, 1991.

24. Wladimiroff JW, Stewart PA, Reuss A, Sachs ES: Cardiac and extra-cardiac anomalies as indicators for trisomies 13 and 18: a prenatal ultrasound study, *Prenat Diagn* 9:515, 1989.

CHAPTER 16

Evaluation and Management
of Single-Organ Malformations

NANCY C. CHESCHEIR

Prenatal diagnosis is both an art and a science, for when a fetal anomaly is suspected, the parents must be informed about a broad range of medical, embryologic, and genetic data as well as emotional, economic, and legal issues. This complex information must be communicated in a nurturing and supportive manner, and usually in the setting of a busy clinic! The responsibility of making sure that the patient understands the diagnosis ultimately belongs to the patient's prenatal care provider. If unable to complete this task herself or himself, the provider should refer the patient to a center where the relevant expertise exists.

Single-organ malformations can be deceptively complex and challenging. Although ultrasound and karyotyping can frequently help define the abnormality of the involved organ, the practitioner is often unable to determine the extent of the effect on the fetus and also must be cautious about affirming the normality of the other organs. In addition, advances in neonatal surgical and medical care continually improve the prognosis for some of these defects, making it essential for obstetric care providers to stay informed about contemporary management.

❧ Patient Profile: Prenatal diagnosis of a congenital cardiac anomaly

The patient is 27 years old (gravida 3, para 2002). Her two prior pregnancies and children were normal. An ultrasound examination is performed at 24 weeks' gestation to confirm gestational age. The scan shows a singleton fetus whose measurements are compatible with 24 weeks, normal amniotic fluid, and symmetric growth. The patient's obstetrician notes that the fetal heart doesn't seem to point in the correct direction and refers the patient for a targeted ultrasound examination. Three days later, the scan demonstrates normal fetal anatomy except that the heart is deviated so that the apex points to the left axillary line. The atria are symmetric, and the foramen ovale appears patent. The atrioventricular valves move normally, and the ventricles are also symmetric. However, a large ventricular septal defect (VSD) is seen. The pulmonary artery is identified but is much smaller than the aorta, which straddles the ventricular septal defect (Figure 16-1). No pericardial or pulmonary effusion is present. The rhythm is normal, and Doppler measurements confirm flow through both outflow tracts.

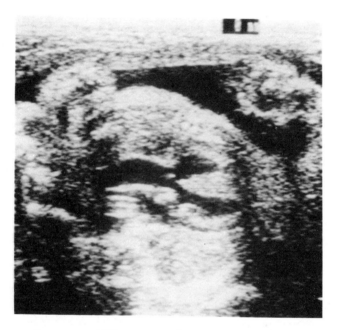

Fig. 16-1 Large outflow tract straddling a ventricular septal defect connected to both the left and right ventricles.

QUESTION 1: WHAT IS THE MOST LIKELY DIAGNOSIS?

The name of this particular defect is relatively unimportant at the beginning of this evaluation. While it is always appealing to be able to categorize disease processes, the important point here is that some cardiac defect is present, with features that include a VSD, an overriding and dilated aorta, and a shifted axis. This heart has abnormalities of both intracardiac and outflow tract structures and therefore has a complex congenital heart defect. Because it is more common, this defect is probably tetralogy of Fallot, although other possibilities include double-outlet left or right ventricle or a truncal abnormality. A complete description of the defect can probably be given after a more detailed fetal echocardiogram is performed, including M-mode to measure vessel and chamber size and contractility and Doppler studies to describe the hemodynamic characteristics of the heart. This study is best performed with the collaboration of a pediatric cardiologist and a fetal echocardiographer.

QUESTION 2: HAVING OBSERVED A COMPLEX CONGENITAL HEART DEFECT, WHAT MORE NEEDS TO BE CONSIDERED?

The diagnosis of an anomaly is only the starting point: many other issues need to be explored and discussed with the family. To provide complete information to the family and to develop a plan with them, a thorough understanding of the fetal condition is essential.

Although most congenital heart defects are isolated anomalies, many are associated with other abnormalities. In a large regional case-control study of liveborn infants known as the Baltimore-Washington Infant Study, investigators found that 73% of infants with cardiovascular defects had isolated heart problems, while 27% also had extracardiac structural or karyotypic abnormalities.[10] The percentage of extracardiac defects reported in the literature ranges from 25% to 44%.[11,20] Even at the lower end of this range, however, the risk that some other defect is present is significant and mandates a careful examination of the fetus and an explanation to the family that other organs may be abnormal.

The converse is also true: the diagnosis of an extracardiac major malformation should prompt a detailed examination of the fetal heart. In a thorough review of the literature, Copel and colleagues[9] discussed the incidence of congenital heart defects in fetuses with noncardiac defects. Overall, the incidence of congenital heart disease in these fetuses is about 7%. For specific anomalies, the range varies considerably: less than 3% of fetuses with Dandy-Walker malformation, gastroschisis, or ureteral obstruction were also found to have a congenital heart defect, whereas at least 30% of fetuses with esophageal atresia, tracheoesophageal fistula, omphalocele, and some renal abnormalities were so affected.

The nonrandom occurrence of groups of defects is known as a *syndrome*. Examples of syndromes that include cardiac defects are listed in the box on the next page. Although the list is not exhaustive, it highlights the spectrum of diagnoses that must be considered.

The four most common aneuploidies seen among liveborn neonates are trisomy 21, trisomy 18, trisomy 13, and monosomy X (45,X).[21] The incidence of congenital heart defects among infants with these karyotypes is 50%, 99%, 84%, and 35%, respectively.[18,21] The relevant clinical question for the woman and her doctor after a fetal congenital heart defect has been identified is, "What is the incidence of karyotypic abnormalities among fetuses with heart defects?" Among liveborn infants with heart defects, the rate of aneuploidy is 12.5%.[8] Allan and associates[2] reported a 16% rate of karyotypic abnormalities among 124 consecutive fetuses with cardiac defects. In a smaller number of patients, Copel and colleagues[9] reported a 32% rate of aneuploidy among fetuses with heart defects. Despite the wide discrepancies in these numbers, even the lower range represents a markedly increased risk of aneuploidy relative to the background population. To put this into a more familiar context, the maternal age-related risk of having a liveborn infant with a clinically significant chromosome abnormality at age 35, the standard age at which prenatal karyotyping is routinely offered, is 5.6 in 1000 and does not reach 150 in 1000 (15%) until age 49![12]

The technique chosen to obtain the fetal karyotype if the woman elects to undergo invasive fetal testing will depend on gestational age, maternal choice, and technical factors, such

---

EXAMPLES OF SYNDROMES KNOWN TO INCLUDE CARDIAC DEFECTS

Pentalogy of Cantrell:

Includes cardiac defects, sternal clefting, diaphragmatic defects, pericardial defects, and omphalocele.

Noonan syndrome:

Autosomal dominant. Includes short stature and short neck, chest deformity, typical facies, mild mental retardation in 35%, and cardiac abnormalities, such as pulmonary stenosis, atrial septal defect, ventricular septal defect, and patent ductus arteriosus.

Fetal alcohol syndrome:

Includes low birthweight, hypotonia, microcephaly, thin upper lip, typical facies, and cardiac defects in 50% (ventricular septal defect, tetralogy of Fallot, and atrial septal defect are common).

Maternal phenylketonuria (PKU):

Microcephaly, intrauterine growth retardation (IUGR), mental retardation, seizures, congenital heart disease, cleft palate, and clinodactyly.

VACTERL* association:

Sporadic occurrence. Includes vascular, anorectal, cardiac, tracheoesophageal, and renal abnormalities.

---

*Acronym for *v*ertebral, *a*nal, *c*ardiac, *t*racheal, *e*sophageal, *r*enal, and *l*imb.

as placental position and maternal obesity. Rapid karyotyping should be offered if pregnancy termination is a potential option and the legal limit for termination is close.

A complete medical history of the mother should be obtained. Historical risk factors include exposure to certain chemicals and drugs and the presence of some maternal metabolic diseases. Preexisting diabetes mellitus is known to increase the risk of fetal structural malformations to two to three times that of the background incidence. Data from the Collaborative Perinatal Project reported by Mitchell and colleagues[17] indicate that the infant of a diabetic mother has a 25.4 in 1000 risk of congenital heart disease, compared with an 8.1 in 1000 rate among infants of nondiabetic mothers. Successful treatment of childhood phenylketonuria has resulted in an increasing number of women with PKU who become pregnant. In the National Maternal Phenylketonuria Collaborative Study, undertaken by the National Institute of Child Health and Human Development, 6 of 69 women (8.7%) who had maternal phenylalanine levels above 600 μmol/L (>10 mg/dl) had fetuses with congenital heart defects.[19] Any woman whose fetus has such a defect should be questioned directly about PKU and about whether she remembers following a special diet during childhood.

The practitioner should also ask the patient directly about ingestion of certain drugs and chemicals. While central nervous system abnormalities and growth retardation are well-known components of fetal alcohol syndrome, about 50% of affected children will also have structural heart disease. Some researchers estimate that as many as 5% of congenital heart defects are caused by maternal alcohol abuse.[15]

Table 16-1   Recurrence risk for congenital heart defect when a first-degree relative is affected[6]

	Mother affected	Father affected	One sibling affected	Two siblings affected
Aortic stenosis	13%-18%	3%	2%	6%
Atrial septal defect	4%-4.5%	1.5%	2.5%	8%
Atrioventricular canal defect	14%	1%	*	*
Coarctation of the aorta	4%	2%	2%	6%
Pulmonary stenosis	4%-6.5%	2%	2%	6%
Ventricular septal defect	6%-10%	2%	3%	10%
Tetralogy of Fallot	2.5%	1.5%	2.5%	8%

*Data not available.

Despite efforts by the manufacturer of isotretinoin (Accutane) to educate women about the risks of becoming pregnant while taking the drug, some women will conceive while using the medication for treatment of cystic acne. Isotretinoin is a potent teratogen. In one study that examined both retrospectively and prospectively identified cases, 18 of 45 exposed fetuses (40%) had malformations, 12 of which were cardiac defects.[14]

The medical history should include questioning the patient about symptoms of infection during the early prenatal period. Although rubella syndrome is relatively rare now because of widespread vaccination efforts, it does still occur. In addition, cytomegalovirus and syphilis both can cause congenital heart defects. Appropriate serologic studies should be performed, especially if the history is suggestive of such an infection.

A complete family history for both parents should be obtained. The presence of structural heart disease in either parent or in a sibling of the fetus increases the risk of congenital heart disease in the offspring. Commonly quoted recurrence risks are given in Table 16-1. However, a recurrent heart defect may be of a different type than that of the previously affected family member.[18]

Having made these efforts to diagnose the cause of the cardiac defect and to rule out as much as possible the existence of other fetal abnormalities, a frank discussion between the patient and a pediatric cardiologist or cardiothoracic surgeon is important. The purpose of this meeting is to give the family a thorough understanding of the possible diagnostic and treatment plans after birth and an idea of the long-term prognosis. By including the pediatric specialists early, the parents are generally more prepared for the potentially difficult decisions they may need to make postnatally.

QUESTION 3: HOW DOES THE PRESENCE OF A CONGENITAL HEART DEFECT ALTER THE MANAGEMENT OF THE REMAINDER OF THE PREGNANCY?

Perinatal management will differ according to the specific details of the pregnancy. Especially with complex congenital heart defects that carry a poor prognosis, such as hypoplastic left heart syndrome, some women after counseling will choose to undergo pregnancy termination if that option is legally available to them at the gestational age at which the diagnosis is made. For those who continue their pregnancies, the rate of stillbirth is increased. In one study, 27.5 per 1000 stillborn fetuses were found at necropsy to have a congenital heart defect (frequently not isolated), while the rate of identified congenital heart disease among liveborn infants in that same study was 7.7 per 1000.[16] These deaths are largely unpreventable, but the patient should be apprised of the possibility of such an outcome. Few isolated structural heart defects will cause the development of nonimmune hydrops if it is not present at the time of the original diagnosis. Even so, limited serial ultrasound for surveillance of hydrops, interval growth monitoring, and parental reassurance is reasonable.

While some structural heart defects, such as ventricular septal defects and even hypoplastic heart defects, may be asymptomatic at birth, the presence of such a defect may impair the normal transition from fetal to neonatal circulation. If the defect is one that may produce cyanosis or other distress at birth, or if a complete diagnosis of the defect has not been made, it is appropriate to recommend that the infant be delivered at a hospital that offers tertiary neonatal and pediatric cardiac care. Many children with heart defects will do well if appropriate care is provided early to prevent the development of hypoxia and acidosis. In some cases, such as in neonates with duct-dependent lesions, an infant will need to be given an intravenous prostaglandin infusion immediately after birth.

Except for the hydropic fetus, the choice of route of delivery should depend on the usual obstetric factors. Even fetuses with hypoplastic left heart syndrome tolerate labor well.[13] If the defect has caused a significant arrhythmia, cesarean delivery may be necessary because of the inability to monitor the infant's status during labor. However, cesarean delivery should not be offered solely because a heart defect is present.

It is important to remember that perinatal management and prenatal care should continue to address the many issues that arise in "normal" pregnancies; it is easy to focus medical attention only on what is abnormal and to neglect the more routine issues.

QUESTION 4: WHICH PATIENTS SHOULD BE REFERRED FOR TARGETED ULTRASOUND EXAMINATION OF THE FETAL HEART?

Many risk factors for congenital heart disease exist (see the box at the top of p. 122), and women with any of these factors should be offered targeted fetal echocardiography. Nonetheless, the group for whom fetal echocardiography is most valuable is those women who have an abnormal screening ultrasound view known as the *four-chamber view*. To identify patients who should be referred for echocardiography, then, a four-chamber view should be included in all second- and third-trimester scans.[2,3,4,9]

The four-chamber view can reliably be obtained transabdominally after 18 weeks' gestation in most women.[10] The view is obtained by angling cephalad to the fetus from the scan plane at which the abdominal circumference is measured. Another technique is to align the transducer with the full length of one of the fetal ribs and slide the transducer to "step off"

INDICATIONS FOR REFERRAL FOR FETAL ECHOCARDIOGRAPHY*

Abnormal ultrasound screening result   Known fetal aneuploidy
Prior affected child or fetus   Maternal diabetes
Family history of congenital heart defects Maternal alcohol abuse
Sustained fetal arrhythmia   Maternal collagen vascular disease
Nonimmune hydrops fetalis   Maternal phenylketonuria
Polyhydramnios

*Reference 22.

into the intercostal space. The four-chamber heart view is considered normal if all of the criteria listed in the box below are met. Approximately 50% of fetuses in whom a four-chamber view was abnormal actually had a congenital heart defect, whereas between 40% and 92% of fetuses with a congenital heart defect will have an abnormal four-chamber view.[1,5,8] Women must be aware that a normal screening view does not guarantee the absence of a congenital heart defect. If other risk factors are present, more extensive echocardiography should be offered.

CRITERIA FOR A NORMAL FOUR-CHAMBER SCREENING VIEW OF THE FETAL HEART

Heart occupies one third to one half of fetal chest
Apex points to left side of fetal chest
A-P line from spine to sternum crosses right ventricle
Atria are symmetric
Septum secundum moves into left atrium
Foramen ovale is visible
Ventricles are symmetric
Atrioventricular valves are symmetric or insertion of tricuspid valve is dislocated a little toward
    apex relative to mitral valve
Rhythm is regular (120-160 bpm)
Ventricular contractility is equal

REFERENCES

1. Achiron R, Glaser J, Gelernter I et al: Extended fetal echocardiographic examination for detecting cardiac malformations in low-risk pregnancies, *Br Med J* 304:671, 1992.
2. Allan LD, Sharland GK, Chita SK et al: Chromosomal anomalies in fetal congenital heart disease, *Ultrasound Obstet Gynecol* 1:8, 1991.
3. American College of Obstetricians and Gynecologists Committee on Obstetrics: Maternal and Fetal Medicine: *Ultrasound imaging in pregnancy*, Number 96, August 1991.
4. American Institute of Ultrasound in Medicine: *Guidelines for performance of the antepartum obstetrical ultrasound examination*, Rockville, Md, 1991, AIUM.
5. Bromley B, Estroff J, Sanders S et al: Fetal echocardiography: accuracy and limitations in a population at high and low risk for heart defects, *Am J Obstet Gynecol* 166:1473, 1992.

6. Callan NA, Maggio M, Steger S, Kan JS: Fetal echocardiography: indications for referral, prenatal diagnoses and outcomes, *Am J Perinatol* 8:390, 1991.

7. Copel J, Cullen M, Green J et al: The frequency of aneuploidy in prenatally diagnosed congenital heart disease: an indication for fetal karyotyping, *Am J Obstet Gynecol* 158:409, 1988.

8. Copel JA, Pilu GA, Green J et al: Fetal echocardiographic screening for congenital heart disease: the importance of the four chamber view, *Am J Obstet Gynecol* 157:648, 1987.

9. Copel J, Pilu GL, Kleinman C: Congenital heart disease and extracardiac anomalies: associations and indications for fetal echocardiography, *Am J Obstet Gynecol* 154:1121, 1986.

10. Ferencz C, Rubin JD, McCarter RJ et al: Cardiac and non-cardiac malformations: observations in a population-based study, *Teratology* 35:367, 1987.

11. Greenwood RD, Rosenthal A, Parisi L et al: Extracardiac abnormalities in infants with congenital heart disease, *Pediatrics* 55:485, 1975.

12. Hook EB: Rates of chromosome abnormalities at different maternal ages, *Obstet Gynecol* 58:282, 1981.

13. Jackson GM, Ludmir J, Castelbaum A et al: Intrapartum course of fetuses with isolated hypoplastic left heart syndrome, *Am J Obstet Gynecol* 165:1068, 1991.

14. Lammar EJ, Chen DT, Hoar RM et al: Retinoic acid embryopathy, *N Engl J Med* 313:837, 1985.

15. Lipson T: Fetal alcohol syndrome, *Aust Fam Physician* 17:385, 1988.

16. Mitchell SC, Korones SB, Berendes HW: Congenital heart disease in 56,109 births: incidence and natural history, *Circulation* 43:323, 1971.

17. Mitchell SC, Sellmann AH, Westphal MC et al: Etiologic correlates in a study of congenital heart disease in 56,109 births, *Am J Cardiol* 28:653, 1971.

18. Nora JJ, Nora AH: Update on counseling the family with a first-degree relative with a congenital heart defect, *Am J Med Genet* 29:137, 1988.

19. Platt LD, Koch R, Azen C et al: Maternal phenylketonuria collaborative study, obstetric aspects and outcome: the first 6 years, *Am J Obstet Gynecol* 166:1150, 1992.

20. Wallgren EI, Landtman B, Rapola J: Extracardiac malformations associated with CHD, *Eur J Cardiol* 7:15, 1978.

21. Warkany J, Passarge E, Smith LB: Congenital malformations in autosomal trisomy syndrome, *Am J Dis Child* 112:502, 1966.

22. Winter RM, Baraitser M: In *Multiple congenital anomalies: a diagnostic compendium*, London, 1991, Chapman & Hall Medical.

CHAPTER 17

Intrauterine Growth Retardation

WENDY F. HANSEN

The fetus has a genetically predetermined growth potential that is affected by a host of factors: the mother's health, placental function, drugs, nutrition, and perinatal infection. When fetal growth is compromised by one of these factors, the fetus has a physiologic and metabolic response that is only partially understood. When fetal growth falls below the 10th percentile for gestational age, intrauterine growth retardation (IUGR) is considered to be present. The identification, evaluation, antenatal management, and safe delivery of the affected fetus present one of the greatest challenges in perinatal medicine.

❖ Patient Profile: Evaluation and management of the growth-retarded fetus

A 41-year-old white married woman (gravida 1, para 0000), at 25 weeks' gestation by known last menstrual period and first-trimester ultrasound examination, is transferred for management of IUGR. Maternal history is negative for infectious or drug exposures. Her medical history is remarkable for intermittent symptoms and signs suggestive of an autoimmune disease, although an extensive rheumatologic evaluation was negative. Her obstetric history is remarkable for a positive maternal serum multiscreen (AFP, hCG, uE₃) for trisomy 21. However, after counseling regarding her age and risk, the patient declined amniocentesis.

On ultrasound evaluation, severe IUGR was noted, with an estimated fetal weight of 475 g, which is slightly below the 10th percentile for 25 weeks. Fetal anatomy appeared normal. Amniotic fluid index was decreased, at 5 cm. Umbilical artery velocity waveform showed absent end-diastolic flow. A biophysical profile showed a fetal heart-rate tracing that had decreased variability and no accelerations, but no decelerations. There was good fetal movement and tone. Consultation with the neonatologist and with the patient was undertaken. Delivery at that time, remote from term, was thought to ensure neonatal death. The decision was made to continue the pregnancy, with intensive antenatal surveillance until at least 28 weeks' gestation, recognizing that intrauterine demise was a strong possibility. If at 28 weeks' gestation there was no interval growth, delivery would be accomplished.

Bed rest and continuous oxygen therapy were maintained, along with intensive antenatal surveillance. At 26.5 weeks, an intrauterine fetal death was noted. Delivery was induced, and birthweight was 410 g. The postmortem examination revealed no abnormalities, and the karotype was 46,XX.

QUESTION 1: WHAT CAUSES INTRAUTERINE GROWTH RETARDATION?

Numerous studies have reported a variety of causes of IUGR. However, ethical constraints have made etiologic scientific studies of human IUGR impossible. Consequently, investigators have developed a number of animal models (Table 17-1).[9] The various methods used to induce IUGR in animals are thought to reflect the various causes seen in the human fetus. These causes are summarized in the box below.

CAUSES OF INTRAUTERINE GROWTH RETARDATION

Constitutional

Seen primarily in small women and in those with low weight gain during pregnancy; results in small but healthy babies

Genetic

Short stature syndromes (e.g., Russell-Silver syndrome)
Aneuploidy (e.g., trisomy 13, trisomy18), polyploidy
Structural defects (e.g., gastroschisis, renal agenesis)

Placental

Structural (e.g., circumvallate, chorioangiomas)
Perfusion abnormalities, infarcts

Maternal disease

Hypertension
Vascular disease
Renal disease
Autoimmune disease
Infection

Environmental

Tobacco, alcohol, other drugs

Seeds[20] reported that 40% of all IUGR is constitutional, whereas 40% is caused by placental insufficiency, 10% by genetic factors, and 10% by perinatal infection.

QUESTION 2: HOW DOES THE FETUS RESPOND TO AN ABNORMAL INTRAUTERINE ENVIRONMENT?

Normal fetal growth is dependent on placental transport of substrates and placental and fetal metabolic functions. When one of these factors is compromised, the fetus must adapt to survive.

Table 17-1   Animal models for etiologic studies of intrauterine growth retardation

Species	Method of inducement
Rats	Interruption of the uterine blood supply
	Selective nutrient deprivation (zinc)
	Extrinsic stress: forced exercise, sham surgeries, hypothermia
	Chronic hypoxia (ambient 9.5% O_2)
Mice	Superovulation with crowding
	Numerous chemical agents
Pigs	Starvation
	Natural occurrence due to high litter rates

Traditionally, IUGR has been divided into two categories: *symmetric*, or type I, and *asymmetric*, or type II.[16] In symmetric IUGR, the underlying cause is thought to begin to affect the fetus during early development and may be chromosomal, genetic, infectious, structural, or teratologic in origin. In this model, all systems are equally affected. Therefore, sonographic biometric measurements generally show a biparietal diameter (BPD), femur length, and abdominal circumference (AC) with a symmetric growth delay. However, this model arose during an era of limited imaging technology, when little was known about the patterns of normal fetal growth. Recent observations show that this model is not precise. For example, certain fetuses with aneuploidy do not show completely symmetric growth delay.

In contrast, asymmetric IUGR is often diagnosed in the middle to late second trimester and is thought to be secondary to placental dysfunction. In this model, the fetus reacts to the nutritional deprivation by redistributing blood flow in favor of the vital organs: brain, heart, and adrenal glands. This redistribution is generally reflected in a decreased abdominal circumference as liver glycogen stores are depleted. Measurements on ultrasound show a BPD appropriate for gestational age, a markedly small AC, and an intermediate femur measurement.

The advent of Doppler ultrasonography in the early 1980s has allowed examination of this model in more detail. Altered Doppler bloodflow-velocity waveforms have been demonstrated in several vascular beds. Fleischer and colleagues[10] were the first to show that the umbilical artery velocity waveforms were abnormal in intrauterine growth–retarded fetuses, reflecting the increased vascular resistance of the placenta. Wladimiroff and associates[27] showed that in growth retarded fetuses increased resistance in the umbilical artery was associated with decreased resistance in the internal carotid artery. This supported evidence in animals of redistribution of bloodflow favoring the brain. Arduini and associates[2] demonstrated increased renal vascular resistance in growth-retarded fetuses. This increased resistance was particularly evident in fetuses with oligohydramnios, supporting the hypothesis that a mechanism of decreased renal perfusion is present. Akalin-Sel and colleagues[1] described the "lower limb reflex" when they investigated the circulatory redistribution of the intrauterine growth–retarded fetus. They found a loss of end-diastolic flow in the abdominal aorta in severe IUGR. This vasoconstriction seen in the abdominal aorta reflects the compensatory response of the fetus, with increased resistance in the vascular beds of the lower limbs, skeletal muscles, skin, and mesentery.

Consistent with this redistribution in bloodflow is a redistribution of fetal cardiac output.[18] The fetal heart is right-side dominant, with a right to left cardiac output ratio of 1.3 to 1. During fetal life, right ventricular output is directed through the ductus arteriosus to the lower body and placenta, while left ventricular output is directed through the ascending aorta and brain. Rizzo and Arduini[18] showed that there is a preferential shift of cardiac output in favor of the left ventricle, leading to improved perfusion of the brain.

In response to this nutritional deprivation, a profound metabolic and hormonal adaptation occurs in the fetus. Supporting evidence comes from direct measurements of fetal plasma levels obtained during percutaneous umbilical blood sampling in both intrauterine growth–retarded and normal-size fetuses. First, there are marked disturbances in carbohydrate, fat, and amino acid metabolism. Specific observations are summarized in Table 17-2. Some intrauterine growth–retarded fetuses are hypoglycemic, with elevated levels of glucagon and lactate.[13] Whether this is caused by impaired placental transfer or by increased glycolysis in anaerobic metabolism of lactate is unknown. There is also a hypoinsulinemia that is more severe than expected, suggesting pancreatic β-cell dysfunction. Plasma triglyceride levels are elevated in some intrauterine growth–retarded fetuses, suggesting either reduced triglyceride oxidation or less incorporation into body fat.[22] Essential amino acids are decreased so that a high ratio of nonessential to essential amino acids, similar to that in children with protein-calorie malnutrition, is seen.[6,8]

The fetal endocrine axis adapts by slowing the fetal basal metabolic rate. Thyroid-stimulating hormone is elevated, and T_3 and T_4 are decreased (Table 17-3).[23] There appears to

Table 17-2   Fetal metabolic alterations in intrauterine growth retardation

Increase	Decrease
Glucagon	Glucose
Triglycerides	Essential amino acids
Nonessential amino acids	
Lactate	

Table 17-3   Fetal hormonal alterations in intrauterine growth retardation

Increase	Decrease
TSH	T_3, T_4
Erythropoietin	Platelets
Erythroblasts	Leukocytes
Growth hormone	
GHRH	
IGF, IGF_2	

TSH, Thyroid-stimulating hormone, T_3, triiodothyronine, T_4, tetraiodothyronine (thyroxine), *GHRH*, growth hormone releasing hormone, *IGF, IGF_2*, insulin-like growth factors.

be a hypersecretion of growth hormone and a hyperresponsiveness to growth hormone releasing hormone (GHRH) that persists for 1 month after birth. Erythropoietin increases in proportion to the degree of fetal acidemia, with a resultant increase in the erythroblast count.[22] In contrast to the response of the red cell line, thrombocytopenia and leukopenia are seen. Whether this is secondary to impaired hematopoiesis or to a consumptive coagulopathy is unknown. Like most disturbances, there is a spectrum of severity. Highly abnormal levels were noted when IUGR was more severe and when it was accompanied by hypoxia.

After birth, the fetus, which was profoundly affected both physiologically and biochemically, must adapt to an extrauterine existence. The first few days of life are often characterized by hypoglycemia and thermoregulatory difficulties.[3] In addition, many infants with IUGR are born prematurely and must cope with the sequelae of prematurity.

QUESTION 3: HOW IS THE INTRAUTERINE GROWTH–RETARDED FETUS IDENTIFIED?

Concern for identification of the growth-retarded fetus predates the ultrasound era. In 1953, Rumbolz and McGoogan[19] showed that reduced growth of the uterine fundus and IUGR were associated. In 1982, Calvert and colleagues[5] confirmed that a simple screening method, measurement of symphysis to fundal height between 20 and 36 weeks' gestation, was useful in the detection of IUGR. They noted that the simplicity and reliability of the method were independent of the clinician's level of experience. They found that a fundal height measurement 3 cm less than the corresponding gestational age had a sensitivity of 64% in detecting IUGR, with a false-positive rate of 71%. Despite its high false-positive rate, use of this simple, inexpensive screening method has become a standard practice in prenatal care.

The era of ultrasonography ushered in the use of this imaging technique both as a screening tool for IUGR and as a diagnostic modality.[20] Many different measurements have been analyzed: BPD, AC, the fetal ponderal index (which describes the relationship between weight and length), mean abdominal diameter-femur length ratio, and head circumference-abdominal circumference ratio. It is known that the BPD by itself is a poor indicator of IUGR. Abdominal circumference is the single best predictor of IUGR, reflecting both the physiologic adaptation of the fetus to deprivation and the decrease in growth seen in symmetric growth delay.

How can these studies be translated into practice? All patients at high risk for having a fetus with IUGR should have an early dating scan before 20 weeks' gestation, when biometric measurements are most accurate. Since measurement of the symphysis to fundal height will miss one third of all intrauterine growth–retarded fetuses, patients at risk should have serial ultrasound examinations to assess growth. At 20 weeks' gestation and thereafter, all patients should have a symphysis to fundal height measurement at each prenatal visit. If a difference of 3 cm or greater is noted, an ultrasound examination should be performed. An estimated fetal weight is determined by analyzing a variety of fetal biometric measurements using a fetal weight chart reflecting the local conditions. If the estimated fetal weight is below the 10th percentile for gestational age, further evaluation and management are dictated by the clinical situation.

QUESTION 4: WHAT ARE THE PREFERRED CLINICAL MANAGEMENT AND EVALUATION WHEN INTRAUTERINE GROWTH RETARDATION IS SUSPECTED?

When growth retardation is identified, its evaluation and management depend on a host of factors: maternal history, gestational age when recognized, pattern of growth delay, and severity. Practically, growth-retarded fetuses can be classified into three groups: (1) those that represent the lower extreme of normal; (2) those with IUGR secondary to genetic, infectious, or teratologic causes; and (3) those with chronic nutritional deprivation secondary to placental dysfunction. Although it is not always possible, evaluation of IUGR should focus on placing the fetus into one of these three groups.

A thorough maternal history is warranted, with special consideration given to medical history, maternal and paternal genetic history, known infectious exposures, and tobacco, alcohol, and other drug use. A detailed ultrasound anatomic survey is needed, along with evaluation of amniotic fluid and Doppler velocity indices of the umbilical artery. Karyotype of the fetus and viral cultures of the amniotic fluid and maternal serum should be considered in all fetuses thought to be at risk. Maternal serum TORCH* titers, although often performed, are generally of minimal benefit. A thorough investigation will not always reveal a cause, and these fetuses with IUGR of unknown origin must be managed with intensive antenatal surveillance, much as the nutritionally deprived fetus is managed.

The intrauterine growth–retarded fetus is at high risk for perinatal morbidity and mortality and is perhaps more susceptible to the effects of hypoxia on long-term neurodevelopment than fetuses with normal growth. Therefore, conventional management of the intrauterine growth–retarded fetus is based on three principles: optimizing the fetal environment, providing intensive fetal surveillance, and determining optimal timing of delivery.

The practitioner's ability to optimize the fetal environment is limited, and current treatment modalities are controversial. First, control of the underlying maternal disease, insofar as this is possible, is imperative. Examples include discontinuation of cigarettes in smokers and control of blood pressure in severely hypertensive patients. Next, all women with intrauterine growth–retarded fetuses should be placed on some form of bed rest to maximize placental perfusion. The role of maternal hyperoxygenation is unclear. Most recently, Battaglia and colleagues[4] studied 36 pregnant women carrying fetuses with severe IUGR; 17 women were treated with 55% oxygen at a rate of 8 L/min by face mask 24 hours a day.[4] The control group consisted of 19 women with similar characteristics who received conventional treatment and no oxygen. Three patients in the treated group showed significant improvement in umbilical artery Doppler indices, and there were no intrauterine deaths. Three patients in the control group

---

*Toxoplasmosis, other (infections), rubella, cytomegalovirus, and herpes simplex.

showed worsening Doppler indices, and there was one intrauterine death. No difference in birthweight was found between the two groups. This improvement in Doppler velocity indices in the treated group was accompanied by a statistically significant improvement in fetal cord gases at delivery and an overall decrease in perinatal death and neonatal complications. The long-term significance of these findings is currently unknown.

The role of antiplatelet therapy as both prevention and therapy for IUGR is evolving. Initial studies in the late 1980s using aspirin or aspirin and dipyridamole were promising, showing significant reductions in IUGR when the medication was used prophylactically and increases in birthweight when used therapeutically.[24,26] In addition, meta-analysis of several small studies showed that aspirin reduced the risk of both pregnancy-induced hypertension (PIH) and IUGR. However, these studies were small and had widely varying patient selection criteria, and antiplatelet therapy was started at various gestational ages. Since then, four large, multicenter, randomized, double-blind, placebo-controlled trials have been conducted in which the therapeutic and preventive roles of aspirin were examined. The first of these studies took place in France in 1991 and involved 323 women with a history of IUGR, fetal death, or placental abruption.[25] Women were placed into one of three groups between 15 and 18 weeks' gestation: those given aspirin (150 mg/day); those given placebo; and those given aspirin (150 mg/day) plus dipyridamole (225 mg/day). Birthweight was significantly higher (225 g) in both treated groups, compared with the control group. No significant difference was found between the aspirin and aspirin plus dipyridamole groups. This was the first large study supporting the conclusions drawn earlier that aspirin has a role in the prevention of IUGR.

The Italian Study of Aspirin in Pregnancy, conducted in 1993, assessed the efficacy of low-dose aspirin in women judged to be at moderate risk for both IUGR and preeclampsia.[15] A total of 1106 women were placed into one of two groups: those given aspirin (50 mg/day) and those given placebo. Surprisingly, this was the first large study in which no difference in birthweight or incidence of IUGR was found between groups. This study did not support the conclusion drawn by previous studies that the use of aspirin is beneficial in women at moderate risk of PIH or IUGR. Later in 1993, Sibai and associates[21] studied 3135 normotensive, nulliparous, healthy women and placed patients into one of two groups: those given aspirin (60 mg/day) and those given placebo. No significant change was seen in birthweight or incidence of IUGR. In addition, a higher rate of placental abruption was noted in the aspirin group. Most recently, the Collaborative Low-Dose Aspirin Study in Pregnancy (CLASP), conducted in 1994, assessed the efficacy of aspirin therapy in women who had a history of preeclampsia or IUGR, or who had preeclampsia or IUGR in the target pregnancy.[7] A total of 9364 women were placed into one of two groups: those given aspirin (60 mg/day) and those given placebo. No significant difference was seen between groups in the incidence of IUGR or in birthweight.

The findings of recent large trials, then, do not support the use of aspirin in all women at risk of IUGR. This is not surprising, since IUGR has a very heterogeneous etiology. Aspirin's beneficial effect in a subset of women at risk of IUGR has yet to be proved.

The method and intensity of antenatal surveillance depend on the severity of IUGR and on the gestational age of the fetus. Fetal kick counts, nonstress tests, and amniotic fluid assessment are usually the first tests employed in conjunction with serial ultrasound examinations to evaluate growth. Several studies suggest that Doppler flow-velocity waveforms in the umbilical artery are useful in the clinical management of severe IUGR. However, their predictive value remains unclear. It *is* known that fetuses with either absent or reversed end-diastolic flow are at high risk for perinatal morbidity and mortality, including stillbirth. Ribbert and associates[17] completed a retrospective longitudinal assessment of fetal behavior in severe IUGR. They found that umbilical artery velocity waveform patterns become abnormal first, fetal heart-rate variation is reduced next, and fetal body movements and breathing movements become abnormal last.

When the fetus is at term and IUGR is present, conventional wisdom dictates that delivery be accomplished at the first sign of fetal compromise or lack of demonstrable growth. It is those fetuses remote from term with severe IUGR that pose the biggest challenge: the practitioner must decide not only how to follow the pregnancy but also when to deliver the baby. Consultation with a neonatologist is imperative, since the decision is often a balance of risk: when the risk to the fetus in the neonatal intensive care unit is less than the presumed risk to the fetus in utero, delivery is frequently recommended. Delivery is often accomplished by cesarean section because the cervix is frequently unfavorable and the fetus often cannot tolerate the stress of labor.

QUESTION 5: WHAT IS THE LONG-TERM PROGNOSIS FOR THE INTRAUTERINE GROWTH–RETARDED INFANT?

Intrauterine growth retardation may affect neurodevelopment, even when obvious pathology and disability are absent, but this effect has not been clearly defined. The prognosis partially depends on the cause, since IUGR affects a very heterogeneous group of infants. The neonatal period is often complicated by prematurity, with its associated metabolic, cardiorespiratory, and central nervous system complications. In addition, studies are always confounded by the influence of psychosocial factors: education, economics, and family dynamics.

Lowe and colleagues[14] studied 218 high-risk children at birth and at 1, 4, 9, and 11 years of age. Seventy-seven of these 218 children had had birthweights below the 10th percentile for gestational age. Forty-six percent of the term intrauterine growth–retarded infants and 50% of the preterm intrauterine growth–retarded infants had learning deficits as children. Intrauterine growth retardation was the single biologic variable in this study that was associated with learning deficits. However, the findings were complicated by the significant relationship between parental education and learning deficits in these children. It is this complexity that makes this question so difficult to answer.

QUESTION 6: WHICH DIRECTIONS ARE LIKELY TO BE FOLLOWED IN FUTURE RESEARCH OF INTRAUTERINE GROWTH RETARDATION?

During the last decade, several important breakthroughs have been made in the understanding of fetal physiologic and biochemical adaptation to nutritional deprivation. This understanding has sparked interest in feeding the growth-retarded fetus by manipulating the fetal nutrient supply and by manipulating the fetal and placental endocrine status.[12] Early attempts at transamniotic fetal feeding were initially promising but have yet to be proved safe or effective. Manipulation of the fetal endocrine status using intrauterine growth factors is another intriguing possibility, but it remains untested.

From experimental studies in animal models have come some observations that need further explanation, such as the concept of irreversibility.[10] When pregnant sheep are deliberately underfed, a prompt fall in the rate of fetal growth is seen. Re-feeding is usually accompanied by a prompt recovery in fetal growth. However, if underfeeding persists longer than 19 days, fetal growth does not recover, and the IUGR is irreversible. The mechanism underlying this irreversibility and its relationship to the human experience have yet to be described.

Epidemiologic studies have shown a correlation between IUGR and an increased risk of hypertension, non–insulin-dependent diabetes mellitus, and cardiovascular and cerebrovascular diseases in adulthood.[11] The underlying hypothesis is that programming of certain critical axes occurs at vulnerable periods of development. The alteration of this programming has life-long consequences. This hypothesis is being investigated.

Finally, clinical studies are needed concerning the proper management of the intrauterine growth–retarded fetus. Currently, no antenatal tests can predict an acidotic fetus except percutaneous umbilical blood sampling. The role of maternal hyperoxygenation, the role of Doppler ultrasonography, and the role of aspirin remain unclear. Both basic science and clinical research, then, are needed if progress is to be made in improving the management of the growth-retarded fetus.

REFERENCES

1. Akalin-Sel T, Campbell S: Understanding the pathophysiology of intra-uterine growth retardation: the role of the "lower limb reflex" in redistribution of blood flow, *Eur J Obstet Gynecol Reprod Biol* 46:79, 1992.
2. Arduini D, Rizzo G: Fetal renal artery velocity waveforms and amniotic fluid volume in growth-retarded and post-term fetuses, *Obstet Gynecol* 77:370, 1991.
3. Avery GB, Fletcher MA, MacDonald MG: Pathophysiology and management of the newborn. In *Neonatology*, ed 4, JB Lippincott, 1994.
4. Battaglia C, Artini PG, D'Ambrogio G et al: Maternal hyperoxygenation in the treatment of intrauterine growth retardation, *Am J Obstet Gynecol* 167:430, 1992.
5. Calvert JP, Crean EE, Newcombe RG, Pearson JF: Antenatal screening by measurement of symphysis-fundus height, *Br Med J* 285:846, 1982.
6. Cetin I, Marconi AM, Corbetta C et al: Fetal amino acids in normal pregnancies and in pregnancies affected by intrauterine growth retardation, *Early Hum Dev* 29:183, 1992.
7. Collaborative Low-dose Aspirin Study in Pregnancy (CLASP) Collaborative Group: A randomized trial of low-dose aspirin for the prevention and treatment of pre-eclampsia among 9364 pregnant women, *Lancet* 343:619, 1994.
8. Economides DL, Nicolaides KH, Gahl WA et al: Plasma amino acids in appropriate and small-for-gestational-age fetuses, *Am J Obstet Gynecol* 161:1219, 1989.
9. Evans MI, Mukherjee AB, Schulman JD: Animal models of intrauterine growth retardation, *Obstet Gynecol Surv* 38:183, 1983.
10. Fleischer A, Schulman H, Farmakides G et al: Umbilical artery velocity waveforms and intrauterine growth retardation, *Am J Obstet Gynecol* 151:502, 1985.
11. Gluckman PD: Intrauterine growth retardation: future research directions, *Acta Pædiatr Suppl* 388:96, 1993.
12. Harding J, Liu L, Evans P et al: Intrauterine feeding of the growth retarded fetus: can we help? *Early Hum Dev* 29:193, 1992.

13. Hubinont C, Nicolini U, Fisk NM et al: Endocrine pancreatic function in growth-retarded fetuses, *Obstet Gynecol* 77:541, 1991.
14. Low JA, Handley-Derry MH, Burke SO et al: Association of intrauterine fetal growth retardation and learning deficits at age 9 to 11, *Am J Obstet Gynecol* 167:1499, 1992.
15. Parazzini F, Benedetto C, Frusca T et al: Low-dose aspirin in prevention and treatment of intrauterine growth retardation and pregnancy-induced hypertension, *Lancet* 341:396, 1993.
16. Pollack RN, Divon MY: Intrauterine growth retardation: definition, classification, and etiology, *Clin Obstet Gynecol* 35:99, 1992.
17. Ribbert LM, Visser GA, Mulder EH et al: Changes with time in fetal heart rate variation, movement incidences and hæmodynamics in intrauterine growth retarded fetuses: a longitudinal approach to the assessment of fetal well being, *Early Hum Dev* 31:195, 1993.
18. Rizzo G, Arduini D: Fetal cardiac function in intrauterine growth retardation, *Am J Obstet Gynecol* 165:876, 1991.
19. Rumbolz WL, McGoogan LS: Placental insufficiency and the small undernourished full-term infant, *Obstet Gynecol* 1:294, 1953.
20. Seeds JW: Impaired fetal growth: definition and clinical diagnosis, *Obstet Gynecol* 64:303, 1984.
21. Sibai BM, Caritis SN, Thom E et al: Prevention of preeclampsia with low-dose aspirin in healthy, nulliparous pregnant women, *N Engl J Med* 329:1213, 1993.
22. Soothill PW, Ajayi RA, Nicolaides KN: Fetal biochemistry in growth retardation, *Early Hum Dev* 29:91, 1992.
23. Thorpe-Beeston JG, Nicolaides KH, Snijders RJM et al: Relations between the fetal circulation and pituitary-thyroid function, *Br J Obstet Gynæcol* 98:1163, 1991.
24. Trudinger BJ, Cook CM, Thompson RS et al: Low-dose aspirin therapy improves fetal weight in umbilical placental insufficiency, *Am J Obstet Gynecol* 159:681, 1988.
25. Uzan S, Beaufils M, Breart G et al: Prevention of fetal growth retardation with low-dose aspirin: findings of the EPREDA trial, *Lancet* 337:1427, 1991.
26. Wallenburg HS, Rotmans N: Prevention of recurrent idiopathic fetal growth retardation by low-dose aspirin and dipyridamole, *Am J Obstet Gynecol* 157:1230, 1987.
27. Wladimiroff JW: A review of the etiology, diagnostic techniques, and management of IUGR, and the clinical application of Doppler in the assessment of placental blood flow, *J Perinat Med* 19:11, 1991.

PART FIVE

INVASIVE TESTING

CHAPTER 18

Amniocentesis

MICKI L. CABANISS

Although amniocentesis was first performed in 1882 by Schatz for management of hydramnios,[20,26] it was not until the 1960s that the technique was used regularly to evaluate isoimmunized pregnancies. Initially, fetal position was determined by palpation, and placental position was determined by auscultation of the maternal souffle or even by x-ray.[18] Safety has been improved by incorporating ultrasound guidance of needle placement, making amniocentesis more acceptable to both patients and health care providers.

Cytogenetic and molecular genetics studies are commonly performed using cells (amniocytes) obtained from the amniotic fluid. Biochemical analysis of the fluid permits the detection of open neural tube defects and fetal pulmonary maturity. Intrauterine infection can be assessed by various bacterial and viral studies. Amniocentesis also allows injection of fluid, contrast agents, and medications. For instance, amnioinfusion in the presence of severe oligohydramnios improves fetal sonographic visualization and allows demonstration of pre-existing occult rupture of the membranes.

Amniocentesis classically refers to the insertion of a needle into the amniotic space to remove fluid; however, it is also the fundamental technique on which percutaneous umbilical blood sampling, fetoscopy, and other fetal biopsy methods are based. By providing access to the fetus, amniocentesis has opened the door to medical care of the fetus. Improvement of noninvasive procedures, such as maternal serum testing and harvesting of fetal cells in the maternal circulation, may eventually make the traditional procedure of amniocentesis obsolete. Should it be superseded, however, the important role that amniocentesis has played in the evolution of modern fetal diagnosis and therapy cannot be overlooked.

❦ Patient Profile: Abnormal karyotype detected at amniocentesis

A 38-year-old woman (gravida 1, para 0000) seeks prenatal care at 7 weeks' gestation, at which time she is informed about the indications and options for prenatal diagnosis. After genetic counseling, the patient elects to undergo amniocentesis at 15 weeks' gestation. The karyotype of the fetus is reported as 47,XY,+13 (male fetus with trisomy 13). The patient experiences intense grief and requests pregnancy termination.

QUESTION 1: WHAT ARE THE PRIMARY INDICATIONS FOR SECOND-TRIMESTER DIAGNOSTIC AMNIOCENTESIS?

The most common indication for performance of amniocentesis during the midtrimester is to obtain fetal cells for cytogenetic evaluation. Because of the risks and costs involved in amniocentesis, the procedure has traditionally been reserved for women thought to be at significantly increased risk for fetal aneuploidy. Because early experience resulted in a pregnancy loss rate of approximately 1 in 200 (0.5%), a "significant risk" of aneuploidy was thus considered to be about 1 in 200. Consequently, the maternal age of 35 at the time of delivery became the standard age at which amniocentesis was first offered.

Many forces are working to alter this traditional thinking, but they often lead in opposite directions. On the one hand, safety of the procedure has improved so that some centers now quote a procedure-related loss rate of 1 in 400. Following the earlier logic, perhaps these centers should offer the procedure to women for whom the midtrimester risk for aneuploidy is approximately 1 in 400. On the other hand, sonographic identification of fetal phenotypes suggestive of abnormal karyotypes and maternal serum screening for aneuploidy have improved so much that some argue that, regardless of maternal age, only women with abnormal findings in these studies should be offered amniocentesis. Third-party and public health policymakers are intensely interested in this shifting debate and will likely further attempt to regulate use of fetal karyotyping.

All patients must be advised of their risk for fetal chromosome abnormalities and of the screening and diagnostic tests available to them. The box below contains a list of indications for offering second-trimester fetal karyotype analysis.

INDICATIONS FOR SECOND-TRIMESTER FETAL KARYOTYPE ANALYSIS

Maternal age ≥35 at delivery
Two or more unexplained spontaneous abortions
Known parental balanced translocation
Previous aneuploid offspring
Previous child with birth defect and unknown karyotype
Dysmorphology found on fetal ultrasound examination
Increased risk for aneuploidy demonstrated by maternal serum screening results

---

Increasingly, genetic disorders are detectable by studying fetal cells obtained through amniocentesis. DNA testing using linkage analysis, direct gene identification techniques, or mutation analysis is available for a rapidly expanding list of genetic disorders. Indications for this type of testing include the previous birth of an affected child, family history of an inherited genetic condition, known carrier status of either parent for an inherited genetic condition, and ethnic ancestry that indicates an increased risk of having an affected fetus. It is important to communicate with the DNA laboratory to determine the sample type and quantity of amniotic fluid needed and to determine whether modification of the sample collection technique is necessary. In some instances, larger volumes of fluid are needed or special media or other forms of special handling are required.

Biochemical markers for fetal disorders can be measured in the amniotic fluid. For instance, elevated levels of amniotic fluid α-fetoprotein with detection of an acetylcholinesterase band will be found in 99.1% of fetuses with an open neural tube defect.[7] Thus, amniocentesis may be beneficial to a woman who is at increased risk for having a fetus with an open neural tube defect. Weighing the risks of the procedure against the adjusted risk obtained by performing a targeted ultrasound examination allows the patient to be involved in the decision regarding whether to perform amniocentesis in this setting.

QUESTION 2: WHAT ARE THE TECHNICAL CONCERNS WHEN PERFORMING AN AMNIOCENTESIS?

The most serious complications of amniocentesis are predominantly related to pregnancy loss. This risk has diminished during the three decades of experience with the procedure. The degree of risk, however, is difficult to ascertain from the literature because of differences in research design, gestational age, maternal age, indication for the procedure, definition of procedure-related loss, and level of experience of the operators reported in the various studies. For example, the incidence of spontaneous loss increases with increasing maternal age; therefore, a study consisting predominantly of older women will likely demonstrate a higher loss rate than one in which the women are younger.

Generalizing the risk data from published reports also requires strict attention to how different investigators define a procedure-related loss. *Total pregnancy loss,* for research purposes, is typically defined as any failure of the pregnancy to result in a surviving newborn, even if the pregnancy is terminated because the fetus is found to be abnormal and even if death occurs during the newborn period.

An estimated procedure-related loss risk of approximately 0.5% (1 in 200) was derived from a National Institutes of Health study in which a 0.3% loss rate difference was reported between amniocentesis patients and control patients (3.5% and 3.2%, respectively), although this was not a statistically significant difference.[20] Subsequent collaborative studies suggest a risk of 1% to be more accurate, although this estimate antedated modern high-resolution, sonographically directed procedures.[6] Clinical experience has led practitioners skilled in amniocentesis to estimate a lowered risk of pregnancy loss after midtrimester amniocentesis (0.3% to 0.5%).

Postamniocentesis transvaginal leakage of fluid has been reported in about 1.2% of genetic amniocenteses.[12,20] Reported incidence may vary with such factors as needle size and gestational age.[28] Resealing of the needle puncture site occurs in most of these instances. Ruptured membranes may be prevented by using a small-gauge needle, such as a 20 or 22 gauge, and by minimizing the number of intraamniotic needle passes. If leakage occurs, it is reasonable, although of unproved benefit, to recommend pelvic rest and decreased activity until the situation resolves itself. The use of antibiotics in this situation is of unproved benefit.

In a National Institutes of Health study of 1000 women, the incidence of possible procedure-related infection as a cause of pregnancy loss was 0.1%.[20] Excellent sterile technique cannot prevent tracking some bacteria from the maternal skin to the amniotic space. Nonetheless, cleansing the maternal skin with an adequate antiseptic preparation is critical. Even in patients at increased risk of subacute bacterial endocarditis, antibiotics are not indicated for routine genetic amniocentesis. The presence of a maternal skin infection in the area of the proposed needle insertion site is a contraindication to the procedure.

Many vascular structures are encountered as the needle traverses the maternal abdominal wall, the uterus, and the placenta. Nevertheless, postprocedure bleeding is not commonly observed by sonography. Significant fetal-maternal hemorrhage as measured by a rising red cell antibody titer was demonstrated in 1.9% of isoimmunized women even when ultrasound was used to avoid placental needle contact.[5] Thus, it is recommended that known Rh-negative women receive Rh immune globulin after amniocentesis. Transient elevation of maternal serum α-fetoprotein (MSAFP) levels after amniocentesis is additional evidence of a fetal-maternal hemorrhage and is a well-documented occurrence.[22] For this reason, MSAFP testing should never be performed immediately after amniocentesis.

Next to loss of the entire pregnancy, women seem most concerned about the potential for fetal trauma during the amniocentesis. While certainly a theoretic problem, ultrasound guidance has decreased the likelihood of such an occurrence. Careful selection of the needle insertion site is important to prevent fetal injury, ensure collection of fluid, decrease the risk of fetal-maternal hemorrhage, and increase the comfort for the patient. The selection criteria for choosing the needle insertion site ideally include the presence of a relatively large fluid pocket on the opposite side of the uterus from the face and head, with no overlying placenta. Most studies indicate that traversing the placenta during second-trimester amniocentesis does not increase the loss rate associated with the procedure, but it should be avoided if possible.

Intrauterine processes can prevent the easy aspiration of fluid. A localized uterine contraction may occur immediately in response to the presence of the needle.[10] Such a contraction can alter the course of the small-gauge needle or dislodge it from its position, decrease visualization of the needle, or obliterate an optimal fluid pocket. These contractions are unavoidable, and when they occur the operator can either wait for the contraction to pass or remove the needle and readjust its direction. If the contraction has been uncomfortable enough to cause maternal motion, needle removal may be prudent. It is reasonable to warn women before the procedure that such contractions are possible.

Membrane tenting occurs when the amnion is not yet well annealed to the underlying chorion and tends to be a more common problem with early amniocentesis. It is usually easily corrected by advancing the needle to the opposite myometrial wall under ultrasound guidance[4] or by rotating the bevel of the needle.

Obliteration of the targeted fluid pocket can occur in response to a uterine contraction, maternal movement, or fetal movement. If it results from fetal movement, the operator can withdraw the needle to the edge of the amniotic space, awaiting another fetal movement and reaccumulation of fluid under the needle. If the fetus does roll against or brush the needle tip during the procedure, it usually does not cause injury to the fetus. Experience with fetal surgical procedures and skin biopsies has shown that fetal skin injuries generally heal without scarring.[19] While disturbing to watch for both the obstetrician and the parents, adequate counseling before the procedure can frequently assuage the parents' concerns.

The method of fluid removal and aliquoting into transportation tubes is important. Details should be arranged with each cytogenetic laboratory to accommodate their preferences. The first aliquot should be of small volume, perhaps 2 to 3 ml. This small volume should clear the needle of maternal cell contamination and can be sent for amniotic fluid α-fetoprotein testing. After this, it is reasonable at 15 to 20 weeks' gestation to collect another 20 ml of fluid. During these weeks of gestation, the total amniotic fluid volume has been measured at 240 ml, so this amount represents less than 10% of the normal volume.[25] To minimize risk of loss or contamination of the entire specimen, some prefer to collect the 20 ml in two aliquots, using different syringes, while others split a single syringe collection into two transport tubes. In either case, strict attention to sterile technique is important.

If bloody fluid is obtained during the fluid collection, it is important to add a small amount (0.1 ml) of heparin to the fluid specimen as quickly as possible to prevent clotting of the cells with trapping of the amniocytes in the clot. Bright red blood in the fluid is usually the result of uterine wall or placental bleeding, and if it occurs suddenly during the procedure, ultrasound guidance usually allows the operator to redirect the needle into better position. Dark or discolored fluid is noted with an approximate 2% incidence in second-trimester procedures. A brown discoloration may indicate fetal death, an open fetal defect, or, more commonly, a previous intraamniotic hemorrhage.[17] Discolored fluid indicates a higher-than-average pregnancy loss rate, no doubt related to the underlying cause of the discoloration and not to the procedure itself. In 1986, Hess and colleagues[14] reviewed 12 series spanning the decade between 1976 and 1986 and found an average 12.1% pregnancy loss rate associated with discolored fluid. Allen[1] studied 4709 consecutive cases from 1978 to 1983 and found a 5.06% fetal loss rate associated with fluid discoloration. This finding should be documented in the procedure note, and it is reasonable to advise the patient and referring physician of this higher loss rate.

Another important concern for parents and physicians alike is making sure that the specimens do not become mislabeled. Strict attention to detail in the fluid collection and labeling is mandatory. No specimen should be removed from the procedure room without being labeled and accompanied by appropriate laboratory requisitions. Before discharging the patient from the room, it is helpful to have her and her partner confirm that the name and identification number attached to each of the transport tubes are indeed the patient's own.

QUESTION 3: HOW IS AMNIOCENTESIS PERFORMED IN MULTIFETAL PREGNANCIES, AND WHAT IS THE LOSS RATE?

Twins or higher-order gestations present a unique challenge. For most amniocentesis indications, it is essential to obtain fluid from all fetuses. Zygosity cannot always be definitively diagnosed in utero, so the genetic makeup of a presumed monozygotic co-twin cannot be confidently studied by sampling only one fetus. When obtaining multiple fetal fluid specimens, it is important to verify that separate sacs have been entered. The clinician should document the findings in such a way that should an abnormal result occur, accurate assignment of the information to the appropriate fetus can be made. A thorough diagram should be made in the patient's chart of the fetal and placental positions and of any discordancy in sex or anatomy visible by ultrasound (Figure 18-1).

To confirm that different sacs have been sampled, a variety of techniques have been employed. The traditional method is a two-needle insertion technique that involves the instillation of a dye into the amniotic cavity after aspiration of fluid from the sac of the first fetus. If clear fluid is aspirated from the second sac, resampling of the first sac has been excluded. Indigo carmine and Evans blue dye are currently used for this purpose because of the possible association of fetal hemolytic anemia, intestinal atresia, and methemoglobinemia with the use of methylene blue.[21,24,29] A newer method of ensuring sampling of different sacs includes simultaneous documentation of needle insertion into separate sacs.[3] While the needle used for the first procedure remains in the amniotic sac of the first twin, the second needle is placed in the sac of the other fetus with ultrasound documentation of the intervening membrane.

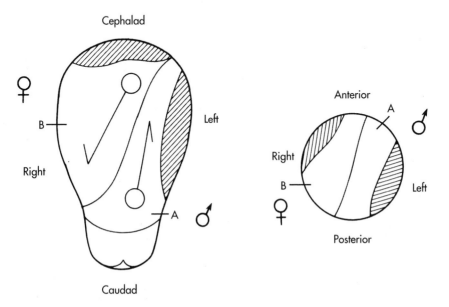

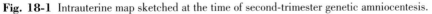

Fig. 18-1 Intrauterine map sketched at the time of second-trimester genetic amniocentesis.

Jeanty and associates[15] describe the use of a single needle insertion with transmembrane entry into the second sac after fluid has been obtained from the first. Perforation of the intervening membrane is presumed to be without risk, although a theoretic concern remains regarding contamination of specimens with fluid and cells from the other amniotic sac, leading to inaccurate interpretation. This method may be necessary when the sac of a dependent twin is inaccessible without traversing the other's sac.

Even with two insertions, risk of amniocentesis in twin pregnancies does not appear to be significantly greater than that in singletons when corrected for the increased risk of pregnancy loss anticipated in multifetal pregnancies.[2,11,24] Ghidini and colleagues[11] compared loss rates in twin pregnancies with and without amniocentesis in a series of 209 patients and found no difference (3.5% and 3.2%, respectively) despite a higher maternal age in the amniocentesis group.[11] Pruggmayer and colleagues[24] studied 528 twin pregnancies and found a pregnancy-loss rate approximately double that of singletons postamniocentesis, but not greater than that predicted for the spontaneous loss of twins.

QUESTION 4: IS EARLY AMNIOCENTESIS DIFFERENT FROM AMNIOCENTESIS PERFORMED AT THE MORE TRADITIONAL TIME, 15 TO 18 WEEKS' GESTATION?

One advantage of early amniocentesis is that it allows a couple to be reassured earlier in the pregnancy of the normality of their fetus. In addition, if a woman elects to undergo pregnancy termination after an abnormal result, early amniocentesis allows this to be done at an earlier gestational age. First- and early second-trimester abortions are technically easier and safer to perform than those performed during the late second trimester and obviate the additional emotional distress of undergoing pregnancy termination after quickening.

Early amniocentesis may be technically more difficult to perform than routine amniocentesis. There is an increased rate of membrane tenting, potentially requiring an increased number of needle insertions and possibly a lower likelihood of resealing of the membranes should fluid leakage occur.[23] Early reports of decreased cell growth and higher reported rates of mosaicism in fluid obtained earlier in gestation have been minimized with improvement in cytogenetic technology.[16] Nomograms for interpretation of amniotic fluid α-fetoprotein levels have been developed and published.[8] However, these nomograms await use in significant numbers of abnormal pregnancies, and the problem remains of false-positive acetylcholinesterase levels in early pregnancies. In addition, each laboratory must establish its own medians at each gestational age to reflect its own experience. Using published nomograms from a different laboratory is insufficient.

Amniotic fluid volumes are lower in these earlier pregnancies, so the volume removed must be of greater concern than with later studies. For example, Penso and associates[23] reported a 6.1% incidence of neonatal pulmonary complications after early amniocentesis. On the other hand, the lower concentration of amniocytes in the early pregnancy fluids may lengthen the time necessary to grow an adequate number of cells to obtain results, potentially decreasing the advantage of the earlier procedure. It has been suggested that the total volume of fluid to be removed during early amniocentesis should be equivalent to 1 ml per week of gestation.[13]

Until the relative safety of early amniocentesis can be established with controlled studies, patients should be advised that the risk, even when corrected for the increased rate of spontaneous abortion with earlier pregnancy, is probably greater than that of more traditional midtrimester amniocentesis. Dunn and Godmillow[9] showed an increased risk of fetal loss in early amniocentesis in comparison with CVS (4.2% and 1.9%, respectively), with traditional amniocentesis producing only a 1.1% loss rate in the same population of older women. Shulman and colleagues[27] reported an increased risk of pregnancy loss in early amniocentesis in comparison with CVS (3.8% and 2.1%, respectively) in a nonrandomized series. As with any technique, increased clinical experience appears to lower the risk of an adverse outcome.[13]

REFERENCES

1. Allen R: The significance of meconium in midtrimester genetic amniocentesis, *Am J Obstet Gynecol* 152:413, 1985.
2. Anderson RL, Goldberg JD, Golbus MS: Prenatal diagnosis in multiple gestation: 20 years' experience with amniocentesis, *Prenat Diagn* 11:263, 1991.
3. Bahado-Singh R, Schmitt R, Hobbins JC: New techniques for genetic amniocentesis in twins, *Obstet Gynecol* 79:304, 1992.
4. Bowerman RA, Barclay ML: A technique to overcome failed second-trimester amniocentesis due to membrane tenting, *Obstet Gynecol* 70:806, 1987.
5. Bowman JM, Pollock JM: Transplacental fetal hemorrhage after amniocentesis, *Obstet Gynecol* 66:749, 1985.
6. British Collaborative Study: An assessment of the hazards of amniocentesis, *Br J Obstet Gynæcol* 85:1, 1978.
7. Crandall BF, Matsumoto M: Risks associated with an elevated amniotic fluid alpha-fetoprotein level, *Am J Med Genet* 39:64, 1991.
8. Drugan A, Syner FN, Greb A et al: Amniotic fluid alpha-fetoprotein and acetylcholinesterase in early genetic amniocentesis, *Obstet Gynecol* 72:35, 1988.
9. Dunn LK, Godmillow L: A comparison of loss rates for first-trimester chorionic villus sampling, early amniocentesis and mid-trimester amniocentesis in a population of women of advanced age, *Am J Hum Genet* 47:A273, 1990.
10. Finberg HJ, Frigolitto FD: Sonographic demonstration of uterine contraction during amniocentesis, *Am J Obstet Gynecol* 139:740, 1981.
11. Ghidini A, Lynch L, Hicks C et al: The risk of second-trimester amniocentesis in twin gestations: a case control study, *Am J Obstet Gynecol* 78:623, 1991.
12. Gold RB, Goyert GL, Schwartz DB et al: Conservative management of second trimester post-amniocentesis fluid leakage, *Obstet Gynecol* 74:745, 1989.
13. Hanson FW, Happ RL, Tennant FR: Ultrasonography-guided early amniocentesis in singleton pregnancies, *Am J Obstet Gynecol* 162:1376, 1990.
14. Hess LW, Anderson RL, Golbus MS: Significance of opaque discolored amniotic fluid at second-trimester amniocentesis, *Obstet Gynecol* 67:44, 1986.
15. Jeanty P, Shah D, Roussis P: Single needle insertion in twin amniocentesis, *J Ultrasound Med* 9:511, 1990.
16. Jorgensen FS, Bang J, Lind AM et al: Genetic amniocentesis at 7-14 weeks of gestation, *Prenat Diagn* 12:277, 1992.
17. Legge M: Dark brown amniotic fluid: identification of contributing pigments, *Br J Obstet Gynæcol* 88:632, 1981.
18. Liley AW: Amniocentesis (current concepts), *Am J Obstet Gynecol* 272:731, 1965.
19. Longaker MT, Harrison MR, Crombleholme TM et al: Studies in fetal wound healing: I. A factor in fetal serum that stimulates deposition of hyaluronic acid, *J Pediatr Surg* 24:789, 1989.
20. *The safety and accuracy of mid-trimester amniocentesis*, DHEW Publication No. (NIH) 78-190, 1-22, 1978.

21. McEnerney JK, McEnerney LN: Unfavorable neonatal outcome after intraamniotic injection of methylene blue, *Obstet Gynecol* 61:35S, 1983.

22. Mennuti MT, Brummond W, Crombleholme WR: Fetal-maternal bleeding associated with genetic amniocentesis, *Obstet Gynecol* 55:48, 1980.

23. Penso CA, Sandstrom MM, Garber M-F et al: Early amniocentesis: report of 407 cases with new-born follow-up, *Obstet Gynecol* 76:1032, 1990.

24. Pruggmayer MRK, Jahoda MGJ, Van der Pol JG et al: Genetic amniocentesis in twin pregnancies: results of a multicenter study of 529 cases, *Ultrasound Obstet Gynecol* 2:6, 1992.

25. Queenan JT, Thompson W, Whitfield CR, Shah SI: Amniotic fluid volumes in normal pregnancies, *Am J Obstet Gynecol* 114:34, 1972.

26. Schatz F: Eine besondere Art von einseitiger Polyhydramnie mit anderseitiger Oligohydramnie bei eineiigen Zwillingen, *Arch Gynäk* 19:329, 1882.

27. Shulman LP, Elias S, Phillips OP et al: Amniocentesis performed at 14 weeks' gestation or earlier: comparison with first-trimester transabdominal chorionic villus sampling, *Obstet Gynecol* 83:543, 1994.

28. Teramo K, Sipinen S: Spontaneous rupture of fetal membranes after amniocentesis, *Obstet Gynecol* 52:272, 1978.

29. Van der Pol JG, Wolf H, Boer K et al: The use of methylene blue in genetic amniocentesis in twins, *Br J Obstet Gynæcol* 99:141, 1992.

CHAPTER 19

Chorionic Villus Sampling

JEFFREY A. KULLER

Chorionic villus sampling (CVS) is a technique that has moved prenatal diagnosis into the first trimester. In 1983, after preliminary data from Italy on this new procedure were published, interest in CVS blossomed in this country. To assess the safety and efficacy of CVS, the National Institute of Child Health and Human Development (NICHD) sponsored a seven-center study.[10]

Chorionic villus sampling offers several advantages to women who seek prenatal testing. Since chorionic villus sampling is performed at 10 to 12 weeks' gestation, pregnancy is not yet physically apparent. In patients in whom CVS indicates an abnormal fetus, complications related to pregnancy termination are significantly less serious if the procedure is performed early in gestation. Because CVS offers information to patients earlier than does amniocentesis, it has been chosen with increasing frequency. Many centers in this country now perform more CVS procedures than amniocenteses.

❧ Patient Profile: Counseling for chorionic villus sampling

A 37-year-old woman (gravida 2, para 0010) seeks obstetric consultation at 7 weeks' gestation. In her last pregnancy, 2 years earlier, she underwent amniocentesis at 16 weeks' gestation because of increased maternal age. Her fetus was diagnosed with trisomy 21 (Down syndrome). At 18 weeks' gestation, she underwent pregnancy termination with prostaglandin E_2 suppositories. She was in the hospital for 3 days and continues to be very distressed about this experience. She and her husband wish to know more about the benefits and risks of CVS.

QUESTION 1: HOW DOES THE LOSS RATE OF CHORIONIC VILLUS SAMPLING COMPARE WITH THAT OF AMNIOCENTESIS?

Large studies comparing transcervical CVS and amniocentesis have recently been published. A randomized study conducted by the Canadian Collaborative Group recruited over

1000 patients for each study arm.[1] The multicenter United States trial conducted by the NICHD recruited approximately 3000 patients.[10] The loss rate of CVS exceeded that of amniocentesis by 0.6% in the Canadian study and by 0.8% in the U.S. study, differences that were not statistically significant. The Medical Research Council of the United Kingdom found a 3.8% greater loss rate from CVS when compared with amniocentesis.[8] The main difference between this study and the U.S. and Canadian trials was that it included a large number of participating centers, with varying levels of experience and widely varying degrees of participation. It appears, then, that the loss rate of CVS, when performed by an experienced operator, is not notably different from that of amniocentesis.

QUESTION 2: HOW DOES CHORIONIC VILLUS SAMPLING COMPARE WITH EARLY AMNIOCENTESIS?

Early amniocentesis is defined as an amniocentesis performed at less than 15 weeks' gestation. The technique requires minor modifications of an already familiar procedure. However, with early amniocentesis, a short, vigorous thrust of the needle aids in accomplishing the procedure, since tenting of the amnion occurs more frequently than in midtrimester procedures. Although several reports have now been published on early amniocentesis, there is a paucity of data on procedures performed at 10 to 12 weeks' gestation, when CVS is normally performed. Hanson and associates[4] reported the findings of a relatively large study of over 900 early amniocenteses performed at or before 12.8 weeks. Spontaneous abortion occurred between the time of procedure and 28 weeks in 2.9% of tested pregnancies. Amniotic fluid leakage occurred in 1.1% of the sampled population, 40% of whom lost the pregnancy. A direct comparison of early and mid–second trimester amniocenteses performed by one operator revealed a statistically significant higher rate of pregnancy loss within 4 weeks of the diagnostic procedure in the early amniocentesis group. Data are insufficient to reach conclusions regarding the incidence of respiratory and orthopedic complications attributable to early amniocentesis. Early amniocentesis has the advantage of allowing measurement of α-fetoprotein (AFP) and acetylcholinesterase (AChE) in amniotic fluid. However, only preliminary normative data exist for amniotic fluid AFP values from 10 to 15 weeks. Therefore, AFP and AChE values in early amniocentesis should be interpreted with caution. When further data are available, it may prove to be an accurate means of diagnosing neural tube and ventral wall defects.

Early amniocentesis is advantageous in that it is a technique with which many obstetricians already feel comfortable. However, the exact loss rate from the procedure is still uncertain, especially when performed before 13 weeks' gestation. This is in contrast to CVS, for which significantly more data are now available. The results of a large randomized trial comparing CVS and early amniocentesis in over 1000 women were recently published. In women randomized to early amniocentesis or CVS at 10 to 13 weeks' gestation, the spontaneous loss (intrauterine and neonatal death) rate was significantly higher after early amniocentesis (5.3%) than after CVS (2.3%).[9]

QUESTION 3: WHAT ARE THE ADVANTAGES AND DISADVANTAGES OF CHORIONIC VILLUS SAMPLING IN COMPARISON TO AMNIOCENTESIS?

Every patient who is a candidate for amniocentesis is also a candidate for CVS except when the primary indication is diagnosis of a neural tube defect. The greatest advantage of CVS is that it can provide information early to patients who want to make reproductive decisions. It allows accurate diagnosis of chromosomal and mendelian disorders. In the U.S. NICHD collaborative study of over 11,000 CVS procedures, a successful cytogenetic diagnosis was obtained in 99.7% of cases.[7] A total of 1.1% of patients had to have a second procedure (CVS or amniocentesis) because of maternal cell contamination, mosaicism, or laboratory failure. Mosaicism (two or more cell lines that differ genetically but are derived from a single zygote) was observed in 0.8% of cases, while pseudomosaicism (a single cell with an abnormality or two or more cells that have identical abnormalities but are confined to one culture flask) was observed in 1.6% of cases. The overall rate of maternal cell contamination was 1.8% for the culture method. However, maternal cell contamination did not contribute to diagnostic error in any case. Chorionic villus sampling is generally not recommended in the isoimmunized patient because sensitization may be enhanced by the procedure; overall, amniocentesis is preferable in such a patient. Finally, CVS offers no information about AFP. Therefore, patients who undergo CVS should be offered maternal serum AFP screening or a detailed fetal ultrasound examination of the neural tube, or both, at 16 weeks' gestation. Amniocentesis is the preferred mode of prenatal diagnosis if the primary indication is testing for neural tube defects.

QUESTION 4: DOES CHORIONIC VILLUS SAMPLING CAUSE LIMB REDUCTION DEFECTS?

In 1991, Firth and colleagues[3] in the United Kingdom reported that five infants had limb reduction defects among 289 pregnancies in which transabdominal CVS was performed at 8 to 9.5 weeks' gestation. Four of the five infants had oromandibular-limb hypogenesis syndromes, a group of syndromes with varying degrees of limb deficiency, hypoglossia, and micrognathia.[3] This series prompted a flurry of brief reports from other centers worldwide. Of particular concern was a small cluster of limb reductions reported by a highly experienced center in Milan when sampling was performed before the eighth completed gestational week. In contrast, many other reports of large series showed no statistically significant increase in limb abnormalities.

The largest available study on the background incidence of limb abnormalities in the general population is the British Columbia Registry, which found an incidence of 5.42 per 10,000 live births. In over 80,000 CVS procedures reported to the CVS registry at Jefferson Medical College in Philadelphia, most of which were performed between 9 and 12 weeks' gestation, the total incidence of limb reduction defects was 6.0 per 10,000, not significantly different from the baseline incidence in the general population.[6]

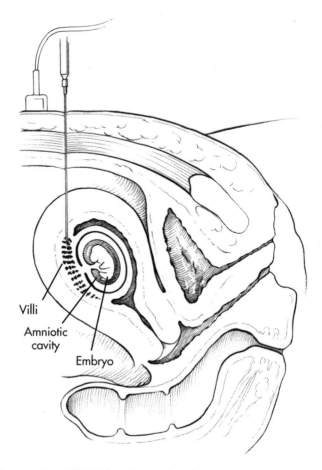

Villi

Amniotic
cavity

Embryo

Fig. 19-1 Transabdominal approach to CVS. Under ultrasound guidance, a long 20-gauge needle is inserted through the abdomen into villous tissue. (From Chueh J, Golbus MS: Fetal invasive procedures. In Plauche WC, Morrison JC, Sullivan MJ, editors: *Surgical obstetrics*, Philadelphia, 1992, WB Saunders.)

If CVS causes limb reduction defects, there are a number of possible causal mechanisms. The most widely held hypothesis is that a vascular accident results from decreased perfusion in distal limbs or from thrombosis at the sampling site, with subsequent embolization. Another theory is that inadvertent amnion puncture may occur, resulting in either amniotic bands or loss of amniotic fluid, with subsequent compression and deformity.

There is no evidence to suggest an increased risk of congenital malformation when CVS is performed after the eighth completed week. Chorionic villus sampling should be performed at 9 to 12 weeks' gestation in an experienced center in which at least 200 to 250 procedures have been performed.

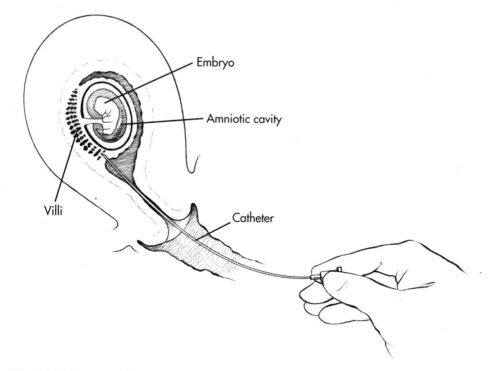

Embryo

Amniotic cavity

Villi

Catheter

Fig. 19-2 Transcervical approach to CVS. Under ultrasound guidance, a malleable catheter is inserted through the cervix into villous tissue. (From Chueh J, Golbus MS: Fetal invasive procedures. In Plauche WC, Morrison JC, Sullivan MJ, editors: *Surgical obstetrics,* Philadelphia, 1992, WB Saunders.)

QUESTION 5: IS A TRANSABDOMINAL ROUTE OR A TRANSCERVICAL ROUTE SAFER?

In a second NICHD study, almost 4000 patients were randomized to transcervical or transabdominal sampling. The loss rate was equal through 28 weeks of pregnancy after either transcervical (2.5%) or transabdominal (2.3%) CVS. A transcervical approach generally allows slightly more tissue to be obtained, but the amount of tissue should not affect the ability to obtain an accurate karyotype.[5]

Ideally, practitioners should be well versed in both methods of sampling (Figures 19-1 and 19-2).[2,6] Transcervical procedures are generally easier in patients with posterior placentas and in patients with retroverted uteri. Transabdominal sampling is generally easier in patients with anterior placentas and is the method of choice in patients with active herpes lesions.

REFERENCES

1. Canadian Collaborators CVS-Amniocentesis Clinical Trial Group: Multicentre randomized clinical trial of chorion villus sampling and amniocentesis, *Lancet* 1:1, 1989.
2. Chorionic villus sampling (CVS): World Health Organization European Regional Office (WHO/EURO) meeting statement on the use of CVS in prenatal diagnosis, *J Assist Reprod Genet* 9:299, 1992.
3. Firth HV, Boyd PA, Chamberlain P et al: Severe limb abnormalities after chorion villus sampling at 56 to 66 days' gestation, *Lancet* 337:762, 1991.
4. Hanson FW, Tennant F, Hune S et al: Early amniocentesis: outcome, risks and technical problems at ≤ 12.8 weeks, *Am J Obstet Gynecol* 166:1707, 1992.
5. Jackson LG, Fowler SE, Zachery JM et al: A randomized comparison of transcervical and transabdominal chorionic villus sampling, *N Engl J Med* 327:594, 1992.
6. Kuliev AM, Modell B, Jackson L et al: Risk evaluation of CVS, *Prenat Diagn* 13:197, 1993.
7. Ledbetter DH, Martin AO, Verlinsky Y et al: Cytogenetic results of chorionic villus sampling: high success rate and diagnostic accuracy in the United States collaborative study, *Am J Obstet Gynecol* 162:495, 1990.
8. Medical Research Council Working Party: Medical Research Council European trial of chorionic villus sampling, *Lancet* 337:1491, 1991.
9. Nicolaides K, Brizot M, Patel F, Snijders R: Comparison of chorionic villus sampling and amniocentesis for fetal karyotyping at 10-13 weeks' gestation, *Lancet* 344:435, 1994.
10. Rhoads GG, Jackson LG, Schlesselman SE et al: The safety and efficacy of chorionic villus sampling for early prenatal diagnosis of cytogenetic abnormalities, *N Engl J Med* 320:609, 1989.

CHAPTER 20

Percutaneous Umbilical
Blood Sampling

STEVEN A. LAIFER
JEFFREY A. KULLER

Percutaneous umbilical blood sampling (PUBS), also called *cordocentesis* or *funipuncture*, is a technique that allows blood to be obtained directly from the fetal-placental circulation. First described by Bang and colleagues[1] and Daffos and colleagues[3] in the early 1980s, the procedure involves placing a needle under ultrasound guidance into an umbilical vessel and aspirating a sample of blood. This procedure was made feasible by important technologic advances in high-resolution ultrasound and fetal imaging procedures.

Access to the fetal circulation has markedly expanded the ability to assess and evaluate the fetus and has greatly enhanced the ability to treat the fetus in utero through direct intravascular therapy. Percutaneous umbilical blood sampling has revolutionized the management and intrauterine treatment of severe red blood cell alloimmunization and erythroblastosis fetalis.

❦ Patient Profile: Evaluation of fetal hydrops

A 25-year-old Caucasian patient (gravida 1, para 0000) at 26 weeks' gestation is found to have a fundal height of 30 cm. An ultrasound examination reveals polyhydramnios, fetal ascites, bilateral fetal pleural effusions, and fetal skin edema. No structural abnormalities are apparent, the placenta is anterior, and the fetal heart rate is 140 beats per minute. The patient's medical history is unremarkable, and she works as a schoolteacher. Her blood type is A+, her rapid plasma reagin (RPR) serology is nonreactive, and she has immunity to rubella. The Kleihauer-Betke test is negative. Further maternal serologic evaluation reveals negative IgG but positive IgM for parvovirus.

Fetal anemia secondary to acute parvovirus infection is suspected as the cause of fetal hydrops, and after discussion with the patient, a PUBS with possible fetal transfusion is recommended. At the time of fetal blood sampling, the fetal hematocrit is found to be 13% and the fetus is immediately transfused with 40 ml of adult packed red blood cells.

151

During the next several weeks, serial ultrasound evaluation of the fetus reveals resolution of the hydrops. Results of tests on fetal blood obtained during the PUBS procedure reveal positive IgM to parvovirus, parvovirus DNA determined by polymerase chain reaction amplification, and a normal male karyotype. The remainder of the pregnancy is uncomplicated, and the patient delivers an apparently healthy fetus at 39 weeks' gestation.

QUESTION 1: HOW IS PERCUTANEOUS UMBILICAL BLOOD SAMPLING PERFORMED?

The PUBS procedure is generally performed in an outpatient setting. However, when an intravascular fetal transfusion is planned and the pregnancy has reached viability, the procedure is ideally performed in the delivery room, with the patient prepared for an emergency delivery if one becomes necessary. The patient is positioned comfortably, and an ultrasound examination of the uterus, placenta, and fetus is performed.

The preferred site for PUBS is the placental cord insertion site because the cord is best anchored at this site and needle entry is more likely to be successful. Other potential sites for blood sampling include free loops of cord, the fetal abdominal cord insertion site, and the intrahepatic section of the umbilical vein. Free loops of cord tend to move when needle penetration is attempted, and fetal movement is more likely to hinder successful needle insertion at the abdominal insertion site. Although successful procedures have been reported using the intrahepatic section of the umbilical vein,[13] this site has not been widely used in the United States. Intracardiac fetal blood sampling should not be used because of unacceptably high fetal morbidity.

When the optimal site has been identified, the maternal abdominal skin is aseptically prepared and draped in a manner similar to that used for amniocentesis. For diagnostic blood sampling, maternal sedation is unnecessary, but the skin can be infiltrated with a local anesthetic. Continuous ultrasound visualization is required and is most easily accomplished by placing a curvilinear ultrasound transducer in a sterile plastic bag or glove that can remain on the aseptic field during the procedure.

The procedure is ideally carried out by two operators. We prefer the freehand technique, in which one operator simultaneously holds the transducer and continuously images the cord insertion site with one hand while inserting the needle percutaneously with the other hand. A 20- or 22-gauge spinal needle is used; the length of the needle is determined by the distance from the skin to the anticipated umbilical vessel puncture site. The needle is visualized sonographically as it traverses the abdomen and uterus and is directed into an umbilical vessel (Figure 20-1). When the umbilical vessel has been punctured, the assistant can remove the stylet and attach heparinized syringes, which are used for aspiration of blood samples. Some operators prefer to attach a short extension tube to the hub of the needle, which minimizes both movement at the hub and the potential for dislodg-

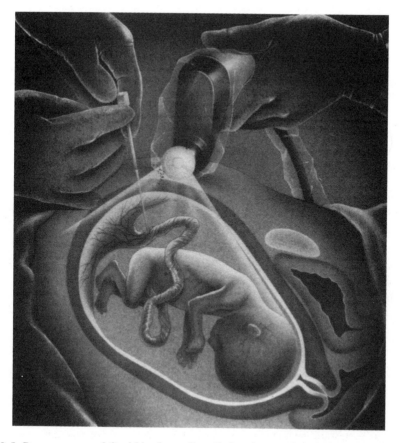

Fig. 20-1 Percutaneous umbilical blood sampling. Under ultrasound guidance, a 22-gauge spinal needle is inserted into the placental insertion site of the umbilical cord. (From Chueh J, Golbus MS: Fetal invasive procedures. In Plauche WC, Morrison JC, Sullivan MJ, editors: *Surgical obstetrics*, Philadelphia, 1992, WB Saunders.)

ment of the needle.[11] Proper positioning and placement of the needle are confirmed with continuous ultrasound imaging. When the necessary amount of blood has been aspirated, the needle is withdrawn.

It is imperative to confirm that the blood specimen is of fetal origin. Purity of fetal blood in the aspirate is suggested immediately by red cell indices showing a high mean corpuscular volume relative to adult red blood cell indices. Other tests that distinguish adult hemoglobin from fetal hemoglobin, such as the Kleihauer-Betke or Apt tests, should be used as well.

When an intravascular transfusion is performed, the needle must remain in the umbilical vessel for the duration of the transfusion. Fetal movement may dislodge the needle, which may prevent completion of the transfusion or traumatize the cord. To avoid this complication, most perinatologists administer neuromuscular blocking agents, such as pancuronium or atracurium, to the fetus intravascularly or intramuscularly immediately before the transfusion. While some centers administer perioperative antibiotics, no convincing data indicate that they decrease the fetal loss rate.

QUESTION 2: WHAT ARE THE LIMITATIONS, RISKS, AND COMPLICATIONS OF PERCUTANEOUS UMBILICAL BLOOD SAMPLING?

The main limitation in performing PUBS is the occasional inability to adequately visualize the cord insertion site to allow the cord to be safely punctured and fetal blood to be aspirated. The procedure can be performed as early as 16 to 18 weeks' gestation and as late as term if an appropriate site is visualized. Although cord vessel diameters enlarge with advancing gestational age, fetal position and movement may interfere with optimal cord visualization and needle placement. Placental position may influence the likelihood of success or determine the complications associated with the procedure. Performing PUBS through an anteriorly positioned placenta involves traversing the placental villi and has the highest probability of causing intermixing of fetal and maternal blood[17]; this may cause or worsen red blood cell alloimmunization. Attempting PUBS with a posteriorly positioned placenta is more likely to be difficult because the interposed fetus may obstruct the optimal pathway for the needle. We have found that using color Doppler ultrasound sometimes facilitates localization of the cord insertion site.

Complications that have been associated with PUBS are listed in the box below. Transient bleeding from the cord puncture site lasting up to 3 minutes is a common occurrence; observation of the bleeding with ultrasound is all that is required and will in most cases demonstrate that the bleeding is self-limited. Fetal bradycardia is usually also transient, but if bradycardia occurs, a period of observation is warranted. Although uterine contractions have been reported to occur after PUBS, the risk of preterm delivery is not increased.

Hickock and Mills[9] reviewed the results of 302 PUBS procedures performed by the Western Perinatal Collaborative Group from 1986 to 1990. Most of the procedures were

---

COMPLICATIONS OF PERCUTANEOUS UMBILICAL BLOOD SAMPLING

Chorioamnionitis
Premature rupture of membranes
Cord hematoma or thrombosis (may obstruct blood flow, causing fetal distress)
Bleeding from the cord puncture site lasting longer than 3 minutes
Bradyarrhythmia (more common after puncture of the umbilical artery)
Placental abruption

performed for evaluation of red blood cell alloimmunization or severe fetal growth retardation. The success rate for accomplishing the procedure was 93.7%. Postprocedural fetal death occurred in six cases, yielding a loss rate of 2.1%. Ludomirski[12] presented data from a North American registry of fetal blood sampling procedures performed between 1987 and 1991. In 6023 patients, 7462 procedures were performed, most of which were for rapid karyotyping and assessment of red cell alloimmunization. The fetal loss rate was 1.12% per procedure. Ghidini and colleagues[6] reviewed the English literature to determine the incidence and significance of complications related to percutaneous fetal blood sampling. They concluded that patients should be counseled that the overall risk of fetal loss from fetal blood sampling is approximately 2.7%.

The loss rate tends to be higher in certain circumstances, such as with genetically and structurally abnormal fetuses and severely growth-retarded fetuses. The results of a large series of PUBS procedures performed in otherwise normal fetuses for the evaluation of fetal infection with toxoplasmosis indicate that the loss rate related to the procedure is closer to 1%.[3] For diagnostic PUBS, we cite a 1% to 2% fetal loss rate when counseling patients.

Complications and the risk of fetal loss from PUBS can be minimized by carefully selecting patients who have appropriate indications. A prudent approach to performing the procedure is also necessary. If adequate imaging of the cord is not possible, the procedure should be postponed for several days or an alternative test selected. Adhering to aseptic technique and limiting the number of attempts to puncture the vessel will also reduce the frequency of complications. Because of the risk of transplacental hemorrhage, nonalloimmunized Rh-negative patients should receive RhoGAM after the procedure.

QUESTION 3: WHAT ARE THE INDICATIONS FOR PERCUTANEOUS UMBILICAL BLOOD SAMPLING?

Fetal blood sampling has been used for a variety of clinical indications. The most common indications for PUBS are rapid karyotype analysis, diagnosis and treatment of fetal anemia, diagnosis of fetal infection, and evaluation of nonimmune hydrops. Less common indications include diagnosis of thrombocytopenia, diagnosis of inherited disorders such as hemophilia, and evaluation of fetal thyroid function. The use of fetal blood sampling for evaluation of fetal oxygenation and acid-base balance remains controversial. Investigational uses include direct fetal therapy and stem cell transplantation (see Chapter 31).

Rapid Karyotyping

Fetal structural anomalies that suggest a lethal chromosome abnormality, such as trisomy 13 or trisomy 18, may be detected sonographically. Knowledge of the fetal karyotype in this situation may provide critical information regarding optimal obstetric management. If these anomalies are detected near term or in the setting of preterm labor, the diagnosis of a lethal chromosome abnormality may help avert a cesarean delivery for fetal distress or malpresentation. Alternatively, the diagnosis of a lethal chromosome abnormality may help the patient decide whether to terminate the pregnancy. Determining a fetal karyotype by conventional amniocentesis may take 10 to 14 days or longer, and the results may not be available in time for clinical decision making. Culturing lymphocytes obtained from a fetal blood sample can provide information on the fetal karyotype in as little as 48 to 72 hours.

In certain situations in which imaging of the cord is difficult (e.g., in the setting of oligohydramnios) and a rapid karyotype is desired, an alternative to fetal blood sampling is placental biopsy. The main disadvantage of this technique is the small potential for placental mosaicism.[10] The technique of fluorescent in situ hybridization (FISH), which involves the use of chromosome-specific DNA probes to detect aneuploidy, has become clinically available. This diagnostic technique is commonly performed on uncultured amniocytes and provides clinical information in 2 to 3 days.[15] The advantage of this procedure is that amniocentesis clearly has a lower risk of fetal loss than PUBS.

Fetal Anemia

Percutaneous umbilical blood sampling has revolutionized the management of red cell alloimmunization during pregnancy. Before the introduction of fetal blood sampling, spectrophotometric analysis of amniotic fluid was the method most commonly used to evaluate the severity of suspected fetal anemia. This method, which is used to measure small quantities of bilirubin in amniotic fluid, is limited because it is only an indirect assessment of anemia, and its accuracy has not been conclusively validated before 26 weeks' gestation. In addition, contaminants such as blood may be present in amniotic fluid and may prevent accurate interpretation of spectrophotometric results.

Fetal blood sampling provides a method of directly assessing fetal anemia, by measuring the fetal hemoglobin and hematocrit. The decision to treat severely anemic fetuses can now be based on confirmation of severe anemia so that only fetuses that truly require intrauterine treatment receive it. Furthermore, intrauterine treatment in the form of red blood cell transfusion can now be administered directly, as an intravascular transfusion, rather than indirectly, as an intraperitoneal transfusion (Figure 20-2). In a case-control study, Harman and colleagues[8] demonstrated that, with respect to the success of the procedures, neonatal outcome, and complications, intravascular intrauterine transfusions were superior to intraperitoneal transfusions for the treatment of fetal anemia secondary to red cell alloimunization. In view of the aforementioned risks associated with PUBS, however, most centers use fetal blood sampling with some combination of indirect techniques, usually amniotic fluid spectrophotometric analysis and ultrasound, to assess fetal anemia in the management of patients with red cell alloimunization.

Nonimmune Hydrops Fetalis

Nonimmune hydrops fetalis (NIHF) is defined as the presence of fluid in more than one fetal body cavity (e.g., pleural effusion, pericardial effusion, ascites, skin edema) and is associated with a very high fetal and neonatal mortality rate. The differential diagnosis of NIHF includes genetic, chromosomal, or structural abnormalities of the fetus, anemia, cardiac dysrhythmias, fetal infections, and lymphatic abnormalities. Percutaneous umbilical

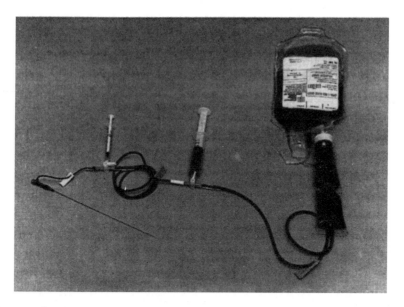

Fig. 20-2 A closed transfusion apparatus for an intravascular fetal transfusion. (From Laifer SA, Kuller JA, Hill LM: In utero intravascular transfusion for treating fetal hemolytic disease, *Surg Gynecol Obstet* 172:312, 1991.)

blood sampling has become a vital component in the evaluation of fetuses with NIHF. Frequently this condition is not reversible in utero, but in the case of fetal anemia, for example, transfusion may be lifesaving and allow for complete resolution of hydrops. As illustrated in the patient profile at the beginning of this chapter, the definitive diagnosis of anemia was made using PUBS, immediate treatment of the fetus was facilitated, and fetal parvovirus infection was confirmed.

Fetal Infection

Fetal viral or bacterial infection may be suspected because of maternal exposure or infection or suspicious findings on fetal ultrasound examination (e.g., NIHF, cerebral or hepatic calcification). The use of fetal blood sampling has proved to be invaluable in the evaluation of suspected fetal infection. Although not all fetuses mount a detectable immune response, the presence of pathogen-specific IgM in the fetal serum is diagnostic of infection.

Furthermore, molecular diagnostic techniques, such as DNA amplification using the polymerase chain reaction,[5] contribute significantly to the diagnosis of infection by detecting the presence of microbial DNA in blood, amniotic fluid, or various tissues. Polymerase chain reaction, for example, has already been used for the detection of cytomegalovirus, parvovirus, and toxoplasmosis DNA in fetal blood or amniotic fluid from affected pregnancies.[4,7,14] In addition to the diagnostic value of PUBS when fetal infection is suspected, the severity of the infection can be ascertained by using blood tests in which fetal blood count, platelet count, and hepatic function are evaluated.[16] If treatment is indicated, as illustrated in the patient profile of NIHF secondary to anemia caused by parvovirus infection, blood can be transfused intravascularly to the fetus.

• • •

The technique of PUBS, which permits direct access to the fetal circulation, has greatly enhanced the ability to evaluate the fetus. Diagnosis of fetal abnormalities and fetal condition is facilitated by PUBS, and evaluation of the red cell alloimmunized pregnancy and treatment of fetal anemia have been optimized by PUBS. An abundance of physiologic information and data regarding the fetus have also been accumulated through PUBS. Access to the fetal circulation has made direct medical treatment of the fetus a reality. As advances continue to be made in the fields of fetal medicine, molecular biology, and genetics, access to the fetal circulation may allow innovative therapies to be used to treat afflicted fetuses. It must be emphasized, however, that PUBS is associated with a significant risk of fetal loss. In clinical practice settings, only patients with clear indications should be selected to undergo the procedure.

REFERENCES

1. Bang J, Bock JE, Trolle D: Ultrasound-guided fetal intravenous transfusion for severe rhesus hæmolytic disease, *Br Med J* 284:373, 1982.
2. Daffos F, Capella-Pavlovsky M, Forestier F: A new procedure for fetal blood sampling in utero: preliminary results of fifty-three cases, *Am J Obstet Gynecol* 146:985, 1983.
3. Daffos F, Cappela-Pavlovsky M, Forestier F: Fetal blood sampling during pregnancy with use of a needle guided by ultrasound: a study of 606 consecutive cases, *Am J Obstet Gynecol* 153:655, 1985.
4. Donner C, Liesnard C, Content J et al: Prenatal diagnosis of 52 pregnancies at risk for congenital cytomegalovirus infection, *Obstet Gynecol* 82:481, 1993.
5. Ehrlich GD, Sirko DA: PCR and its role in clinical diagnostics. In Ehrlich GD, Greenberg SJ, editors: *PCR-based diagnostics in infectious disease*, Boston, 1994, Blackwell.
6. Ghidini A, Sepulveda W, Lockwood CJ, Romero R: Complications of fetal blood sampling, *Am J Obstet Gynecol* 168:1339, 1993.
7. Grover CM, Thulliez P, Remmington JS, Boothroyd JC: Rapid prenatal diagnosis of congenital *Toxoplasma* infection by using polymerase chain reaction and amniotic fluid, *J Clin Microbiol* 20:2297, 1990.
8. Harman CR, Bowman JM, Manning FA, Menticoglou SM: Intrauterine transfusion—intraperitoneal versus intravascular approach: a case-control comparison, *Am J Obstet Gynecol* 162:1053, 1990.
9. Hickock DE, Mills M, Western Collaborative Perinatal Group: Percutaneous umbilical blood sampling: results from a multicenter collaborative registry, *Am J Obstet Gynecol* 166:1614, 1992.
10. Holzgreve W, Tercanli S, Evans MI, Miny P: Late chorionic villus sampling. In Evans MI, editor: *Reproductive risks and prenatal diagnosis*, Norwalk, Conn, 1992, Appleton & Lange.
11. Laifer SA, Kuller JA, Hill LM: In utero intravascular transfusion for treating fetal hemolytic disease, *Surg Gynecol Obstet* 172:319, 1991.
12. Ludomirski A: Intrauterine fetal blood sampling: a multicenter registry evaluation of 7462 procedures between 1987 and 1991, *Am J Obstet Gynecol* (abstract) 168:318, 1993.
13. Nicolini U, Nicolaidis P, Fisk NM et al: Fetal blood sampling from the intrahepatic vein: analysis of safety and clinical experience with 214 procedures, *Obstet Gynecol* 76:47, 1990.
14. Torok TJ, Wang Q-Y, Gary GW: Prenatal diagnosis of intrauterine parvovirus B19 infection by the polymerase chain reaction technique, *Clin Infect Dis* 14:149, 1992.
15. Ward BE, Gersen SL, Carelli MP et al: Rapid prenatal diagnosis of chromosomal aneuploidies by fluorescence in situ hybridization: clinical experience with 4,500 specimens, *Am J Hum Genet* 52:854, 1993.
16. Watt-Morse ML, Laifer SA, Hill LM: The natural history of fetal cytomegalovirus infection as assessed by serial ultrasound and fetal blood sampling, *Prenat Diagn* (in press).
17. Weiner C, Grant S, Hudson J et al: Effect of diagnostic and therapeutic cordocentesis on maternal serum α-fetoprotein concentration, *Am J Obstet Gynecol* 161:706, 1989.

CHAPTER 21

Fetal Tissue Sampling

CHRISTINE R. CADRIN
MITCHELL S. GOLBUS

In utero sampling of fetal skin, liver, and muscle has become an important method of evaluating fetuses at increased risk for congenital abnormalities. In the past, certain genetic disorders, such as X-linked hypohidrotic ectodermal dysplasia, ornithine transcarbamylase deficiency, carbamoyl-phosphate synthetase deficiency, and nonketotic hyperglycinemia, could be diagnosed only by using invasive fetal biopsy techniques. Some of these disorders can now be rapidly diagnosed by enzyme assay or by DNA analysis using amniotic cells or chorionic villi.* However, when meiotic recombination occurs or the results of DNA analysis are uninformative, the direct examination of fetal skin, liver, or muscle may still provide the only means of prenatal diagnosis.

Fetal Skin Biopsy

Genodermatoses are severe and often fatal hereditary skin disorders. Fetal skin sampling is the only method available for prenatal diagnosis of many of these conditions. The first reports of successful prenatal diagnosis by light and electron microscopy of fetal skin biopsy specimens involved fetuses at risk for bullous congenital ichthyosiform erythroderma,[25] harlequin ichthyosis,[17] and the Herlitz syndrome, epidermolysis bullosa letalis.[46] During the last 10 years, more than 200 cases of prenatal diagnosis by fetal skin sampling have been reported.

✤ Patient Profile: Prenatal diagnosis of a hereditary skin disorder by fetal skin biopsy

A 29-year-old Iranian woman (gravida 4, para 3002) was referred at 10 weeks' gestation for prenatal diagnosis. Her previous child died of complications of harlequin ichthyosis congenita

---

*References 12, 29, 43, 50, and 55.

(an autosomal recessive disorder characterized by armor-like scales, with marked ectropion and a degree of eclabium that produces a fish-mouth appearance). This experience was traumatic for the patient, and she continues to be very distressed about it. She and her husband wish to know more about the benefits and risks of fetal skin sampling.

QUESTION 1: WHAT ARE THE INDICATIONS FOR FETAL SKIN SAMPLING?

Genodermatoses that require fetal skin sampling for prenatal diagnosis are those disorders not diagnosable by analysis of chorionic villi or amniotic fluid components (see the box below). In the future, some of these conditions will become detectable by DNA analysis and thereby diagnosable by either chorionic villus sampling (CVS) or amniocentesis. Fetal skin sampling would then be required only if the results of the DNA analysis were uninformative.

GENODERMATOSES DIAGNOSABLE BY FETAL SKIN SAMPLING

Anhidrotic ectodermal dysplasia	Epidermolysis bullosa letalis
Bullous congenital ichthyosiform erythroderma	Harlequin ichthyosis
	Hypohidrotic ectodermal dysplasia
Nonbullous ichthyosiform erythroderma	Oculocutaneous albinism
Epidermolysis bullosa dystrophica	Sjögren-Larsson syndrome

QUESTION 2: HOW IS FETAL SKIN BIOPSY PERFORMED?

Fetal skin biopsy was initially performed by fetoscopy[18,19,31,39]; the specimen is now most frequently obtained by percutaneous insertion of a biopsy forceps under continuous ultrasound guidance.[36] Before any fetal skin sampling procedure, the mother undergoes a preliminary ultrasound examination to confirm gestational age, determine fetal viability, diagnose multifetal pregnancy, diagnose fetal structural abnormalities, determine fetal lie, and locate the placenta.

Fetal skin sampling is optimally performed between 17 and 20 weeks' gestation, depending on the indication. The patient is usually premedicated with 5 to 10 mg of intravenous diazepam (Valium). The abdomen is prepared with an iodine-based solution and alcohol and is draped in a sterile manner. The skin is infiltrated with 1% lidocaine (Xylocaine) for local anesthesia. A trocar is then introduced into the uterus, and a biopsy forceps is passed through the cannula to obtain an approximately 2 mm specimen of skin, preferably from the thorax, back, buttocks or, for certain diagnoses (e.g., oculocutaneous albinism), the scalp. The entire procedure is performed under continuous ultrasound guidance. An ultrasound examination is performed immediately after the procedure to assess fetal viability and any residual bleeding. After sampling, the tissue is placed in an appropriate fixative in preparation for electron and light microscopy. The methods used to evaluate fetal skin for various prenatal diagnoses have been well described (Figures 21-1 and 21-2).*

QUESTION 3: HOW DOES THE LOSS RATE OF FETAL SKIN BIOPSY PERFORMED USING FETOSCOPY COMPARE WITH THE LOSS RATE OF FETAL SKIN SAMPLING PROCEDURES PERFORMED UNDER ULTRASOUND GUIDANCE?

In experienced centers, the incidence of fetal loss from fetoscopy and fetal skin biopsy is less than 5%.[48] Principal risks include spontaneous abortion; amniotic fluid leakage; infection; premature labor and delivery; hemorrhage from injury to the anterior abdominal wall, uterus, or placenta; maternal and fetal injuries; and cosmetic or functional injuries. To date, too few fetal skin sampling procedures have been performed by ultrasound-guided skin biopsy to draw any firm conclusions regarding safety in comparison with the fetoscopy method.

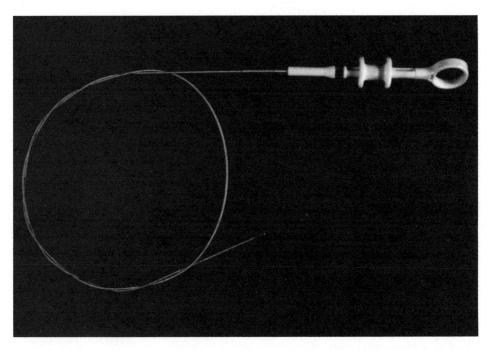

Fig. 21-1 Under direct ultrasound guidance, the flexible sterile biopsy forceps is passed through a trocar sleeve (not shown) to sample the fetal skin.

---

*References 2, 3, 14, 17, 18, 20, 25, 37-39, and 46.

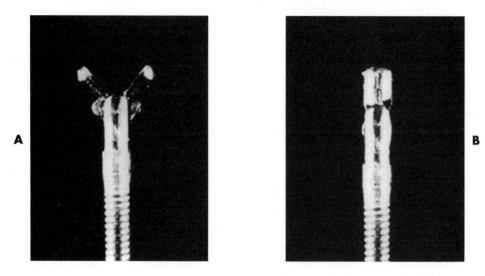

Fig. 21-2 Close-up view of the biopsy forceps used for fetal skin sampling. **A,** Open. **B,** Closed.

QUESTION 4: HOW ACCURATE IS FETAL SKIN SAMPLING?

Too few fetal skin samples, whether obtained by fetoscopy or by ultrasound-guided biopsy, have been recovered to assess the prenatal diagnostic accuracy for any given disorder. These diagnoses generally depend on electromicroscopic studies of fetal skin ultrastructure or on use of immunohistochemical probes. In addition, specific diagnostic testing of each fetal skin sample depends on which genodermatosis the proband is at risk of inheriting; too few prenatal diagnoses of each genodermatosis have been performed to assess accuracy of diagnostic results.

Between January 1979 and May 1993, fetal skin sampling was carried out for prenatal diagnosis in 25 pregnancies at the University of California–San Francisco.[11,27] Satisfactory samples were obtained in 24 cases. Of the 25 fetuses, five were delivered preterm. Another patient had a spontaneous abortion associated with chorioamnionitis 2 days after the sampling procedure. The prenatal diagnosis was confirmed after delivery or termination in 19 cases. In one case in which sampling was performed on a fetus at risk for ichthyosiform erythroderma, although the results of the sampling were normal, the infant was found after delivery to be mildly affected. Five patients were lost to follow-up.

Fetal Liver Biopsy

Most inborn errors of metabolism can be diagnosed by analysis of amniotic fluid constituents or chorionic villi; however, some liver enzyme abnormalities are not currently diagnosable by DNA analysis. Fetal liver biopsy then becomes the only method available for prenatal diagnosis of these conditions. The first reports of successful prenatal diagnosis by fetal liver biopsy involved pregnancies at risk for ornithine transcarbamylase deficiency (OTCD).[32,47] During the last 10 years, 19 cases of prenatal diagnosis using fetal liver biopsy have been reported.*

❧ Patient Profile: Prenatal diagnosis of ornithine transcarbamylase deficiency by fetal liver biopsy

A 33-year-old Caucasian woman (gravida 3, para 2001) was referred at 8 weeks' gestation for prenatal diagnosis. Her previous son died during the newborn period of complications of OTCD, a urea cycle disorder inherited as an X-linked trait in which affected male children generally die during the newborn period secondary to complications of hyperammonemia. The diagnosis of OTCD was confirmed clinically and by liver biopsy. Amniocentesis at 15 weeks' gestation in the current pregnancy revealed a male fetus. A liver biopsy at 19 weeks' gestation indicated that the fetus had less than 1% of ornithine transcarbamylase activity and normal carbamoyl-phosphate synthetase activity. The parents elected to terminate the pregnancy, which was accomplished with a combination of laminaria cervical dilation and surgical evacuation. The prenatal diagnosis was confirmed postabortum by biochemical and histochemical analysis.

QUESTION 1: WHAT ARE THE INDICATIONS FOR FETAL LIVER SAMPLING?

Recent advances in DNA technology have allowed mutations to be identified in the ornithine transcarbamylase gene[12,23,43] and in the carbamoyl-phosphate synthetase gene,[28]

INDICATIONS FOR FETAL LIVER BIOPSY

Ornithine transcarbamylase (OTC) deficiency

A urea cycle deficiency inherited as an X-linked trait; affected male children usually die during the newborn period secondary to complications of hyperammonemia[32,47]

Carbamoyl-phosphate synthetase (CPS) deficiency

A urea cycle deficiency inherited as an autosomal recessive trait; affected children usually have acute neonatal hyperammonemia[41,45]

Von Gierke disease (glycogen storage disease, type 1A)

An autosomal recessive disorder of glycogen metabolism that causes hypoglycemia, lactic acidemia, hyperuricemia, hyperlipidemia, engorgement of hepatocytes with glycogen, and platelet dysfunction[26]

---

*References 11, 26, 27, 32, 41, 45, and 47.

permitting prenatal diagnosis to be performed by DNA analysis of amniotic fluid cells or chorionic villi. However, fetal liver biopsy is still needed for cases in which DNA analysis is not informative for the detected mutations (see the box on p. 163).

QUESTION 2: HOW IS FETAL LIVER BIOPSY PERFORMED?

Similar to fetal skin sampling, fetal liver biopsy requires a preliminary ultrasound examination. The procedure is optimally performed between 17 and 20 weeks' gestation. If desired, the patient is premedicated with 5 to 10 mg of intravenous diazepam, and a 1% lidocaine solution is injected for local anesthesia. A 16.5-gauge thin-walled needle is introduced into the amniotic cavity under continuous ultrasound guidance. The biopsy needle is then directed below the right costal margin and into the fetal liver. Once the needle is within the liver parenchyma, a syringe is attached to exert constant negative pressure and aspirate fetal liver into the biopsy needle. The tissue is removed from the needle by flushing with saline solution.[27] The specimen is then processed for appropriate enzyme assays.* An ultrasound examination is performed immediately after the procedure to assess fetal status.

QUESTION 3: WHAT IS THE COMPLICATION RATE FOR FETAL LIVER BIOPSY?

Complications that may arise from fetal liver biopsy are similar to those associated with fetal skin sampling (see the discussion under Question 3 on p. 161). Too few fetal liver biopsies have been performed to cite an accurate complication rate for the procedure.

QUESTION 4: HOW ACCURATE IS FETAL LIVER SAMPLING?

Too few fetal liver biopsies have been performed to assess the prenatal diagnostic accuracy of the procedure. Patients should be informed of the investigational nature of this procedure. During the last 10 years, 17 fetal liver biopsies were performed at the University of California–San Francisco,[11,27] and satisfactory samples were obtained in all but one case. There were no spontaneous abortions or preterm deliveries. All diagnoses were confirmed after delivery or on termination of the pregnancy. One patient was lost to follow-up.

Fetal Muscle Biopsy

Duchenne muscular dystrophy (DMD) is a progressive, degenerative muscle disease that is inherited as an X-linked recessive trait. Prenatal diagnosis and carrier detection for this disorder can usually be performed using DNA analysis. The first successful prenatal

---

*References 26, 32, 41, 45, and 47.

diagnosis by dystrophin analysis of fetal muscle biopsy was performed by Evans and colleagues[21] in 1991.

❧ Patient Profile: Prenatal diagnosis of Duchenne muscular dystrophy by fetal muscle biopsy

The patient is a 37-year-old Caucasian woman (gravida 4, para 2012) with one DMD-affected 14-year-old son. She has no other affected male relatives. She has a normal creatinine kinase (CK) value of 61 mIU/ml (creatinine kinase is a particularly sensitive indicator of muscle damage and is elevated in patients with DMD and in most carriers of this condition). DNA analysis of the DMD gene in the affected child failed to demonstrate a deletion. Chorionic villus sampling performed at 12 weeks' gestation revealed a male fetus. DNA analysis using 11 restriction fragment length polymorphisms had previously been performed on the patient, her affected son, her daughter, her parents, and three of her siblings. Linkage analysis indicated that the fetus had inherited the same X chromosome as the affected son. The risk for the fetus to be affected with DMD was 33%. At 22 weeks' gestation, the patient underwent fetal muscle biopsy, and three gluteal biopsies were performed. No complications resulted from the procedure. The presence of dystrophin was identified by immunofluorescence studies. At delivery, the cord CK was 35 mIU/ml, which was within normal limits.

QUESTION 1: WHAT ARE THE INDICATIONS FOR FETAL MUSCLE BIOPSY?

Indications for fetal muscle biopsy include risk for DMD. Prenatal diagnosis and carrier detection for DMD can usually be performed using DNA analysis. However, fetal muscle biopsy is still needed when recombination occurs within the DMD gene, when carrier status cannot be ascertained, or when DNA analysis is not informative for the detected mutations. Other indications for fetal muscle biopsy include risk for Becker muscular dystrophy (a form of the disease similar to but not as severe as DMD) and risk for mitochondrial myopathies.

QUESTION 2: HOW IS FETAL MUSCLE BIOPSY PERFORMED?

After a preliminary ultrasound examination, the woman is sedated to reduce fetal movement, and the skin is infiltrated with a 1% lidocaine solution. Fetal muscle is obtained at 16 to 22 weeks' gestation by directing a 14-gauge (Tru-Cut) biopsy needle through the maternal abdomen and obliquely into the fetal gluteal region. Real-time sonography is used to provide continuous visualization. After sampling, the presence of muscle fibers in the specimen is verified, and immunoblotting or immunofluorescence is used to determine whether dystrophin is present (Figure 21-3).[35] An ultrasound examination is performed immediately after the procedure to assess fetal status.

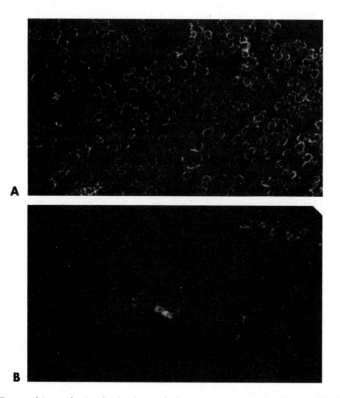

Fig. 21-3 Dystrophin analysis of a fetal muscle biopsy specimen. **A,** A normal fetal muscle sample shows normal dystrophin. **B,** Dystrophin immunofluorescence of fetal muscle in an affected fetus shows dystrophin deficiency.

QUESTION 3: WHAT IS THE COMPLICATION RATE FOR FETAL MUSCLE BIOPSY?

Too few fetal muscle biopsies have been performed to assess the safety of the procedure. Possible complications include spontaneous abortion, leakage of amniotic fluid, fetal or maternal hemorrhage, fetal or maternal injury, infection, prematurity, and cosmetic or functional fetal injury.

QUESTION 4: HOW ACCURATE IS FETAL MUSCLE SAMPLING?

Too few fetal muscle biopsies have been performed to assess the accuracy of the procedure. Patients should be informed of the investigational nature of this procedure.

Fetal muscle biopsy was recently used at the University of California–San Francisco for prenatal diagnosis in seven pregnant women.[11,35] The indication for six of the seven fetal muscle sampling procedures was DMD. One fetal muscle biopsy was performed for a fetus at risk for an autosomal recessive mitochondrial myopathy. Satisfactory specimens were obtained in all but one case. Immunofluorescence studies verified the presence of normal dystrophin in four cases and the absence of normal dystrophin in one other case. No diagnosis could be made for the fetus at risk for the mitochondrial myopathy because of lack of muscle fibers in the biopsy material. Of the seven pregnancies, one ended in spontaneous abortion 3 weeks after the sampling and another ended in spontaneous abortion associated with chorioamnionitis a few days after the procedure. The prenatal diagnosis was confirmed after delivery or termination in six cases.

The Future of Fetal Tissue Sampling

During the last decade, significant advances in invasive prenatal diagnostic techniques, such as fetal skin sampling, fetal liver biopsy, and fetal muscle biopsy, have made possible the diagnosis of congenital disorders not diagnosable using amniocentesis or CVS. In the next few years, many of these conditions will certainly become detectable by DNA analysis, and therefore the need for these procedures may decrease dramatically. Other invasive prenatal techniques, such as fetal kidney biopsy, might become available in the near future. Finnish nephrosis suspected because of excessive elevation of amniotic fluid α-fetoprotein (AFAFP) could potentially be diagnosed prenatally using this technique. Continuing animal research on fetal hematopoietic stem cell transplantation might allow fetal liver biopsy to be used for therapeutic applications of gene transfer.[13,22,40,53]

REFERENCES

1. Aivazian AA, Bakharev VA, Karetnikova NA: The prenatal diagnosis of Herlitz's borderline epidermolysis bullosa letalis, *Vestn Dermatol Venerol* 1:11, 1990.
2. Anton-Lamprecht I: Prenatal diagnosis of genetic disorders of the skin by means of electron microscopy, *Hum Genet* 59:392, 1981.
3. Anton-Lamprecht I, Rauskolb R, Jovanovic V et al: Prenatal diagnosis of epidermolysis bullosa dystrophica Hallopean-Siemens with electron microscopy of fetal skin, *Lancet* 2:1077, 1981.
4. Anton-Lamprecht I: Genetically induced abnormalities of epidermal differentiation and ultrastructure in ichthyoses and epidermolyses: pathogenesis, heterogeneity, fetal manifestations, and prenatal diagnosis, *J Invest Dermatol* 81:149s, 1983.
5. Arnold ML, Rauskolb R, Anton-Lamprecht I et al: Prenatal diagnosis of anhidrotic ectodermal dysplasia, *Prenat Diagn* 4:85, 1984.
6. Bakharev VA, Karetnikova NA, Mordovtsev VN et al: Prenatal diagnosis of several hereditary skin diseases, *Akush Ginekol* (Mosk) 1:53, 1989.
7. Bauer EA, Ludman MD, Goldberg JD et al: Antenatal diagnosis of recessive dystrophic epidermolysis bullosa: collagenase expression in cultured fibroblasts as a biochemical marker, *J Invest Dermatol* 87:597, 1986.
8. Blanchet-Bardon C, Dumez Y, Lab F et al: Prenatal diagnosis of harlequin fetus (letter), *Lancet* 1:132, 1983.
9. Blanchet-Bardon C, Dumez Y: Prenatal diagnosis of a harlequin fetus, *Semin Dermatol* 3:225, 1984.
10. Blanchet-Bardon C, Dumez Y, Lab F et al: Diagnostic prénatal par microscopie électronique d'un fœtus Arlequin, *Ann Pathol* 3:321, 1989.
11. Cadrin C, Golbus MS: Fetal tissue sampling: indications, techniques, complications, and experience with sampling of fetal skin, liver, and muscle. In *Fetal Medicine* (special issue), *West J Med* 159:269, 1993.
12. Chadefaux B, Rabier D, Kamour P: Prenatal diagnosis of enzymopathies of the urea cycle, *Ann Biol Clin* (Paris) 46:471, 1988.

13. Clapp DW, Dumenco LL, Hatzoglou M et al: Fetal liver hematopoietic stem cells as a target for in utero retroviral gene transfer, *Blood* 78:1132, 1991.

14. Dale BA, Perry TB, Holbrook KA et al: Biochemical examination of fetal skin specimens obtained by fetoscopy: use of the method for analysis of keratins and filaggrin, *Prenat Diagn* 6:37, 1986.

15. Eady RAJ, Gunner DB, Garner A et al: Prenatal diagnosis of oculocutaneous albinism by electron microscopy of fetal skin, *J Invest Dermatol* 80:210, 1983.

16. Eady RA, Gunner DB, Carbone LD et al: Prenatal diagnosis of bullous ichthyosiform erythroderma: detection of tonofilament clumps in fetal epidermal and amniotic fluid cells, *J Med Genet* 23:46, 1986.

17. Elias S, Mazur M, Sabbagha R et al: Prenatal diagnosis of harlequin ichthyosis, *Clin Genet* 17:275, 1980.

18. Elias S, Esterly NB: Prenatal diagnosis of hereditary skin disorders, *Clin Obstet Gynecol* 24:1069, 1981.

19. Elias S: Use of fetoscopy for the prenatal diagnosis of hereditary skin disorders. In Gedde-Dahl T, Wuepper KD, editors: *Prenatal diagnosis of heritable skin diseases*, Basel, Switzerland, 1987, Karger.

20. Esterly NB, Elias S: Antenatal diagnosis of genodermatoses, *J Am Acad Dermatol* 8:655, 1983.

21. Evans MI, Greb A, Kunkel LM et al: In utero fetal muscle biopsy for the diagnosis of Duchenne muscular dystrophy, *Am J Obstet Gynecol* 165:728, 1991.

22. Flake AW, Harrison MR, Adzick NS et al: Transplantation of fetal hematopoietic stem cells in utero: the creation of hematopoietic chimeras, *Science* 233:776, 1986.

23. Fox J, Hack AM, Fenton WA et al: Prenatal diagnosis of ornithine transcarbamylase deficiency with use of DNA polymorphisms, *N Engl J Med* 315:1205, 1986.

24. Gilgenkrantz S, Blanchet-Bardon C, Nazzaro V et al: Hypohidrotic ectodermal dysplasia: clinical study of a family of 30 over three generations, *Hum Genet* 81:120, 1989.

25. Golbus MS, Sagebiel RW, Filly RA et al: Prenatal diagnosis of congenital bullous ichthyosiform erythroderma (epidermolytic hyperkeratosis) by fetal skin biopsy, *N Engl J Med* 302:93, 1980.

26. Golbus MS, Simpson TJ, Koresawa M et al: The prenatal determination of glucose-6-phosphatase activity by fetal liver biopsy, *Prenat Diagn* 8:401, 1988.

27. Golbus MS, McGonigle KF, Goldberg JD et al: Fetal tissue sampling: the San Francisco experience with 190 pregnancies, *West J Med* 150:423, 1989.

28. Haraguchi Y, Uchino T, Takiguchi M et al: Cloning and sequence of a cDNA encoding human carbamyl phosphate synthetase I: molecular analysis of hyperammonemia, *Gene* 107:335, 1991.

29. Hayasaka K, Tada K, Fueri N et al: Prenatal diagnosis of nonketotic hyperglycinemia: enzymatic analysis of the glycine cleavage system in chorionic villi, *J Pediatr* 116:444, 1990.

30. Heagerty AH, Eady RA, Kennedy AR et al: Rapid prenatal diagnosis of epidermolysis bullosa letalis using GB3 monoclonal antibody, *Br J Dermatol* 117:271, 1987.

31. Hogge WA, Golbus MS: Surgical management of fetal malformations. In Evans MI, Fletcher JC, Dixler AO, Shulman JD, editors: *Fetal diagnosis and therapy: science, ethics, and the law*, Philadelphia, 1989, Lippincott Harper.

32. Holzgreve W, Golbus MS: Prenatal diagnosis of ornithine transcarbamylase deficiency utilizing fetal liver biopsy, *Am J Hum Genet* 36:320, 1984.

33. Jurkovic D, Kurjak A: Prenatalna dijagnostika epidermolysis bullosa hereditaria ultrazvucno vodenum biopsijom fetalne koze, *Lijec Vjesn* 111:60, 1989.

34. Kousseff BG, Matsuoka LY, Stenn KS et al: Prenatal diagnosis of Sjögren-Larsson syndrome, *J Pediatr* 101:998, 1982.

35. Kuller JA, Hoffman EP, Fries MH, Golbus MS: Prenatal diagnosis of Duchenne muscular dystrophy by fetal muscle biopsy, *Hum Genet* 90:34, 1992.

36. Kurjak A, Alfirevic Z, Jurkovic D: Ultrasonically guided fetal tissue biopsy, *Acta Obstet Gynecol Scand* 66:523, 1987.

37. Löfberg L, Gustavii B: Technical difficulties in fetal skin sampling, *Acta Obstet Gynecol Scand* 61: 505, 1982.

38. Löfberg L, Anton-Lamprecht I, Michalsson G et al: Prenatal exclusion of Herlitz syndrome by electron microscopy of fetal skin biopsies obtained at fetoscopy, *Acta Derm Venereol* 63:185, 1983.

39. Löfberg L, Gustavii B: "Blind" versus direct vision technique for fetal skin sampling in cases for prenatal diagnosis, *Clin Genet* 25:37, 1984.

40. Moen RC: Directions in gene therapy, *Blood Cells* 17:407, 1991.

41. Murotsuki J, Uehara S, Okamura K et al: Prenatal diagnosis of carbamoyl phosphate synthetase deficiency by fetal liver biopsy, *Nippon Sanka Fujinka Gakkai Zasshi (Acta Obstet Gynæcol Japan)* 43:1613, 1991.

42. Nazzaro V, Nicolini U, Ermacora E et al: Prenatal diagnosis of a case of Hallopeau-Siemens recessive dystrophic epidermolysis bullosa, *G Ital Dermatol Venereol* 124:1, 1989.
43. Nussbaum RL, Boggs BA, Beaudet AL et al: New mutation and prenatal diagnosis in OTC deficiency, *Am J Hum Genet* 38:149, 1986.
44. Perry TB, Holbrook KA, Hoff MS et al: Prenatal diagnosis of congenital non-bullous ichthyosiform erythroderma (lamellar ichthyosis), *Prenat Diagn* 7:145, 1987.
45. Piceni-Sereni L, Bachmann C, Pfister U et al: Prenatal diagnosis of carbamoyl-phosphate synthetase deficiency by fetal liver biopsy, *Prenat Diagn* 8:307, 1988.
46. Rodeck CH, Eady RAJ, Gosden CM: Prenatal diagnosis of epidermolysis bullosa letalis, *Lancet* 1:949, 1980.
47. Rodeck CH, Patrick AD, Pembrey ME et al: Fetal liver biopsy for prenatal diagnosis of ornithine carbamoyl transferase deficiency, *Lancet* 2:297, 1982.
48. Rodeck CH, Nicolaides KH: Fetoscopy and fetal tissue sampling, *Br Med Bull* 39:332, 1983.
49. Rosenmann A, Levin A, Neeman Z et al: Prenatal diagnosis of albinism, *Harefuah* 120:703, 1991.
50. Rozen R, Fox J, Fenton WA et al: Gene deletion and restriction length polymorphisms at the human ornithine transcarbamylase locus, *Nature* 313:815, 1985.
51. Shimizu H, Schofield OM, Eady RA: Prenatal diagnosis of lethal junctional epidermolysis bullosa by fetal skin biopsy, *Nippon Hifuka Gakkai Zasshi (Jpn J Dermatol)* 101:539, 1991.
52. Suzumori K, Kanzaki T: Prenatal diagnosis of harlequin ichthyosis by fetal skin biopsy: report of 2 cases, *Prenat Diagn* 11:451, 1991.
53. Touraine JL, Raudrant D, Royo C et al: In utero transplantation of stem cells in bare lymphocyte syndrome (letter), *Lancet* 1:1382, 1989.
54. Trepeta R, Stenn KS, Mahoney MJ: Prenatal diagnosis of Sjögren-Larsson syndrome, *Semin Dermatol* 3:221, 224, 1984.
55. Zonana J, Schinzel A, Upadhyaya M et al: Prenatal diagnosis of X-linked hypohidrotic ectodermal dysplasia by linkage analysis, *Am J Med Genet* 35:132, 1990.

PART SIX

FETAL TREATMENT

CHAPTER 22

Medical Fetal Therapy

STEPHEN K. HUNTER
JEROME YANKOWITZ

The advent of maternal-fetal medicine coupled with the advances made in prenatal diagnostic technology during the last decade has allowed more direct access to the fetus and, consequently, more accurate diagnoses. This access has also led to a better understanding of fetal physiology and of the pathophysiology of certain fetal diseases. With these advances, the perception of the fetus as a patient has become a reality and fetal therapy has become a new and exciting field. Fetal therapy can be classified as either medical or surgical. In this chapter, currently available medical fetal therapies will be discussed and potential future therapies, including gene therapy, will be examined.

✤ Patient Profile: Fetal therapy to prevent virilization of female genitalia caused by congenital adrenal hyperplasia

A 27-year-old patient (gravida 2, para 1001) underwent chorionic villus sampling (CVS) at 10 weeks' gestation 1 week ago. Her previous pregnancy resulted in the term delivery of a severely virilized female infant. Diagnostic evaluation of the infant showed that she had salt-wasting congenital adrenal hyperplasia (CAH). The child underwent surgical repair of her virilized genitalia and has done well on long-term steroid therapy. In this pregnancy, the patient was started on dexamethasone therapy at 5 weeks' gestation pending CVS results. Genetic and metabolic results from CVS show this fetus to be a female who also exhibits 21-hydroxylase deficiency. Dexamethasone therapy is thus continued throughout the pregnancy.

QUESTION 1: CAN CONGENITAL ADRENAL HYPERPLASIA BE TREATED EFFECTIVELY IN UTERO?

Congenital adrenal hyperplasia, an autosomal recessive disorder, results in varying degrees of virilization of the external genitalia of affected females (Figure 22-1). The disorder is caused, in most cases, by 21-hydroxylase deficiency. This enzyme is necessary for the

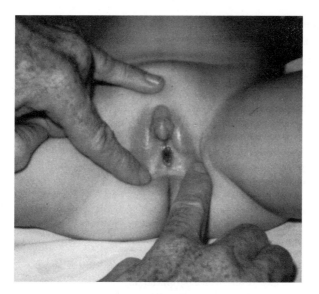

Fig. 22-1 Virilized female infant with congenital adrenal hyperplasia, demonstrating clitoral hypertrophy and mild labial fusion.

conversion of progesterone and 17-hydroxyprogesterone to 11-deoxycorticosterone and 11-deoxycortisol, respectively. Lack of this enzyme results in decreased cortisol production, leading to a compensatory increase in adrenocorticotropic hormone (ACTH) secretion, which in turn leads to elevated androgen production.

David and Forest[8] first reported the treatment of two patients with fetuses at risk for CAH. Each patient had previously had an affected infant. One patient received hydrocortisone, 40 mg/day, starting at 9.4 weeks. Amniocentesis at 18 weeks documented an affected female infant. Amniotic fluid 17-hydroxyprogesterone, androstenedione, and testosterone levels were still elevated at the time of amniocentesis, so the hydrocortisone dosage was increased to 50 mg/day. At birth, the infant had mild clitoral hypertrophy and slight posterior labial fusion. The second patient received 0.5 mg dexamethasone twice daily starting at 5 weeks' gestation. Amniocentesis at 15 weeks also revealed an affected female infant; in addition, low to normal 17-hydroxyprogesterone and androstenedione levels were documented, suggesting fetal adrenal suppression. Only extremely mild posterior labial fusion was present at birth. Evans and colleagues[10] later documented that fetal adrenal steroid levels in maternal urine decreased after initiation of maternal dexamethasone treatment. Since these initial reports, several investigators[11,24] have reported varying degrees of success, using several different treatment protocols.

Despite inconsistent results, in utero treatment of fetuses at risk for CAH is still recommended and remains a model for fetal therapy. Currently it is recommended that steroid therapy be started early in gestation (before CVS diagnosis is made) in any pregnancy in which the fetus is known to be at risk for CAH, to decrease the risk of virilization. Steroid therapy is either continued or stopped based on the CVS or amniocentesis results. Determination of whether the fetus is affected can be made using CVS or amniocentesis. Fetal cells can be tested by restriction fragment length polymorphism (RFLP) analysis and other molecular DNA techniques, including mutation analysis. Virilization is probably present by 10 to 14 weeks' gestation, so steroid treatment should probably not be initiated later than this time. Ideally, preconceptional counseling will help to ensure optimal prenatal treatment for this potentially congenitally and psychologically damaging condition.

QUESTION 2: CAN ANY OTHER METABOLIC DISORDERS BE TREATED IN UTERO?

In utero treatment of two other metabolic disorders has been reported in the literature: cobalamin deficiency and biotin deficiency, both inherited as autosomal recessive disorders. Cobalamin (vitamin B_{12}), in its coenzymatically activated form, is required for the conversion of methylmalonyl coenzyme A (CoA) to succinyl CoA. Defects in the production of this coenzyme, which is essential in the degradation of several amino acids and fatty acids, result in methylmalonic acidemia in affected infants, a life-threatening condition characterized by vomiting, failure to thrive, hepatomegaly, lethargy, and ketoacidosis. Morrow and associates[20] first reported the prenatal diagnosis of this condition by the detection of elevated methylmalonic acid in the amniotic fluid and maternal urine in a pregnancy in which the fetus was affected.

Ampola and colleagues[1] first described the prenatal treatment of a cobalamin-deficient fetus. The woman's first child died at the age of 3 months, and a diagnosis of cobalamin deficiency was made postmortem. In the second pregnancy, increased maternal urinary excretion of methylmalonic acid was noted during the second trimester. Amniocentesis was also remarkable for elevated methylmalonic acid in the amniotic fluid. At 32 weeks' gestation, maternal oral administration of cyanocobalamin, 10 mg/day in divided doses, was initiated. Intramuscular injections of cyanocobalamin, at a dosage of 5 mg/day, were given during the last 7 weeks of gestation. Maternal serum vitamin B_{12} levels were markedly elevated on this regimen, and urinary methylmalonic acid levels decreased significantly. Postnatal evaluation of neonatal fibroblasts confirmed the diagnosis of cobalamin deficiency. At 19 months of age, the infant was described as developmentally and neurologically normal. Rosenblatt and colleagues[29] subsequently reported a very similar case. They used intramuscular injections of 1 mg hydroxocobalamin given twice weekly beginning at 25 weeks' gestation. The infant was described as normal at birth.

Biotin deficiency is the other metabolic disorder for which in utero therapy has been reported. Biotin, a water-soluble vitamin B complex, acts as a prosthetic group for three mitochondrial carboxylase enzymes. A deficit of this complex results in multiple carboxylase deficiency. Affected infants present with severe metabolic acidosis, respiratory and eating difficulties, hypotonia, seizures, and dermatitis. If untreated, they become lethargic and then comatose and will eventually die. Prenatal diagnosis is possible by measuring biotinidase activity in amniocytes.

In a case reported by Packman and associates,[25] a woman who had previously had an infant affected with multiple carboxylase deficiency underwent amniocentesis at 17 weeks' gestation in the subsequent pregnancy. Elevated amniotic fluid methylcitrate levels and enzyme assay of the amniocytes, which demonstrated sensitivity to biotin deprivation, suggested the diagnosis of multiple carboxylase deficiency. Maternal biotin administration, 10 mg/day orally, was instituted at 23 weeks' gestation and continued until delivery. Cord blood biotin was 34 times the upper normal neonatal concentration at the time of delivery, and the diagnosis was confirmed with enzyme assay of neonatal skin fibroblasts. Roth and associates[30] described a second case of maternal administration of biotin during a twin pregnancy. This patient previously had two affected children, both of whom died of unremitting metabolic acidosis. In this subsequent twin pregnancy, biotin was administered to the mother, 10 mg/day orally, during the last 4 weeks of gestation. One of the twins was diagnosed postnatally as having multiple carboxylase deficiency.

The efficacy of prenatal versus postnatal treatment for these metabolic conditions has not been assessed. However, preliminary evidence suggests that prenatal treatment is safe for both mother and unaffected fetuses, and restoring normal metabolic status to a presumably affected fetus would seem reasonable, rather than waiting to treat the neonate.

QUESTION 3: WHAT OTHER FETAL CONDITIONS ARE CURRENTLY TREATABLE IN UTERO?

The box below contains a list of fetal disorders whose course can currently be altered by in utero medical therapy (including those already discussed).[38]

Fetal hypothyroidism is usually either congenital or the result of maternal ingestion of antithyroid agents, such as propylthiouracil. Congenital hypothyroidism is relatively common, occurring in about 1 in 3500 liveborn infants.[23] Regardless of the underlying cause, fetal hypothyroidism can lead to fetal goiter formation or developmental deficits, including language, visual-spatial, and perceptual-motor delays.[15,36] Large goiter formation can lead to malpositioning of the fetal head, rendering vaginal delivery traumatic or impossible. In

---

FETAL CONDITIONS TREATABLE IN UTERO

Metabolic disorders

Congenital adrenal hyperplasia
Cobalamin deficiency
Biotin deficiency

Endocrinologic disorders

Thyroid disease
  Hypothyroidism
  Hyperthyroidism

Cardiovascular disorders

Cardiac arrhythmias and dysrhythmias
  Supraventricular tachycardia
  Complete atrioventricular block

Hematologic disorders

Isoimmunization
Alloimmune thrombocytopenia

addition, fetal swallowing may be impaired, resulting in polyhydramnios and an increased rate of preterm labor. Fetal hypothyroidism can be suspected if fetal goiter is seen on ultrasound and is confirmed by evaluation of fetal thyroid hormone levels in fetal blood obtained by percutaneous umbilical blood sampling (PUBS).[9,26,15] Treatment consists of intraamniotic injection of 200 to 500 µg thyroxine every 1 to 2 weeks.

Fetal hyperthyroidism is usually caused by transplacental passage of maternal thyroid-stimulating immunoglobulins (TSI), which then stimulate the fetal thyroid gland. Diagnosis is possible with PUBS,[28,36] and therapy consists of maternal administration of antithyroid agents. Percutaneous umbilical blood sampling can also be used to assess the efficacy of treatment by evaluating fetal thyroid parameters.[28]

In utero congestive heart failure of the fetus is a serious and life-threatening condition that requires aggressive treatment. Supraventricular tachycardia (SVT) and complete atrioventricular block are the most common causes. For the treatment of SVT, digoxin is usually considered the drug of choice, but other medications have been used, including verapamil, procainamide, propranolol, flecainide, and amiodarone.

As gestation advances, digoxin crosses the placenta in increasing concentrations, with a third-trimester cord blood level of 50% to 83% of maternal concentration.[38] A maternal serum digoxin level toward the upper end of the therapeutic range is desired (2 ng/ml) unless signs of digoxin toxicity are evident.[16] Intravenous digoxin loading for the first 24 hours followed by oral maintenance with rather large doses (0.50 to 0.75 mg/day) is recommended. As a cautionary note, the use of digoxin for SVT secondary to Wolff-Parkinson-White (WPW) syndrome may be associated with rapid conduction of atrial fibrillation, resulting in ventricular fibrillation, which may be fatal.[16] In addition, transplacental passage of digoxin may be inefficient if the fetus already exhibits evidence of hydrops. Weiner and Thompson[35] describe a case in which direct fetal therapy with digoxin was used after transplacental therapy with digoxin, verapamil, and procainamide was unsuccessful in a 24-week fetus with SVT. Intramuscular (thigh or buttocks) injections of digoxin and digoxitin were initiated. The calculated half-life of the digoxin was only 15 hours, and repeat dosing intervals of 6 hours were needed to maintain normal fetal heart rate. Percutaneous umbilical blood sampling was performed to monitor fetal digoxin level. Therapy was discontinued after several days, and the fetal heart rate remained in the normal range until delivery at term. At 7 days of life, however, SVT recurred in the neonate but responded rapidly to digoxin therapy.

Complete atrioventricular (A-V) block is associated with structural heart defects in about one half of cases. In the remaining cases, in which cardiac anatomy is normal, most A-V blocks are found in fetuses whose mothers have autoimmune connective tissue disease or antinuclear antibodies. Watson and Katz[34] reported a case in which maternal steroid administration was used to treat a fetus with hydrops associated with antibody-mediated congenital heart block. Fetal ascites and pericardial effusion resolved with prednisone therapy, 10 mg/day, but no change in fetal heart block was observed. Copel and colleagues[4] reported on five cases of congenital heart block treated with dexamethasone, 4 mg/day orally, throughout pregnancy. Hydrops, seen in three fetuses, resolved after therapy was initiated, and the degree of heart block improved in two cases. Preliminary studies suggest that fetal steroid administration may prove to be a useful form of therapy for this condition, but further trials are needed for definitive proof. .

Another relatively common fetal condition requiring therapy is anemia, most commonly caused by hemolytic disease secondary to the transplacental passage of maternal antibodies directed against fetal red blood cell antigens. Therapy for hemolytic disease is given directly to the fetus via PUBS by the infusion of packed red blood cells (PRBCs), and in some instances intraperitoneally. Intrauterine transfusion is discussed in Chapter 20.

Alloimmune thrombocytopenia can be thought of as Rh disease of the platelet. Transplacental passage of maternal antibodies directed against fetal platelet antigens, usually PLA1, destroys the fetal platelets, producing severe thrombocytopenia in the fetus and a high incidence of intracranial hemorrhage (ICH) in utero.[22] This condition is usually diagnosed after the birth of an affected infant. Intravenous administration of large doses of immune globulin (1 g/kg) to the pregnant patient at weekly intervals has been shown to raise the fetal platelet count in 80% of cases.[2] In a report by Lynch and associates,[18] 18 women who had previously delivered infants with severe alloimmune thrombocytopenia were treated with weekly infusions of intravenous gamma-globulin (IVGG) or IVGG and corticosteroids. There were no intracranial hemorrhages in any of the treated fetuses, even when the fetal platelet count was less than 30,000/mm³. Among the previous 21 untreated siblings, 10 had an ICH.

QUESTION 4: ARE FETAL INFECTIONS POTENTIALLY TREATABLE?

An area of medical fetal therapy that has only recently been considered is the treatment of fetal infections. Daffos and colleagues[7] have reported on the prenatal diagnosis and treatment of congenital toxoplasmosis, a disease that is endemic to the French population. They concluded that prenatal diagnosis of congenital toxoplasmosis is practical and that prenatal antibiotic therapy reduces the severity of the disease manifestations.

Parvovirus, a DNA virus, causes a wide spectrum of diseases. Parvovirus can cause an acute aplastic anemia that results in high-output heart failure in the fetus. The most common clinical presentation of parvovirus in a symptomatic infected fetus is nonimmune hydrops (see *Patient Profile: Evaluation of fetal hydrops,* p. 149). Intrauterine transfusions of PRBCs have been successfully used to treat the fetus during the acute crisis.[31]

QUESTION 5: CAN PRECONCEPTIONAL THERAPY PREVENT FETAL MALFORMATION?

A number of preconceptional therapies appear to prevent or reduce the frequency of congenital anomalies. One example is diabetes mellitus, the leading identifiable cause of birth defects in the United states. In humans, the incidence of major congenital malformation in the offspring of diabetic women is two to five times that of nondiabetics. Several studies involving pregnant diabetic women have shown conclusively that preconceptional tight glucose control significantly reduces the incidence of malformation in these fetuses (see Chapter 2).[12,14]

Phenylketonuria (PKU), an autosomal recessive condition caused by a defect in the enzyme phenylalanine hydroxylase, is treated by following a diet low in phenylalanine. This therapy restores homeostatic phenylalanine metabolism and prevents impaired brain development in infants of mothers with poorly controlled PKU. A study by Lenke and Levy[17] found that of the offspring of women who had PKU with elevated antenatal phenylalanine levels of greater than 20 mg/dl, 90% had IQs less than 75, 73% had microcephaly, 17% had congenital heart defects, and approximately 50% had a low birthweight. Because amino acids are maintained against a concentration gradient across the placenta, the fetus is exposed to even higher phenylalanine concentrations than the mother. Other studies have shown that preconceptional treatment resulting in normal phenylalanine levels that are maintained throughout pregnancy significantly reduces or eliminates these effects.[27] These studies also show that therapy begun after conception is of little or no benefit.

The Medical Research Council Working Party on Phenylketonuria has provided guidelines for women with PKU who wish to conceive.[3] They state that phenylalanine concentrations during pregnancy need to be at least as strictly controlled as they were during infancy. Effective contraception should be used until control has been achieved. The goal is to delay pregnancy until a maternal serum phenylalanine concentration of 60 to 250 μmol/l can be maintained. The guidelines recommend that termination of pregnancy be offered to women who conceive while phenylalanine concentrations are 900 μmol/l or above because of the high risk of fetal malformations.

Folic acid has recently been advocated preconceptionally and periconceptionally to reduce the incidence of neural tube defects (NTDs) (see Chapter 1). Several studies address this issue.[5,6,21] Most studies demonstrated a benefit from the use of folic acid supplementation during the preconceptional and periconceptional periods. One retrospective study, though, did not support the finding of a lower incidence of NTDs in folic acid users.[19] However, most patients who participated in this study lived in California, which already has a lower than average NTD incidence, possibly because the diets of many Californians are already high in folic acid. Not only have studies shown a decrease in the recurrence of NTDs, but two recent reports also demonstrate a reduction in the initial occurrence rates.[5] Folate supplementation (0.4 mg/day) is currently recommended to all women at low risk who are attempting conception; a dose of 4 mg/day is recommended to patients who have had a previous pregnancy complicated by a neural tube defect.

QUESTION 6: WHAT IS THE CURRENT STATUS OF GENE THERAPY?

Recent advances in molecular genetics and recombinant DNA technology have made gene therapy a much more likely possibility. Gene therapy can be accomplished with either somatic or germ cell lines. Germ-line gene therapy will most likely be performed in the preimplantation pronucleus or in the very early embryo and therefore will not be discussed as possible in utero fetal therapy. Somatic cell gene therapy, using cells derived from donor bone marrow or liver, would be performed by the introduction of donor genes into a specific cell line. An example would be the transplantation of bone marrow to treat genetic disorders involving the hematopoietic cell lines, including erythroid, myeloid, lymphoid, and thromboid lines. Most of these therapies are now carried out postnatally. However, there have been a few instances in which in utero stem cell therapy has been attempted.[33] Touraine[33] has reported on the in utero transplantation and engraftment of fetal liver stem cells into three human fetuses for conditions such as Rh isoimmunization, thalassemia, and severe combined immunodeficiency disease.[13,37]

An emerging technology that may make in utero gene therapy feasible and would not require somatic cell line replacement or alteration until after delivery is the microencapsulation of recombinant cells within polymeric semipermeable membranes. These encapsulated cells are used as a delivery system for desired proteins. Cells are genetically engineered so that a specific desired protein is produced. The genetically altered cell is then encapsulated within a small microsphere made of a biocompatible polymer. The microsphere is engineered to have pores of a size that will allow the desired protein to diffuse out while preventing immune inactivation or destruction of the altered cell by the host's immune system. Encapsulated mouse fibroblasts containing the human growth hormone (hGH) gene (*Ltk-GH*) have been placed intraperitoneally in mice. There were detectable serum levels of hGH for the duration of the study (115 days). Moreover, encapsulated cells recovered from a recipient 1 year after transplantation continued to secrete high levels of hGH in culture.[32] The topic of stem cell transplantation for the treatment of genetic disease is covered in more detail in Chapter 31.

REFERENCES

1. Ampola MG, Mahoney MJ, Nakamura E, Tanaka K: Prenatal therapy of a patient with vitamin B_{12}–responsive methylmalonic acidemia, *N Engl J Med* 293:313, 1975.
2. Bussel JB, Berkowitz RL, McFarland JG et al: Antenatal treatment of neonatal alloimmune thrombocytopenia, *N Engl J Med* 319:1374, 1988.
3. Cockburn F, Barwell BE, Brenton DP et al: Recommendations on the dietary management of phenylketonuria, *Arch Dis Child* 68:426, 1993.
4. Copel JA, Buyon JP, Kleinman CS: Successful in utero treatment of fetal heart block, *Am J Obstet Gynecol* 170:280, 1994.
5. Czeizel AE, Dudas I: Prevention of the first occurrence of neural-tube defects by periconceptional vitamin supplementation, *N Engl J Med* 327:1832, 1992.
6. Czeizel AE: Prevention of congenital abnormalities by periconceptional multivitamin supplementation, *Br Med J* 306:1645, 1993.
7. Daffos F, Forestier F, Capella-Pavlovsky M et al: Prenatal management of 746 pregnancies at risk for congenital toxoplasmosis, *N Engl J Med* 318: 271, 1988.
8. David M, Forest MG: Prenatal treatment of congenital adrenal hyperplasia resulting from 21-hydroxylase deficiency, *J Pediatr* 105:799, 1984.
9. Davidson KM, Richards DS, Schatz DA, Fisher DA: Successful in-utero treatment of fetal goiter and hypothyroidism, *N Engl J Med* 324:543, 1991.
10. Evans MI, Chrousos GP, Mann DW et al: Pharmacologic suppression of the fetal adrenal gland in utero: attempted prevention of abnormal external genital masculization in suspected congenital adrenal hyperplasia, *JAMA* 253:1015, 1985.
11. Forest MG, David M, Morel Y: Prenatal diagnosis and treatment of 21-hydroxylase deficiency, *J Steroid Biochem Molec Biol* 45:75, 1993.

12. Fuhrmann K, Reiter H, Semmler H et al: Prevention of congenital malformations in infants of insulin-dependent diabetic mothers, *Diabetes Care* 6:219, 1983.

13. Golbus MS, Bauer D: Transplantation of hematopoietic stem cells. In Harrison MR, Golbus MS, Filly RA, editors: *The unborn patient*, ed 2, Philadelphia, 1990, WB Saunders.

14. Goldman JA, Dicker D, Feldberg D et al: Pregnancy outcome in patients with insulin–dependent diabetes mellitus with preconceptional diabetic control: a comparative study, *Am J Obstet Gynecol* 155:293, 1986.

15. Kirsch M, Josefsberg Z, Schoenfeld A et al: Congenital hereditary hypothyroidism—prenatal diagnosis and treatment, *Prenat Diagn* 10:491, 1990.

16. Kleinman CS, Copel JA: In utero cardiac therapy in fetus and mother. In Reece EA, Hobbins JC, Mahoney MJ, Petrie RH, editors: *Medicine of the fetus and mother*, Philadelphia, 1992, JB Lippincott.

17. Lenke RR, Levy HL: Maternal phenylketonuria and hyperphenylalaninemia, *N Engl J Med* 303:1202, 1980.

18. Lynch L, Bussel JB, McFarland JG et al: Antenatal treatment of alloimmune thrombocytopenia, *Obstet Gynecol* 80:67, 1992.

19. Mills JL, Rhoads GG, Simpson JL et al: The absence of a relation between the periconceptional use of vitamins and neural-tube defects, *N Engl J Med* 321:430, 1989.

20. Morrow G, Schwarz RH, Hallock JA, Barness LA: Prenatal detection of methylmalonic acidemia, *J Pediatr* 77:120, 1970.

21. MRC Vitamin Study Research Group: Prevention of neural tube defects: results of the medical research council vitamin study, *Lancet* 338:131, 1991.

22. Mueller-Eckhardt C, Grubert A, Weisheit M et al: 348 cases of suspected neonatal alloimmune thrombocytopenia, *Lancet* 2:363, 1989.

23. New England Congenital Hypothyroidism Collaborative Study: Characteristics of infantile hypothyroidism discovered on neonatal screening, *J Pediatr* 104:593, 1984.

24. New MI: Prenatal diagnosis and treatment of adrenogenital syndrome (steroid 21-hydroxylase deficiency), *Dev Pharmacol Ther* 15:200, 1990.

25. Packman S, Cowan MJ, Golbus MS et al: Prenatal treatment of biotin-responsive multiple carboxylase deficiency, *Lancet* 1:1435, 1982.

26. Perelman AH, Johnson RL, Clemens RD et al: Intrauterine diagnosis and treatment of fetal goitrous hypothyroidism, *J Clin Endocrinol Metab* 71:618, 1990.

27. Platt LD, Koch R, Azen C et al: Maternal Phenylketonuria Collaborative Study, obstetric aspects and outcome: the first 6 years, *Am J Obstet Gynecol* 166:1150, 1992.

28. Porreco RP, Bloch CA: Fetal blood sampling in the management of intrauterine thyrotoxicosis, *Obstet Gynecol* 76:509, 1990.

29. Rosenblatt DS, Cooper BA, Schmutz SM et al: Prenatal vitamin B_{12} therapy of a fetus with methylcobalamin deficiency (cobalamin E disease), *Lancet* 1:1127, 1985.

30. Roth KS, Yang W, Allan L et al: Prenatal administration of biotin in biotin responsive multiple carboxylase deficiency, *Pediatr Res* 16:126, 1982.

31. Sahakian V, Weiner CP, Naides SJ et al: Intrauterine transfusion treatment of nonimmune hydrops fetalis secondary to human parvovirus B19 infection, *Am J Obstet Gynecol* 164:1090, 1991.

32. Tai IT, Sun AM: Microencapsulation of recombinant cells: a new delivery system for gene therapy, *FASEB J* 7:1062, 1993.

33. Touraine JL: In utero transplantation of stem cells in humans, *Nouv Rev Fr Hematol* 32:441, 1990.

34. Watson WJ, Katz VL: Steroid therapy for hydrops associated with antibody-mediated congenital heart block, *Am J Obstet Gynecol* 165:553, 1991.

35. Weiner CP, Thompson MIB: Direct treatment of fetal supraventricular tachycardia after failed transplacental therapy, *Am J Obstet Gynecol* 158:570, 1988.

36. Wenstrom KD, Weiner CP, Williamson RA, Grant SS: Prenatal diagnosis of fetal hyperthyroidism using funipuncture, *Obstet Gynecol* 76:513, 1990.

37. Westgren M, Brubakk AM, Bui TH et al: Fetal stem cell transplantation in fetal α and β-thalassemia (abstract), *Am J Obstet Gynecol* 170:398, 1994.

38. Yankowitz J, Golbus MS: Fetal treatment. In Simpson JE, Elias S, editors: *Essentials of prenatal diagnosis*, New York, 1993, Churchill Livingstone.

CHAPTER 23

Surgical Fetal Therapy

JEROME YANKOWITZ

A.W. Liley's work[19] during the 1950s and 1960s in treating hydrops fetalis by intrauterine transfusion is often cited as the first example of fetal therapy. Today, a few conditions are known to be improved by in utero surgical treatment. For a condition to be considered for this type of intervention, several criteria must be fulfilled. First, there must be a comprehensive understanding of the natural history and pathophysiology of the disorder. Second, it must be known from evaluation in animal models that the treatment is safe and feasible. Third, it must be established that the condition is not irreversibly lethal in utero or soon after delivery. Finally, it must be known that in utero treatment improves outcome or allows survival, whereas delaying treatment until delivery results in a poor prognosis. Conditions that are currently thought to meet these criteria include obstructive uropathy, acardiac twinning, cystic adenomatoid malformation, fetal hydrothorax, and congenital diaphragmatic hernia. A review of surgical fetal therapy has recently been published.[34]

❧ Patient Profile: Prenatal diagnosis and treatment of congenital diaphragmatic hernia

A 22-year-old patient (gravida 2, para 1001) undergoes an ultrasound examination at 19 weeks' gestation. The examination confirms gestational age. A stomach bubble is seen in the fetal thorax adjacent to the bowel, and peristalsis of the bowel within the thorax is seen during the ultrasound examination (Figure 23-1). The liver appears to be in the abdominal cavity. No other abnormalities are seen. The patient is told that her fetus has a diaphragmatic hernia, and she is given information about this condition. She is appropriately distraught but also wants to gather as much information as possible about the implications of this diagnosis.

QUESTION 1: WHAT IS THE INCIDENCE OF CONGENITAL DIAPHRAGMATIC HERNIA, AND WHAT SYNDROMES ARE ASSOCIATED WITH IT?

Congenital diaphragmatic hernia (CDH) is a defect in development of the diaphragm and occurs in 0.033% to 0.05% of births. This figure was confirmed by a recent study of over

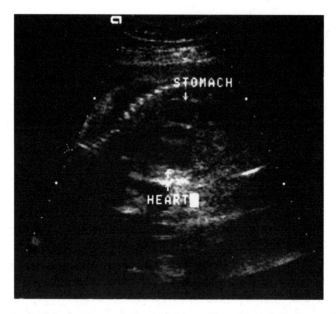

Fig. 23-1 Longitudinal fetal ultrasound view of a fetus with congenital diaphragmatic hernia. The fetal stomach is visualized in the chest, which is pathognomonic for this condition.

700,000 births in California from 1983 to 1987, which showed an incidence of 3.3 per 10,000 births.[30] An incidence of 2.7 per 10,000 births was shown in the Iowa Birth Defects Registry, in which data were evaluated for over 240,000 births between 1983 and 1988.[32] The incidence of CDH is higher prenatally, since in utero and neonatal deaths are not included in incidence figures. Among 20,000 fetuses assessed by ultrasound examination at a large referral center, 19 cases of CDH were found.[3] The defect can have a variety of causes and has been associated with Beckwith-Wiedemann syndrome, Fryns syndrome, Simpson-Golabi-Behmel syndrome, de Lange syndrome, Marfan sydrome, DiGeorge sequence, and chromosome abnormalities, such as trisomy 13 and trisomy 18.[15] Therefore, whenever CDH is seen, a karyotype is recommended to rule out chromosome abnormalities. Thorough ultrasound and fetal echocardiographic examinations should be performed to search for other anomalies that may point to a syndromic cause for the defect.

QUESTION 2: WHAT IS THE PROGNOSIS FOR A FETUS WITH PRENATALLY DIAGNOSED CONGENITAL DIAPHRAGMATIC HERNIA?

For the neonate who has survived life in utero, the main cause of death is respiratory failure due to pulmonary hypoplasia. Persistent pulmonary hypertension is also a significant concern and is seen because the development of the pulmonary vasculature parallels that of the airways. During the 13 years since the initial use of extracorporeal membrane oxygenation (ECMO) for this condition, appropriate neonatal surgical management and use of ECMO have resulted in a reported survival rate of over 70%.[13] Use of high-frequency ventilation and nitric oxide (a potent vasodilator) may also be beneficial. Others have reported a higher mortality rate for this condition, but a 50% likelihood of survival for a liveborn neonate with CDH seems to be a fair prediction.[30,33]

Adzick and colleagues[1] and Benacerraf and Adzick[3] have reported a much lower survival rate for cases diagnosed prenatally. Harrison and associates[11] have attributed this difference to "hidden mortality." They argue that only milder cases of CDH are seen in tertiary care centers; the more severe cases, they believe, are lost through stillbirth, early neonatal death, and failed resuscitations at birth, before diagnosis. In contrast, Thorpe-Beeston and colleagues[29] reported a 60% rate of survival among fetuses with isolated CDH (no other structural anomalies and a normal karyotype) diagnosed by ultrasound examination between 18 and 36 weeks' gestation. A similar higher rate of survival was seen in a small cohort from Iowa.[32]

In cases of isolated CDH, there are no ultrasound findings that have been shown to have a consistent predictive value in separating a high-risk from a low-risk group. Given the range in predicted mortality rates for prenatally diagnosed cases of CDH, a survival rate of about 50% again appears to be a fair figure to use for counseling purposes.

QUESTION 3: CAN CONGENITAL DIAPHRAGMATIC HERNIA BE SURGICALLY CORRECTED IN UTERO?

Harrison and colleagues[12] have attempted in utero surgical correction of this disorder in over 20 human cases. The surgery involves a laparotomy and hysterotomy on the pregnant patient, partial removal of the fetus from the uterus, abdominal and thoracic incisions into the fetus, repair of the CDH, and placement of Gore-Tex grafts for repair of the diaphragmatic and abdominal incisions. Unfortunately, survival of these fetuses has been disappointingly low—20% at best. This figure is lower than any published figures for survival without surgery. In addition, the procedure causes significant morbidity for the pregnant woman, including a need for cesarean sections for that pregnancy and for all future deliveries due to the hysterotomy. Preterm labor and premature rupture of the membranes associated with the performance of the hysterotomy on the gravid uterus are also significant problems. Certainly, at this time, fetal surgery for CDH must be considered investigational.

QUESTION 4: HAS FETAL SURGERY BEEN ATTEMPTED FOR OTHER PULMONARY CONDITIONS?

Congenital cystic adenomatoid malformation (CCAM) is a rare pulmonary malformation characterized by overgrowth of the terminal bronchioles. The lesions are classified according to the relative amount of cystic and solid components. These masses can cause mediastinal shift with pulmonary, esophageal, and vena caval compression, leading to polyhydramnios and fetal hydrops. As a result, the clinical presentation can range from in utero death with nonimmune hydrops to incidental discovery during childhood. Lesions have been noted to regress over time.[16] The overall prognosis for fetuses with antenatally discovered lesions appears to depend on whether the condition progresses to hydrops, which portends a very poor outcome. Polyhydramnios does not appear to be a useful prognostic indicator. Fetal surgery in several high-risk cases resulted in liveborn infants discharged to home.[2,17] This successful outcome represents a marked improvement over the nearly uniform fatality associated with development of hydrops. The rare patient carrying a fetus with CCAM and hydrops should be counseled about the probability of intrauterine or neonatal death. Patients should be aware that fetal surgery is an experimental option but also that in a minority of cases even mild hydrops has resolved, resulting in a liveborn infant.[23,24]

Fetal hydrothorax has also been treated in utero.[27] This condition, as with the other fetal pulmonary abnormalities, causes morbidity and mortality by compressing the developing fetal lung, resulting in pulmonary hypoplasia. The lesion can also cause generalized hydrops by mass effect and vascular compression. A complete evaluation for fetal and chromosome abnormalities should be performed, and a search for an immune or infectious cause should be undertaken. Fetuses with unilateral hydrothorax and hydrothorax without hydrops have virtually uniform survival and should not be treated in utero. Development of hydrops portends a 50% or lower rate of survival.[31] Needle drainage and percutaneous placement of a thoracoamniotic or pleurocutaneous shunt have yielded only modest results, with a 50% to 75% survival rate. This has been due to rapid reaccumulation of fluid, necessitating multiple drainage procedures; blockage or dislodging of shunts; and pulmonary hypoplasia despite apparently adequate drainage.

QUESTION 5: HAS FETAL SURGERY BEEN USED FOR NONPULMONARY CONDITIONS?

The obstructive uropathies, whether caused by posterior urethral valves or by other factors, have received attention as defects that may be successfully treated in utero. As with the pulmonary lesions, the most serious concern is pulmonary hypoplasia as a result of urinary tract obstruction leading to oligohydramnios. Fetal therapy is reserved for cases in which obstruction is bilateral, amniotic fluid is decreased but not absent, gestational age is less than 30 weeks, and no other anomalies are present.[10] The fetus with unilateral obstruction or mild disease with normal amniotic fluid volume does not require invasive therapy. The fetus with severely dysplastic kidneys and no amniotic fluid early in gestation has irreversible disease and pulmonary hypoplasia and will not benefit from invasive in utero therapy. When the fetus that may benefit from in utero intervention has been identified,[10] the fetal bladder can be decompressed by placement of a vesicoamniotic shunt or a suprapubic vesicostomy.

Objective criteria have been developed for evaluating fetal urinary electrolyte values to identify the group of fetuses most likely to benefit from in utero therapy.[6] Poor renal function was predicted for the fetus with hypertonic urine evidenced by a urinary sodium level above 100 mEq/ml, a chloride level above 90 mEq/ml, or osmolarity above 210 mOsm. Good renal function was predicted for fetuses with values lower than these cut-offs. However, the predictive value of urinary electrolyte patterns has not been as reliable when evaluated by others.[33] Review of the UCSF Fetal Treatment Program's results shows that urine electrolyte values were not predictive of survival or renal status after delivery.[8] Assessment of fetal urinary amino acids[18] and evaluation of the microproteins β_2-microglobulin and α_1-microglobulin have been suggested as diagnostic tools for determining whether a fetus should undergo in utero therapy.[4,14] The prognostic value of these measurements has not been definitively shown.

Over 70 cases of fetuses with obstructive uropathy treated with placement of a vesicoamniotic shunt have been reported.[20] There was a 41% survival rate and a procedure-related death rate of 4.6%. Complications of catheter use included chorioamnionitis, displacement, and clogging. Open fetal surgery to marsupialize the fetal bladder has been undertaken in at least five cases at the University of California–San Francisco.[5] Two of these fetuses died after delivery due to pulmonary hypoplasia, one died at 9 months from complications of gastrointestinal malformations not diagnosed antenatally, one required renal transplantation at 2.5 years of age, and another had chronic renal insufficiency. Clearly, better criteria by which to choose appropriate candidates for intervention must be established and the final cost-benefit analysis of in utero intervention must be addressed before this therapy can move beyond the experimental stages.

Fetal surgical treatment has also been used in cases of acardiac twinning, a rare complication of monozygotic twin pregnancies. It occurs in about 1% of these pregnancies and in about 1 in 35,000 pregnancies overall. Acardiac twinning can lead to congestive heart failure of the pump (normal) twin, polyhydramnios, and preterm delivery. Likelihood of survival of the normal twin is about 50% to 60%.[22] Percutaneous placement of a thrombogenic coil into the umbilical cord of the acardiac twin at 24 weeks has resulted in delivery of the healthy pump twin at 39 weeks.[25] Hysterotomy with removal of the acardiac twin has been performed in at least seven cases at three institutions, with six surviving infants.[7,9,26]

QUESTION 6: ARE ANY OTHER AREAS OF POSSIBLE SURGICAL FETAL INTERVENTION ON THE HORIZON?

Treatment of complications of multifetal pregnancies has been attempted, with promising results. Percutaneous selective reduction of multifetal pregnancies has been performed for a variety of indications and appears to be relatively safe in experienced hands (see Chapter 24).[34] Use of invasive procedures to treat twin-to-twin transfusion has been reported, with good outcomes.[34]

Fetal surgery certainly promises to be beneficial in treating a variety of other conditions, but in each of these instances there has been little or no experience. At least two attempts at in utero correction of fetal aortic stenosis have been reported, both with a poor outcome.[21] Some investigators have even suggested the possibility of in utero repair of fetal cleft lip and palate.[28]

Overall, surgical fetal therapy is a fascinating and exciting area that is only beginning to be explored. The etiology and natural history of each disorder must be more precisely described before this very invasive treatment modality can be appropriately applied.

REFERENCES

1. Adzick NS, Harrison MR, Glick PL et al: Diaphragmatic hernia in the fetus: prenatal diagnosis and outcome in 94 cases, *J Pediatr Surg* 20:357, 1985.

2. Adzick NS, Harrison MR, Flake AW et al: Fetal surgery for cystic adenomatoid malformation of the lung, *J Pediatr Surg* 28:806, 1993.

3. Benacerraf BR, Adzick NS: Fetal diaphragmatic hernia: ultrasound diagnosis and clinical outcome in 19 cases, *Am J Obstet Gynecol* 156:573, 1987.

4. Burghard R, Pallacks R, Gordjani N et al: Microproteins in amniotic fluid as an index of changes in fetal renal function during development, *Pediatr Nephrol* 1:574, 1987.

5. Crombleholme TM, Harrison MR, Langer JC et al: Early experience with open fetal surgery for congenital hydronephrosis, *J Pediatr Surg* 23:1114, 1988.

6. Crombleholme TM, Harrison MR, Golbus MS et al: Fetal intervention in obstructive uropathy: prognostic indicators and efficacy of intervention, *Amer J Obstet Gynecol* 162:1239, 1990.

7. Fries MH, Goldberg JD, Golbus MS: Treatment of acardiac-acephalus twin gestations by hysterotomy and selective delivery, *Obstet Gynecol* 79:601, 1992.

8. Fries M, Norton M, Goldberg J et al: Renal function after in utero intervention for fetal obstructive uropathy, *Am J Obstet Gynecol* 166:357, 1992.

9. Ginsberg NA, Applebaum M, Rabin SA et al: Term birth after midtrimester hysterotomy and selective delivery of an acardiac twin, *Am J Obstet Gynecol* 167:33, 1992.

10. Golbus MS, Harrison MR, Filly RA: Prenatal diagnosis and treatment of fetal hydronephrosis, *Semin Perinatol* 7:102, 1983.

11. Harrison MR, Bressack MA, Churg AM, De Lorimer AA: Correction of congenital diaphragmatic hernia in utero. II. Simulated correction permits fetal lung growth with survival at birth, *Surgery* 88:260, 1980.

12. Harrison MR, Adzick NS, Longaker MT et al: Successful repair in utero of a fetal diaphragmatic hernia after removal of herniated viscera from the left thorax, *N Engl J Med* 322:1582, 1990.

13. Heiss K, Manning P, Oldham KT et al: Reversal of mortality for congenital diaphragmatic hernia with ECMO, *Ann Surg* 209:225, 1989.

14. Holzgreve W, Lison A, Bulla M: SDS-PAGE as an additional test to determine fetal kidney function prior to intrauterine diversion of urinary tract obstruction, *Fetal Ther* 4:93, 1989.

15. Jones KL, editor: *Smith's recognizable patterns of human malformation*, ed 4, Philadelphia, 1988, WB Saunders.

16. Kuller JA, Laifer SA, Tagge EP et al: Diminution in size of a fetal intrathoracic mass: caution against aggressive in utero management, *Am J Perinatol* 9:223, 1992.

17. Kuller JA, Yankowitz J, Goldberg J et al: Outcome of antenatally diagnosed cystic adenomatoid malformations, *Amer J Obstet Gynecol* 167:1038, 1992.

18. Lenz S, Lund-Hansen T, Bang J, Christensen E: A possible prenatal evaluation of renal function by amino acid analysis on fetal urine, *Prenat Diagn* 5:259, 1985.

19. Liley AW: Intrauterine transfusion of fœtus in hæmolytic disease, *Br Med* 2:1107, 1963.

20. Manning FA, Harrison MR, Rodeck C, Members of the International Fetal Medicine and Surgery Society: Catheter shunts for fetal hydronephrosis and hydrocephalus: report of the International Fetal Surgery Registry, *N Engl J Med* 315:336, 1986.

21. Maxwell D, Allan L, Tynan MJ: Balloon dilatation of the aortic valve in the fetus: a report of two cases, *Br Heart J* 65:256, 1991.

22. Moore TR, Gale S, Benirschke K: Perinatal outcome of forty-nine pregnancies complicated by acardiac twinning, *Am J Obstet Gynecol* 163:907, 1990.

23. Morris E, Constantine G, McHugo J: Cystic adenomatoid malformation of the lung: an obstetric and ultrasound perspective, *Eur J Obstet Gynecol Reprod Biol* 40:11, 1991.

24. Neilson IR, Russo P, Laberge J-M et al: Congenital adenomatoid malformation of the lung: current management and prognosis, *J Pediatr Surg* 26:975, 1991.

25. Porreco RP, Barton SM, Haverkamp AD: Occlusion of umbilical artery in acardiac, acephalic twin, *Lancet* 337:326, 1991.

26. Robie GF, Payne GG, Morgan MA: Selective delivery of an acardiac, acephalic twin, *N Engl J Med* 320:512, 1989.

27. Rodeck CH, Fisk NM, Fraser DI, Nicolini U: Long-term in utero drainage of fetal hydrothorax, *N Engl J Med* 319:1135, 1988.

28. Strauss RP, Davis JU: Prenatal detection and fetal surgery of clefts and craniofacial abnormalities in humans: social and ethical issues, *Cleft Palate J* 27:176, 1990.

29. Thorpe-Beeston JG, Gosden CM, Nicolaides KH: Prenatal diagnosis of congenital diaphragmatic hernia: associated malformations and chromosomal defects. *Fetal Ther* 4:21, 1989.

30. Torfs CP, Curry CJR, Bateson TF, Honore LH: A population-based study of congenital diaphragmatic hernia, *Teratology* 46:555, 1992.

31. Weber AM, Philipson EH: Fetal pleural effusion: a review and meta-analysis for prognostic indicators, *Obstet Gynecol* 79:281, 1992.

32. Wenstrom KD, Weiner CP, Hanson JW: A five-year experience with congenital diaphragmatic hernia, *Am J Obstet Gynecol* 165:838, 1991.

33. Wilkins IA, Chitkara U, Lynch L et al: The nonpredictive value of fetal urinary electrolytes: preliminary report of outcomes and correlations with pathologic diagnosis, *Amer J Obstet Gynecol* 157:694, 1987.

34. Yankowitz J, Golbus MS: Fetal Treatment. In Simpson JL, Elias S, editors: *Essentials of prenatal diagnosis*, New York, 1993, Churchill Livingstone.

CHAPTER 24

Multifetal Pregnancy Reduction

NANCY C. CHESCHEIR

Multifetal pregnancies pose special challenges to women, families, obstetric care providers, and the fetuses themselves. The incidence of high-order multifetal pregnancies (in excess of two fetuses) is increasing as the application of assisted reproductive technology becomes more widespread. To improve the outcomes of selected pregnancies complicated by multiple fetuses, a procedure known variably as *multifetal pregnancy reduction (MFPR)* or *selective reduction* has evolved. Using this procedure, the number of living fetuses in a multifetal pregnancy is reduced to a number thought to be more compatible with healthy outcomes for the greatest number of fetuses. Multifetal reduction generally has one of five therapeutic goals: (1) to decrease the risk of severe prematurity and its attendant morbidity and mortality in a high-order multifetal pregnancy; (2) to diminish the risk of premature birth, even in a twin pregnancy, in a woman with significant *a priori* risk factors for prematurity (e.g., in a woman with a history of in utero DES exposure, previous premature birth of a singleton, and a multiply scarred uterus); (3) to accommodate parental choices regarding the number of children resulting from a pregnancy; (4) to reduce the risk of morbidity and mortality in women with preexisting severe chronic renal disease or hypertension in whom the risk of preeclampsia is already increased; and (5) to avoid the delivery of an infant with a significant structural or karyotypic abnormality when there is a normal co-twin.

❧ Patient Profile: Second-trimester multifetal pregnancy reduction

A couple seeks infertility therapy after 3 years of primary infertility. He is 39 and she is 38 years old. They ultimately conceive twins, using gamete intrafallopian transfer (GIFT) technology and their own gametes. The first trimester of pregnancy is uncomplicated. At 15 weeks' gestation, ultrasound examination and amniocentesis are performed because of increased maternal age. The ultrasound scan demonstrates discordant twins separated by a thick membrane. The placentas are on opposite sides of the uterus. The fetus on the maternal right and inferior in the uterus (fetus A) has symmetric measurements consistent with 15 weeks' gestation. Nuchal skinfold thickness is 3 mm. The heart and the other anatomic features appear normal. Fetus B occupies the superior portion of the left side of the uterus. This fetus has measurements consistent with a head size of 14 weeks, an abdomen of 13 weeks, and femur and humerus measurements of 13 weeks. The nuchal skinfold measurement is 6 mm. The fetus has bilateral pleural effusions. An amniocentesis of fetus A shows a normal female karyotype, 46,XX, while fetus B is a male with trisomy 21. These results are available to the family at 16.5 weeks' gestation. The family undergoes extensive genetic and obstetric counseling. After much consideration, they request selective reduction of the affected twin. The procedure is performed transabdominally, using intrathoracic potassium chloride–induced asystole, and is aided by the uterine map and careful description that was made at the time of the amniocentesis. As well, the phenotype of the affected fetus is clearly male, and the growth asymmetry is more apparent at the time of the procedure, at 17.5 weeks. Upon completion of the selective reduction, before the needle is removed from the sac, a confirmatory amniocentesis is obtained. The woman delivers a healthy girl at 38 weeks' gestation without complications.

QUESTION 1: UNDER WHAT CIRCUMSTANCES IS SELECTIVE REDUCTION OF AN ABNORMAL FETUS A REASONABLE OPTION?

The appropriateness of selective reduction for a given woman hinges not only on medical criteria but also on the woman's moral and ethical beliefs. As with induced abortion, there is no universally accepted set of criteria that will satisfy all health care providers or all patients. Some general guidelines, however, can be set forth.

In the case described here, the first question that should be addressed is the certainty of the diagnosis. The obstetric care provider should discuss with the patient not only the degree of abnormality of the affected twin but also the degree of certainty that the unaffected twin is indeed "normal." Thorough ultrasound examination of both twins is vital. Karyotype examination of both twins should be considered given the phenotypic variablity of the major aneuploidies. Monozygotic twins could be concordant for the trisomy 18 genotype but have widely disparate phenotypic expression such that one of the fetuses appears normal on scan. It cannot be emphasized enough that careful mapping of the uterine contents is vital when invasive procedures are performed in multifetal pregnancies so that if selective reduction is later performed the affected twin can be identified with certainty. Fetal blood sampling should be performed before the selective reduction to document which fetus is karyotypically abnormal if there is any uncertainty. A precise uterine map should be made at the time of the blood sampling in order to guide the procedure once the repeat karyotype is available.

If the abnormal twin is thought to have a clearly lethal malformation, such as renal agenesis or anencephaly, the important effect of the continued in utero survival of the affected fetus is the resultant risk of prematurity to the normal co-twin. If the anomaly is associated with polyhydramnios (e.g., anencephaly) or occurs in a woman who has independent factors that increase the risk of prematurity, selective reduction of a lethally affected fetus may be reasonable. On the other hand, it may also be reasonable to provide expectant management of that pregnancy without having the patient take both the medical and emotional risks of a selective reduction. This approach is especially appropriate if the twins are thought to be monochorionic, since all cases of attempted selective reduction of one of a set of mono-chorionic twins have resulted in the death of the unaffected twin, presumably due to embolic phenomena or to passage of the lethal agent to the unaffected twin.[7,9,19,21] If the abnormal twin is thought to have a potentially morbid but not universally lethal malformation (e.g., Down syndrome) and they are dichorionic, then selective reduction may be appropriate if it does not conflict with the woman's moral and ethical values and is desired by the patient.

QUESTION 2: WHAT ARE THE POTENTIAL COMPLICATIONS OF SELECTIVE REDUCTION PROCEDURES?

In any MFPR, there is the given mortality for the embryos that are killed. This mortality must be included when mortality rates of MFPR are compared with those of nonreduced pregnancies. The literature is more complete regarding the complication rate following first-trimester reduction performed due to high-order multifetal pregnancy than for those typically performed later in the second trimester after the identification of a fetal malformation. The reported rates of complete pregnancy loss after first-trimester MFPR vary widely, ranging from 6% to 15%.*

In an article describing the collective experience in 183 second-trimester selective terminations performed at nine centers in four countries, Evans and colleagues[7] showed a 14.4% loss rate for procedures performed after 16 weeks and a 5.4% loss rate for pro-cedures performed at or before 16 weeks. As with any technically challenging procedure, there appears to be a learning curve along which the loss rate is higher. For instance, Lynch and associates[13] report that six of eight losses in 85 procedures occurred in the first 20 they performed.[13] Pregnancy loss is also related to the background increased rate of loss for multifetal pregnancies, since most are reduced at least to twins. The underlying pathogenic mechanisms for loss of the complete pregnancy include premature rupture of the membranes, chorioamnionitis, premature labor, and incompetent cervix.

Because most MFPRs for high-order multifetal pregnancies are performed by about 11 weeks' gestation, at which time ultrasound evaluation for structural fetal anomalies is less sensitive than later and the rate of malformation in multifetal pregnancies, especially those involving monozygotic twins, is increased relative to singletons, it is important to offer fur-ther evaluation of these pregnancies during the second trimester.[2] There are no reports of any teratogenic effect of the reduction procedure on the surviving embryos.[20] In the case of mono-chorionic twins, as noted earlier, both twins die after the induced death of one. It is theoret-ically possible that if one survived, embolic phenomena could cause porencephaly or other damage. For these reasons, monochorionic twins should be either left alone or both killed. Another option, clearly more invasive and potentially morbid, includes hysterotomy with removal of the affected monochorionic twin. This procedure has been performed in the case of acardiac twins (see Chapter 23).[8]

---

*References 5, 13, 14, 16, 19, 21, and 22.

The literature on first-trimester reduction of high-order multifetal pregnancies indicates the possibility of an increased risk of growth restriction among the fetuses who survive the selective reduction of their co-fetuses. This has not been a universally noted phenomenon and, if it exists, may be related to the altered hormonal milieu that results from infertility therapy.[5,14,16]

Maternal medical complications from MFPR are the same as those for any intraamniotic procedure and are minimal. There is a small risk of chorioamnionitis. Some but not all published protocols call for the prophylactic administration of antibiotics.[3,13,18,21] Theoretically, there is a risk of maternal coagulopathy resulting from a retained dead fetus. However, as shown by Chescheir and Seeds[4] and Mitra and colleagues,[15] the maternal fibrinogen level may fall, but it is unusual for there to be a resultant clinical coagulopathy when the loss occurs early in pregnancy. It seems reasonable to consider this theoretic risk during the preoperative discussions, but the chance is so minimal that it is not cost effective to perform routine coagulation monitoring.

The emotional complications of this procedure are extremely distressing. Whenever a family is faced with the knowledge that their fetus has a malformation, they feel grief and pain. The decision to abort a malformed fetus is understandably a complex one. If the stress of making this decision is compounded by the difficulty of trying to maintain the health of co-fetuses, it is easy to imagine the complex psychologic processes that occur as a woman and her partner must simultaneously feel grief and joy. It is important to discuss this with the woman and her partner during the preoperative discussions and to provide additional support for them.

As with any medical therapy, MFPR carries potential risks and benefits. Despite the highly charged emotional condition of the families after a fetal anomaly is diagnosed in a multifetal pregnancy, it is vital that a frank discussion of the risks and benefits be held. Although the data regarding background rates of complications associated with multifetal pregnancies are variable, this information must be included in the discussion. Even so, selective reduction is a reasonably safe alternative to abortion of the entire pregnancy and offers a choice to families who do not wish to deliver a child known to have a significantly handicapping illness or malformation.

QUESTION 3: HOW IS SELECTIVE REDUCTION PERFORMED?

The selective reduction procedures that have been described in the literature take one of three tacks: (1) removal of embryos from the uterus; (2) destruction of the embryos; or (3) induction of asystole by injection of an arrhythmogenic agent. Most published series now report using either transabdominal or transvaginal injection of potassium chloride into the fetal thorax to induce asytole.

The first reported selective termination of a fetus occurred in 1978, when a twin with Hurler syndrome was given an intracardiac puncture that produce asystole.[1] Later, a hysterotomy for removal of a fetus with trisomy 21 was performed after the operator was unable to grasp and occlude the umbilical cord.[12] In 1986, Dumez and Oury[6] described the transcervical minisuction curettage at 8 to 11 weeks as a method of MFPR. A 50% pregnancy loss rate was associated with this method. In 1988, Itskovitz and colleagues[11] performed transvaginal needle aspiration to reduce a quadruplet pregnancy to twins. Such a procedure would clearly need to be performed extremely early in gestation, or the fetal mass would be too great. One advantage to the patient of waiting until 10 to 11 weeks' gestation is that there is a significant rate of "vanishing embryos," a natural decrease in the number of fetuses in utero, saving the woman and her partner from having to make this difficult decision.

Kerenyi and Chitkara[12] used intracardiac puncture to exsanguinate a 20-week Down syndrome fetus. Boulot and associates[3] used forceps to crush early first-trimester fetuses but abandoned this method in favor of transabdominal potassium chloride injection. Rodeck and colleagues[17] were the first to describe intrafetal injection of arrhythmogenic agents to induce asystole. In 1982, using fetoscopic guidance, they injected air intravascularly. Although successful, this method resulted in very poor visualization of the fetus after the air was injected.

During the first trimester, ultrasound guidance of a 22-gauge needle into the fetal thorax with injection of about 1 mEq potassium chloride will cause asystole. It is important to direct the needle into the thorax and to continue watching for a return of the heart beat for at least 1 minute before removing the needle. In addition, repeat scanning 20 to 30 minutes after presumed completion of the procedure is vital because of the possibility that the heart beat will have resumed.[17] The injection can then be repeated. When the procedure is performed later in gestation, direct intracardiac injection of potassium chloride is required to achieve asystole.

Authorities on this procedure disagree regarding the appropriate route. Some operators believe that the safest approach is the transvaginal route, while others advocate the transabdominal route. In experienced hands, both appear to be safe.*

QUESTION 4: WHAT FOLLOW-UP CARE IS IMPORTANT AFTER A WOMAN UNDERGOES A SELECTIVE REDUCTION PROCEDURE?

If the patient is Rh-negative, Rh immune globulin should be administered on the same day as the MFPR procedure. Ultrasound examination within 2 to 3 days of the procedure is important to document that the fetus or fetuses selected for termination are dead and that the other or others continue to show fetal heart beats. Repeat procedures may be performed expediently if necessary.

The patient may need a considerable amount of support during the weeks following the procedure until it becomes more clear that the likely outcome of the pregnancy will be a good one. Some women may have spotting or cramping after the procedure, and appropriate analgesics will often help. Amniotic fluid or serum may leak, presumably from the involuting sac or sacs. Grau and colleagues[10] have shown that second-trimester MSAFP levels are elevated after first-trimester selective reduction. Thus, MSAFP screening should not be offered to patients who have undergone this procedure.

---

*References 3, 13, 18-20, and 22.

The remainder of the prenatal care should be directed toward addressing normal obstetric and family issues. In the presence of continued multiple fetuses, significant efforts should be made to identify premature labor to prevent premature birth.

REFERENCES

1. Aberg A, Mitelman F, Cantz M, Gehler J: Cardiac puncture of fetus with Hurler's disease avoiding abortion of unaffected co-twin, *Lancet* 2: 990, 1978.
2. Botting BJ, Davies IM, Macfarlane AJ: Recent trends in the incidence of multiple births and associated mortality, *Arch Dis Child* 62:941, 1987.
3. Boulot P, Hedon B, Pelliccia G et al: Multifetal pregnancy reduction: a consecutive series of 61 cases, *Br J Obstet Gynæcol* 100:63, 1993.
4. Chescheir NC, Seeds JW: Spontaneous resolution of hypofibrinogenemia associated with death of a twin in utero, *Am J Obstet Gynecol* 159:1183, 1988.
5. Donner C, De Maertelaer V, Rodesch F: Multifetal pregnancy reduction: comparison of obstetrical results with spontaneous twin gestations, *Eur J Obstet Gynecol* 44:181, 1992.
6. Dumez Y, Oury JF: Method for first trimester selective abortion in multiple pregnancy, *Contrib Gynecol Obstet* 15:50, 1986.
7. Evans MI, Goldberg JD, Dommergues M et al: Efficacy of second trimester selective termination for fetal abnormalities: international collaborative experience among the world's largest centers, *Am J Obstet Gynecol* 171:90, 1994.
8. Fries MH, Goldberg JD, Golbus MS: Treatment of acardiac-acephalus twin gestations by hysterotomy and selective delivery, *Obstet Gynecol* 79:601, 1992.
9. Golbus MS, Cunningham N, Goldberg JD et al: Selective termination of multiple gestations, *Am J Med Genet* 31: 339, 1988.
10. Grau P, Robinson L, Tabsh K, Crandall BF: Elevated maternal serum alpha-fetoprotein and amniotic fluid alpha-fetoprotein after multifetal pregnancy reduction, *Obstet Gynecol* 76:1042, 1990.
11. Itskovitz J, Boldes R, Thaler I et al: Transvaginal ultrasonography-guided aspiration of gestational sacs for selective abortion in multiple pregnancy, *Am J Obstet Gynecol* 160:15, 1989.
12. Kerenyi TD, Chitkara U: Selective birth in twin pregnancy with discordance for Down's syndrome, *N Engl J Med* 304:1525, 1981.
13. Lynch L, Berkowitz RL, Chitkara U, Alvarez M: First-trimester transabdominal multifetal pregnancy reduction: a report of 85 cases, *Obstet Gynecol* 75:735, 1990.
14. Melgar CA, Rosenfeld DL, Rawlinson K, Greenberg M: Perinatal outcome after multifetal reduction to twins compared with nonreduced multiple gestations, *Obstet Gynecol* 78:763, 1991.
15. Mitra AG, Chescheir NC, Tatum BS, Cefalo RC: Spontaneous resolution of hypofibrinogenemia in a triplet gestation associated with second trimester in utero demise of two fetuses, *Am J Perinatol* 10:448, 1993.
16. Porreco RP, Burke MS, Hendrix ML: Multifetal reduction of triplets and pregnancy outcome, *Obstet Gynecol* 78:335, 1991.
17. Rodeck CH, Mibashan RS, Abramowicz J, Campbell S: Selective feticide of the affected twin by fetoscopic air embolism, *Prenat Diagn* 2:189, 1982.
18. Tabsh KMA: Transabdominal multifetal pregnancy reduction: report of 40 cases, *Obstet Gynecol* 75:739, 1990.
19. Timor-Tritsch IE, Peisner DB, Monteagudo A et al: Multifetal pregnancy reduction by transvaginal puncture: evaluation of the technique used in 134 cases, *Am J Obstet Gynecol* 168:799, 1993.
20. Vauthier-Brouzes D, Lefebvre G: Selective reduction in multifetal pregnancies: technical and psychological aspects, *Fertil Steril* 57:1012, 1992.
21. Weinblatt V, Wapner R, Davis G et al: Fetal reduction and selective termination in multifetal pregnancy: outcomes, ethical and counseling issues, March of Dimes Birth Defects Foundation, *Birth defects: original article series* 26:81, 1990.
22. Yovel I, Yaron Y, Amit A et al: Embryo reduction in multifetal pregnancies using saline injection: comparison between the transvaginal and the transabdominal approach, *Hum Reprod* 7:1173, 1992.

CHAPTER 25

Pregnancy Termination

NANCY C. CHESCHEIR

Prenatal diagnosis conveys specific information to couples about the health of their potential child. Providers are usually able to reassure patients that the fetus does not have the disorder or disorders for which testing has been performed. Reassurance, in fact, is the primary reason, according to Farrant,[2] that women request prenatal diagnostic services. Nonetheless, abnormal results of prenatal testing are all too frequently found, and the parents are forced to decide between continuing the pregnancy and terminating it if it is early enough in the pregnancy for abortion still to be a legal option. Because a small number of women who undergo prenatal testing ultimately elect to terminate the pregnancy, abortion counseling and services must be readily available.

❧ Patient Profile: Pregnancy termination after diagnosis of a lethal condition

A 25-year-old woman (gravida 1, para 0000) is referred at 18 weeks' gestation for prenatal diagnosis because her testing results indicate elevated MSAFP, at 3.7 MoM. The ultrasound examination confirms the gestational age in this singleton pregnancy, but visualization is hampered by the lack of amniotic fluid. Large multicystic masses are present in the fetal abdomen, and no bladder is seen. The cysts are clustered on both sides of the midabdomen and are of various sizes. The fetal chest is quite small relative to the size of the heart. The diagnosis of bilateral multicystic kidney disease is made, and the patient is apprised of the lethality of this condition. She elects to terminate the pregnancy. The patient is given the option of either dilation and evacuation (D & E) or induced labor with urea and prostaglandin suppositories; she elects to undergo D & E.

QUESTION 1: WHAT INFORMATION SHOULD A PATIENT BE GIVEN ABOUT A FETAL DISORDER TO ALLOW HER TO MAKE AN EDUCATED DECISION ABOUT PREGNANCY MANAGEMENT?

The informing interview is emotional, complex, and critically important, since patients must hear and assimilate very difficult information and then make an irrevocable decision

194

based on this information. This "interview" may in fact take place over several days, with a variety of counselors and physicians providing the information. Unfortunately, because of late gestational age at the time of the diagnosis or because of geographic constraints, the ideal process of information assimilation frequently must be abbreviated drastically. Nonetheless, the following kinds of information must be conveyed.

Medical Information

Unless the patient has previously had an affected child or relative or is herself a health care provider, she probably began the process of prenatal diagnosis naïve about the many medical conditions that may affect the fetus (see the box below for a list of medical questions that should be discussed during the informing interview). A simple description of the type and severity of the abnormality, including the embryology or pathogenesis, is usually well received by families. It is also vital to gather detailed family history information from both sides of the family and to look for historical information that might implicate an avoidable teratogen. If the abnormality is karyotypic, a brief description of the chromosomes with a pictorial illustration of their fetus's karyotype may help. In addition, photographs or line drawings of fetuses with similar structural abnormalities may improve the family's comprehension of their fetus's health. Consultation with pediatric care providers, such as pediatric surgeons, intensivists, neurologists, or geneticists, may be of additional help.

MEDICAL QUESTIONS TO BE ADDRESSED
DURING THE INFORMING INTERVIEW

What is the nature of the disorder?
How certain is the diagnosis?
What caused the abnormality?
Is the abnormality likely to recur in a future pregnancy?
Is the disorder likely to cause stillbirth or immediate neonatal death?
Will the abnormality cause long-term handicapping illness, or is it completely treatable?
Does the abnormality pose any medical threat to the mother, either antepartum or intrapartum?
Could there be any other problems associated with the disorder?
Is a second opinion available?
Is prenatal treatment available, either locally or at another center?

Psychosocial Information

Grief and guilt are intertwined for families when an abnormality is found by prenatal testing. It may be helpful to recommend that the family take a brief break before they make any decision, to allow them time to recover from any acute remorse, to gather members of their support network, such as extended family, and perhaps to become more receptive to information. It may be helpful to put the patient in touch with another family who has had an affected child, although this step should be undertaken only with caution. The family should be advised that grieving after a "genetic" termination is common (77% to 94%).[1,5] No similar data are available to compare this grieving response to that of women whose newborns are diagnosed with major defects. Some effort should be made to explore the potential implications for the entire family, including older siblings, of choosing to raise a seriously handicapped child. The provider should explore the patient's faith and, if reasonable, recommend that she discuss some of these issues with a trusted clergy member or counselor.

Legal Information

Abortion and treatment laws as they apply to the woman's particular situation should be discussed. The provider of this information must be knowledgeable and provide accurate information regarding the relevant laws.

All of this information ideally should be conveyed in a nondirective manner, with respect for the woman's needs for support and time. If the patient ultimately elects to terminate the pregnancy, additional information about the medical aspects of the abortion procedure should be shared.

QUESTION 2: WHICH PROCEDURE IS BETTER: DILATION AND EVACUATION OR INDUCTION OF LABOR?

There is no clear-cut answer to the question of which method of pregnancy termination is preferred. With the exception of abnormalities that are diagnosable by first-trimester ultrasound examination or chorionic villus sampling, most abnormal prenatal diagnoses are made during the second trimester.

One of the criteria by which each method of termination should be judged is whether the abortion provider is more skilled in one method than another. If so, she or he may have a bias toward that procedure. Dilation and evacuation in skilled hands and with special preparation of the patient, including overnight hydrophilic dilator placement, has been proved to have few maternal complications.[3,7] The use of ultrasound guidance with demonstration of a clear uterine stripe at presumed conclusion of the procedure diminishes the risk of retained products. This method has the advantage of any outpatient procedure, is quick, and fulfills many women's wish to "get it over with." However, this detachment may impair the grieving process, and for some, the opportunity to see and hold the fetus if an induction procedure is employed will militate against a D & E. Confirmation of structural abnormalities and diagnosis of unsuspected additional problems may be impaired by the relative unfamiliarity of most surgical pathologists with diagnostic pathology of fetal fragments. On the other hand, Shulman[6,7] reports adequate confirmation of diagnoses by motivated, skilled pathologists and by confirmatory karyotype and DNA analysis. Molecular, genetic, and karyotypic analyses can be made and confirmed on D & E specimens.

Induction of labor usually results in an intact fetus, allowing for more complete autopsy evaluation. This method also affords a more "normal" grieving ritual, with the possibilities of taking photographs, holding the fetus, collecting mementos, such as footprints and locks of hair, and arranging for funeral services. Many women and their families find these options useful and important at this time, as with other perinatal losses. Some families also find it helpful to confirm for themselves the physical defect heretofore visualized only on ultrasound and about which they may have had some doubts. Induction of labor usually requires a 24-hour hospitalization, with hydrophilic dilators placed on the day before admission. The potential dilemma posed by the live birth of an abortus, with its enormous emotional effect on the woman and her medical attendants, although less likely to occur with intraamniotic instillation of urea, can be avoided altogether by interfetal injection of a lethal dose of digoxin or intracardiac potassium chloride.[3,4] If this procedure is not performed, the patient and all concerned should be informed of the possibility of a live birth, and an appropriate ethical plan of management should be developed.

Hysterotomy is a technique used only infrequently for genetic termination. Compared with the other two aforementioned methods of pregnancy termination, it carries greater immediate surgical risk. Because of the frequent necessity of placing the uterine incision into the thick portion of the endometrium, hysterotomy usually requires that all subsequent deliveries be by cesarean section. Higher hospitalization costs will also be incurred with this method. Because intraperitoneal surgery is performed, the risk of postoperative adhesive disease is also significant. Hysterotomy should, therefore, be considered only if the other alternatives are not available or are otherwise contraindicated. Sterilization at the time of genetic termination is contraindicated under most circumstances and certainly is not adequate justification for offering hysterotomy as a first choice for method of termination.

QUESTION 3: WHAT FOLLOW-UP CARE SHOULD THE PATIENT RECEIVE AFTER PREGNANCY TERMINATION?

Appropriate aftercare and counseling for women terminating abnormal fetuses have not been thoroughly studied. However, White-Van Mourik and colleagues' report[8] of the care given to 166 women before and after pregnancy termination for neural tube defects between 1983 and 1985 is an excellent description of an inadequate system. Of these women, 81% received no discharge information about posttermination sequelae, such as breast engorgement (experienced by 60% for at least 5 days), vaginal bleeding, altered sexuality, and conflicting emotions. Both White-Van Mourik and colleagues[8] and Lloyd and Lawrence[5] suggest that comprehensive genetic counseling, discussions of family history, recurrence risk, possible preventive strategies, and prenatal diagnosis in future pregnancies should be delayed for 6 to 12 weeks after termination. A letter of summary for the woman and her partner is also helpful.

Assessment of the patient's psychologic status after termination is important. Contact by the primary physician, nurse, or trained counselor either by telephone or in person during the days and weeks following discharge conveys to the woman one's concern, shows her that emotional support is available, and allows the health-care provider to assess her psychologic well-being.

Advice regarding when a woman should consider another pregnancy is largely based on folklore. Although pregnancy outcome, in general, is improved with an optimal interconceptional interval, "optimal" is variably defined.[9] It seems prudent to recommend that families wait until all laboratory and autopsy results are available in case important information about preventive strategies is obtained. It also seems wise to advise patients that some emotional healing should occur before another pregnancy is undertaken, although the time needed for this varies greatly among individuals.

REFERENCES

1. Blumberg BD, Golbus MS, Hanson KH: The psychological sequelae of abortion performed for a genetic indication, *Am J Obstet Gynecol* 122:799, 1975.
2. Farrant W: Who's for amniocentesis? The politics of prenatal screening. In Homans H, editor: *The sexual politics of reproduction,* London, 1985, Gower.
3. Hern WM, Zen C, Ferguson K et al: Outpatient abortion for fetal anomaly and fetal death from 15-34 menstrual weeks' gestation: techniques and clinical management, *Obstet Gynecol* 81:301, 1993.
4. Isada NB, Pryde PG, Johnson MP et al: Fetal intracardiac potassium chloride injection to avoid the hopeless resuscitation of an abnormal abortus: I. Clinical issues, *Obstet Gynecol* 80:296, 1992.
5. Lloyd J, Lawrence KM: Sequelae and support after termination of pregnancy for fetal malformation, *Br Med J* 290:907, 1985.
6. Shulman LP, Ling FW, Meyers CM et al: Dilation and evacuation for second-trimester genetic pregnancy termination: update on a reliable and preferable method, *Am J Gynecol Health* 5:11, 1991.
7. Shulman LP, Ling FW, Meyers CM et al: Dilation and evacuation for second trimester genetic pregnancy termination, *Obstet Gynecol* 75:1037, 1990.
8. White-Van Mourik MCA, Connor JM, Ferguson-Smith MA: Patient care before and after termination of pregnancy for neural tube defects, *Prenat Diagn* 10:497, 1990.
9. Winikoff B: The effects of birth spacing on child and maternal health, *Studies Fam Plann* 14:231, 1983.

PART SEVEN

TERATOLOGY

CHAPTER 26

Viral Infections in Pregnancy

M. CATHLEEN McCOY

Viral infections in pregnancy can range from a simple maternal upper respiratory infection with little fetal consequence to an infection that is deadly for both mother and baby. When teratogenic fetal infections in pregnancy are discussed, the TORCH acronym comes immediately to mind. *TORCH* stands for *t*oxoplasmosis (caused by the protozoan *Toxoplasma gondii*); *o*ther infections (namely, syphilis, caused by the spirochete *Treponema pallidum*); *r*ubella; *c*ytomegalovirus (CMV); and *h*erpes simplex virus. However, these are no longer the only infections with known fetal effects. Several other viruses, including parvovirus B19, varicella zoster, coxsackievirus, and adenovirus, have been associated with fetal and neonatal abnormalities.

Definitive diagnosis of a potentially teratogenic viral infection in the mother may be difficult. The determination of fetal infection may require invasive testing, with its associated risks to the pregnancy and sometimes uncertain results. Molecular testing, coupled with the invasive techniques of amniocentesis, chorionic villus sampling (CVS), and percutaneous umbilical blood sampling, has made possible the present but continually evolving evaluation of a fetus with a possible congenital infection.

❧ Patient Profile: Prenatal diagnosis of hydrocephalus secondary to viral infection

A 24-year-old nursing student (gravida 3, para 1011) comes for a routine office visit at 28 weeks' gestation. Her pregnancy has been uncomplicated to date, but she reports decreased fetal movement. Her fundal height is 24 cm. She called the practice nurse 1 month ago complaining of myalgia and a fever lasting for 3 days. These symptoms resolved with fluids and rest after 1 week. An ultrasound examination performed for decreased fundal height reveals fetal biometric measurements consistent with 25 weeks. Hydrocephalus is noted, with a posterior lateral atrial measurement of 18 mm (normal <10 mm). She is appropriately distressed and wants to know the implications of these findings.

QUESTION 1: SHOULD ROUTINE PRENATAL SCREENING FOR VIRAL INFECTION OR IMMUNITY BE PERFORMED?

The choice to screen prenatally for immunity to a virus should depend on the planned use of these results. Currently the only viral screen routinely performed in most obstetric practices is the rubella titer. This serologic test should be repeated with every pregnancy because the immunologic memory can decrease over time. Foreknowledge of a nonimmune result allows for a more meaningful follow-up maternal serologic study should exposure occur or a fetal abnormality be identified. Most nonimmune women are not exposed to rubella during pregnancy, and rubella vaccine is administered postpartum to these women.

The optimal time for rubella screening is at a family planning or preconceptional visit. Rubella vaccine is a live attenuated virus that causes nasopharyngeal shedding for several weeks after vaccination. Conception should be avoided during the 3 months after the vaccination. However, to date, no babies have been born with congenital rubella syndrome when conceived within 3 months of the vaccination.[2]

Prenatal screening for viral infection is most controversial for CMV. Known immunity, although it decreases the risk and severity of congenital CMV, is not completely protective. Congenital CMV affects approximately 1% of neonates, or about 35,000 newborns annually in the United States. There is a 25% incidence of sequelae in neonates of mothers with primary infection, versus 8% in neonates of mothers with recurrent infection.[7] Routine screening for viral immunity to CMV is not recommended. Instead, vigorous handwashing and even gloves should be used by women in high-exposure situations, such as day-care workers, dialysis technicians, or other health-care personnel. A live attenuated vaccine for CMV is being developed. This vaccine is thought to be cost beneficial in preventing congenital CMV but requires further testing.[15]

Parvovirus immunity assessment is recommended only with a close contact or maternal symptoms. At least 50% of pregnant women exhibit serologic evidence of prior infection with parvovirus B19.[16] For women who have negative IgG antibodies after an exposure, parvovirus IgM can be drawn up to 8 weeks later. If the IgM is still negative, acute infection is unlikely. If maternal seroconversion occurs, the risk of fetal death is approximately 5%.[16]

With almost 90% of reproductive-age women immune to varicella zoster virus, it is rare to find a pregnant woman without antibodies even if she has no recall of infection. Like parvovirus, only with a close contact or maternal rash are varicella IgG and IgM antibodies assessed. These recommendations may change, since the varicella vaccine has now been approved by the FDA for general use. As with rubella, women of reproductive age may be tested for varicella immunity and vaccinated before pregnancy or postpartum.

Pregnant women are not routinely screened for adenovirus and coxsackievirus because, as with CMV, most patients have antibodies. However, reinfection can occur and may occasionally be the cause of fetal disease. Screening for herpes simplex is not cost effective, particularly because of the rarity of fetal effects.

QUESTION 2: WHAT MATERNAL SYMPTOMS SHOULD PROMPT AN ASSESSMENT FOR CONGENITAL VIRAL INFECTION?

Rubella

The symptoms of rubella infection include fever, postauricular or suboccipital lymphadenopathy, arthralgia, and a transient erythematous rash. In a known nonimmune patient, acute and convalescent titers should be drawn. Maternal infection is indicated by a fourfold rise in IgG titer. Enders and colleagues[5] showed that if the rubella rash appeared before or within 11 days after the last menstrual period, no fetal infection occurred. After a first-trimester maternal rubella exposure, approximately 85% of fetuses are infected. Eighty-five percent of these fetuses are found to have sequelae.[5]

Cytomegalovirus

About 50% of women of reproductive age are susceptible to CMV, depending on the socioeconomic class studied.[4] Almost all maternal infections are asymptomatic. However, a small percentage of women will exhibit malaise, myalgia, and fever, which may be accompanied by a lymphocytosis and elevated liver function studies.

Varicella zoster

Varicella infection is usually evident from the classic skin lesions that progress from macules and papules to vesicles and pustules. If a pregnant woman is exposed to varicella and does not have antibodies, she should receive varicella zoster immune globulin (VZIG) within 96 hours. The goal of VZIG use is to decrease maternal clinical manifestations, particularly pneumonia. Although pneumonia is not more common among pregnant adults with varicella, the severity and mortality rate are probably higher during pregnancy. When respiratory symptoms are present, intravenous acyclovir is recommended.[19] There is no known fetal benefit from administration of VZIG once a maternal infection has been documented.

Parvovirus B19

The most common clinical manifestation of parvovirus B19 is erythema infectiosum. Although infected adults are usually asymptomatic, the symptoms may include fever, adenopathy, arthralgia, and mild arthritis. The classic "slapped cheek" rash commonly seen in children is not usually found in adults.

Adenovirus and coxsackievirus

Adenovirus symptoms are the common cold symptoms of rhinorrhea, cough, and sore throat. Coxsackievirus group B infection can cause pleurodynia, meningoencephalitis, and myocarditis.

Herpes simplex virus

Herpes has both a primary and a secondary pattern. Primary infections have many systemic symptoms, such as fever, headache, and adenopathy, as well as the raised tender ulcerative lesion or lesions. Secondary infections are usually less severe, with fewer systemic symptoms and fewer perineal lesions. Most, but not all, perinatal infections are acquired by vaginal exposure during delivery, especially at the time of primary infection.

QUESTION 3: WHICH FETAL ULTRASOUND FINDINGS SUGGEST VIRAL INFECTION? WHAT FOLLOW-UP IS ADEQUATE TO DETERMINE WHETHER THE FETUS HAS BEEN AFFECTED?

One of the more frequent findings that raises concern about a possible fetal viral infection is symmetric growth retardation. Intrauterine death and hydrops are the other findings that prompt an evaluation for intrauterine infection.

In general, a detailed ultrasound examination should be performed before the limits of pregnancy termination have been reached in one's state so that parents can choose whether to continue the pregnancy with the most complete information possible about the fetus. After viability, diagnosis of a fetal abnormality may influence delivery location or timing. Certainly, many congenital features caused by most of the viruses are not visible by ultrasound examination. Often the ultrasound examinations are provided to reassure parents who are concerned about their baby's normality.

Rubella

Findings more specific to rubella are cataracts and cardiac lesions, such as pulmonary stenosis. Serial ultrasound examinations performed during the second and third trimesters usually allow the visible effects of rubella infection to be detected.

Cytomegalovirus

Findings more specific to CMV are microcephaly, hydrocephalus (as described in the patient profile) with possible periventricular calcification, and hepatosplenomegaly with possible intraabdominal calcification or ascites. Oligohydramnios is a common feature and may require serial sonographic assessment of amniotic fluid volume.[12] There have also been reports of myocarditis with CMV, which can manifest as heart block or supraventricular tachycardia.[6,11] In the absence of oligohydramnios and cardiac manifestations, serial ultrasound examinations usually allow detection of the visible effects of CMV infection. In most children, sequelae of CMV are not evident at birth but become apparent during the next several years.[7]

Herpes simplex virus

The anomalies associated with herpes simplex fetal infection are similar to those associated with CMV. Skin vesicles or scarring at birth and destructive vascular brain lesions, such as hydranencephaly, are more specific to HSV.[10,8] One or two third-trimester ultrasound examinations generally allow detection of visible HSV-related fetal abnormalities.

Varicella zoster

Fetal abnormalities caused by varicella zoster infection are less common (fewer than 10%) than once projected.[1,13,14] Fetal abnormalities described are similar to those associated with CMV. However, cutaneous scars, limb hypoplasia, and rudimentary digits are the more classic malformations of chickenpox that might be visualized by ultrasound. Serial second- and third-trimester ultrasound examinations often allow detection of microcephaly, growth retardation, or many of the other findings present in fetuses with varicella infection.

Parvovirus B19

To date, the only fetal abnormalities clearly associated with parvovirus B19 are isolated ascites and hydrops. There have also been reports of cardiomyopathy and growth deficiency associated with parvovirus.[21] Once maternal IgM antibodies have been identified, sonographic examinations should be performed at 1- to 2-week intervals for approximately 8 weeks. If at that point no sonographic evidence of fetal infection is found, a reasonable follow-up study would be one third-trimester examination to assess growth. Some investigators also perform serial assessments of maternal serum α-fetoprotein (MSAFP) levels. Preliminary reports suggest that fetal infection with parvovirus may cause an elevation in MSAFP.

Coxsackievirus

Infection with coxsackievirus B during the first trimester has been associated with urogenital malformations, such as epispadias and cryptorchidism, that would not likely be identified by fetal ultrasound. Coxsackievirus infection is also associated with myocarditis and could manifest as a fetal arrhythmia.[3] Doppler evaluation of fetal heart tones and a third-trimester ultrasound examination to assess growth are reasonable follow-up studies.

Adenovirus

Adenovirus was recently found by polymerase chain reaction (PCR) of fetal or placental tissue or amniotic fluid in 9 of 33 fetuses with nonimmune hydrops or ascites. Polymerase chain reaction is a technique in which DNA polymerase is used to amplify 10^6 to 10^7 copies of a specific sequence of DNA. This amplification allows identification of viruses when tissue is no longer culturable. Because PCR is such a sensitive technique, it is critical to eliminate sources of maternal contamination that may cause a false-positive result.[20] If nonimmune hydrops develops presumably secondary to adenovirus infection, ultrasound examinations should be performed at approximately 1- to 2-week intervals to assess for worsening or resolution of hydrops.

QUESTION 4: WHICH PROCEDURES AND LABORATORY TESTS ARE MOST ACCURATE IN ASSESSING FETAL VIRAL INFECTION?

Fetal viral testing is still evolving as investigators learn more about PCR. Polymerase chain reaction allows detection of viral genomic material, and although it is very specific, the sensitivity for any given fetal infection is still unclear.

When a fetal abnormality is diagnosed and viral infection is among the differential diagnoses of potential causes, the maternal history of symptoms and exposures should guide viral IgG and IgM testing. Even if the history is negative, initial maternal titers for CMV and parvovirus should be obtained. Rubella titer in a nonimmune patient should also be repeated at this time. It is wise to save 10 ml of blood for other titers that might later be considered necessary.

Amniocentesis is then performed for viral culture. Percutaneous umbilical blood sampling can be performed at this same visit to obtain a complete fetal blood count, which can reveal elevations or decreases in hematologic profiles, including white blood cell count, hematocrit, and platelets. If PUBS is performed, fetal blood gases should be obtained to rule out acidemia. Hepatitis is a frequent fetal finding, evidenced by elevations in lactic dehydrogenase, gamma-glutamyl transpeptidase, transaminases, and even bilirubin. A total IgM level should be determined as well as specific IgG and IgM antibodies to CMV and parvovirus. If possible, 2 ml of fetal blood should be saved for additional tests, such as PCR.

QUESTION 5: WHAT ADVANTAGE IS GAINED BY PRENATALLY DIAGNOSING VIRAL INFECTION?

There are several advantages to pursuing a prenatal diagnosis of viral infection. If results are negative, the obstetrician can reassure the parents that a fetal anomaly or growth retardation is not likely to be related to a viral infection. The family can then be less concerned about a global neurologic insult and focus on the specific abnormality visualized sonographically. If, however, the possibility of infection with one of the more debilitating viruses is raised early in the pregnancy, some parents who are unwilling to tolerate the risk of having a handicapped child may choose to terminate the pregnancy.

If a maternal viral infection has been identified, the fetus can be followed by serial ultrasound examinations to assess for development of abnormalities for which in utero therapy might be appropriate. Fetal therapy, although limited for most viruses, may be possible for parvovirus B19, CMV, or coxsackievirus infection.

Only during the last 10 years has the obstetric literature begun to report an association between nonimmune hydrops and parvovirus B19. Several reports in the last 5 years have documented the use of intrauterine transfusion to treat hydrops caused by parvovirus B19–mediated erythroid suppression.[17,18] However, other reports have also documented spontaneous resolution of hydrops associated with parvovirus.[9] Thus, the role of intrauterine transfusion in preventing fetal death from hydrops and cardiac failure is no longer clear. If isolated ascites is identified, performing serial ultrasound examinations to monitor fetal condition is a reasonable step to take before proceeding to transfusion. Until more data are gathered, the option of in utero transfusion for a fetus with hydrops and severe anemia remains one of the most important reasons for assessing for viral infection during pregnancy.

Both CMV and coxsackievirus fetal infections have been associated with fetal myocarditis and arrhythmia. Drug therapy appropriate for the specific type of arrhythmia may increase fetal survival.

Serial ultrasound examinations may also allow identification of an abnormality that cannot be treated in utero but would benefit from intensive neonatal support. This finding may prompt the obstetrician to change the location of the delivery to a tertiary care center. The timing of delivery may also be changed when a fetal viral infection is known to be the cause of intrauterine growth retardation. If the fetus dies in utero or the immunologic response is not sustained and invasive fetal testing has not been undertaken, it may be more difficult to pinpoint the cause of the fetal abnormality. Only with exact diagnosis can the physician give the parents the most accurate information about the cause of the fetal anomaly and the risk of recurrence.

REFERENCES

1. Balducci J, Rodis JF, Rosengren S et al: Pregnancy outcome following first-trimester varicella infection, *Obstet Gynecol* 79:5, 1992.
2. Bart SW, Stetler HC, Preblud SR et al: Fetal risk associated with rubella vaccine: an update, *Rev Infect Dis* 7:S95, 1985.
3. Brown GC, Karunas RS: Relationship of congenital anomalies and maternal infection with selected enteroviruses, *Am J Epidemiol* 95:207, 1972.
4. Demmler GJ: Infectious Diseases Society of America and Centers for Disease Control and Prevention: summary of a workshop on surveillance for congenital cytomegalovirus disease, *RID* 13:315, 1991.
5. Enders G, Nickerl-Pacher U, Miller E, Cradock-Watson JE: Outcome of confirmed periconceptional maternal rubella, *Lancet* 1:1445, 1988.
6. Filloux F, Kelsey DK, Bose CL et al: Hydrops fetalis with supraventricular tachycardia and cytomegalovirus infection, *Clin Pediatr* 24:534, 1985.
7. Fowler KB, Stagno S, Pass RF et al: The outcome of congenital cytomegalovirus infection in relation to maternal antibody status, *N Engl J Med* 326:663, 1992.
8. Freij BJ, Sever JL: Herpesvirus infections in pregnancy: risks to embryo, fetus, and neonate, *Clin Perinatol* 15:203, 1988.
9. Humphrey W, Magoon M, O'Shaughnessy R: Severe nonimmune hydrops secondary to parvovirus B19 infection: spontaneous reversal in utero and survival of a term infant, *Obstet Gynecol* 78:900, 1991.
10. Hutto C, Arvin A, Jacobs R et al: Intrauterine herpes simplex virus infections, *J Pediatr* 110:97, 1987.
11. Lewis PE, Cefalo RC, Zaritsky AL: Fetal heart block caused by cytomegalovirus, *Am J Obstet Gynecol* 136:967, 1980.
12. Lynch L, Daffos F, Emanuel D et al: Prenatal diagnosis of fetal cytomegalovirus infection, *Am J Obstet Gynecol* 165:714, 1991.
13. Paryani SG, Arvin AM: Intrauterine infection with varicella-zoster virus after maternal varicella, *N Engl J Med* 314:1542, 1986.
14. Pastuszak AL, Levy M, Schick B et al: Outcome after maternal varicella infection in the first 20 weeks of pregnancy, *N Engl J Med* 330:901, 1994.
15. Porath A, McNutt RA, Smiley LM, Weigle KA: Effectiveness and cost benefit of a proposed live cytomegalovirus vaccine in the prevention of congenital disease, *Rev Infect Dis* 12:31, 1990.
16. Rodis JF, Quinn DL, Gary GW et al: Management and outcomes of pregnancies complicated by human B19 parvovirus infection: a prospective study, *Am J Obstet Gynecol* 163:1168, 1990.
17. Sahakian V, Weiner CP, Naides SJ et al: Intrauterine transfusion treatment of nonimmune hydrops fetalis secondary to human parvovirus B19 infection, *Am J Obstet Gynecol* 164:1090, 1991.
18. Schwarz TF, Roggendorf M, Hottenträger B et al: Human parvovirus B19 infection in pregnancy (letter), *Lancet* 2:566, 1988.
19. Smego RA, Asperilla MO: Use of acyclovir for varicella pneumonia during pregnancy, *Obstet Gynecol* 78:1112, 1991.
20. Van den Veyver IB, Ni J, Moise KJ, Towbin JA: Detection of intrauterine viral infection by polymerase chain reaction, *Am J Obstet Gynecol* 170:278 (A31), 1994.
21. Weiner CP, Grose CF, Naides SJ: Diagnosis of fetal infection in the patient with an ultrasonographically detected abnormality but a negative clinical history, *Am J Obstet Gynecol* 168:6, 1993.

CHAPTER 27

Clinical Teratology

MICHAEL J. McMAHON
VERN L. KATZ

Human development is a delicate process that begins with the union of a single egg and sperm. Years ago, the developing fetus was considered to be protected from most external stimuli; birth defects were thought to be primarily of genetic origin. Recent studies, however, have revealed that many external factors, including drugs and medications used by the expectant mother, may pose a threat to the developing fetus. Agents that can cause abnormal development of physical structures in the embryo are called *teratogens*. *Teratology* is the study of abnormal development and congenital malformation.

Throughout pregnancy, the expectant mother is commonly exposed to many drugs and medications. Sound medical judgment dictates that the practitioner should not expose the mother and her developing fetus to potentially harmful drugs or medications. However, from a practical standpoint, it is often necessary to treat problems such as the common cold, hyperemesis, urinary tract infections, sexually transmitted diseases, thromboembolic disease, hypertension, diabetes, epilepsy, and many other conditions. Medical treatment requires the consideration of the mother, her fetus, and the pathophysiology of the disease process. The use of drugs and medications by the mother for many medical conditions, including those listed above, is usually safe. The responsibility, though, for evaluating these conditions and their treatment rests with both the physician and patient.

A preconceptional visit is an excellent time to discuss potential risks of exposure to drugs and medications. In the patient who requires medication for a particular medical condition, preconceptional counseling provides an opportunity to discuss the risks and benefits of the specific medication the patient uses and its potential effects on the developing fetus. This discussion will allow the patient and her partner to make an informed decision concerning future reproduction and to avoid unnecessary anxiety.

Many maternal, fetal, and placental factors influence whether a given drug will have an effect on the developing fetus. Maternal factors include altered physiologic functions, which may affect the absorption, distribution, metabolism, or excretion of specific drugs. For example, intravascular and extravascular volumes change during pregnancy, and renal function is significantly altered.[16] This affects the distribution and elimination patterns of many medications. Gut peristalsis is usually decreased during pregnancy, thus allowing more time for drug absorption and increasing total exposure time. Genetic factors in the fetus often play

207

a significant role in determining whether it will be susceptible to the teratogenic effects of medications and drugs. Placental factors affecting teratogenicity involve transfer across the maternal-fetal interface. Placental transfer of a given drug is dependent on lipid solubility, ionization in the serum, and molecular weight. Most prescribed medications are of low molecular weight and thus are of concern because they are easily transported across the placenta. The placenta allows two-way transfer of most molecules below a molecular weight of 600 Da. Ultimately, the drug concentration in the developing fetus depends on a combination of the aforementioned maternal, fetal, and placental factors.

Most important of all factors, though, is the gestational age at the time of drug exposure. Determining the precise embryonic age is critical in estimating potential effects of a specific drug. In most cases, the preimplantation period is a time during which the developing embryo is protected from the harmful effects of drugs. During this stage of development, drugs are often said to have an "all or nothing" effect: a drug either will induce abortion or will not affect the pregnancy at all.

The period of organogenesis, between 17 and 56 days after fertilization, is the most vulnerable time for the development of the embryo (Table 27-1). During organogenesis, most of the major internal and external structures begin to develop, making the embryo highly susceptible to the teratogenic effects of various drugs. Tissues and organ systems that are developing most rapidly during this time may suffer injury if affected by specific drugs. Between days 15 and 25, central nervous system differentiation occurs. Between days 20 and 30, precursors to the axial skeleton, musculature, and limb buds appear. From days 25 to 40, major differentiation of the eyes, heart, and lower limbs occurs. By day 60, differentiation is complete for many organ systems and well under way in the rest.

Day 60, by definition, is the beginning of the fetal period. During this period of development, little susceptibility to structural congenital malformation exists. However, the organs are still growing in size. Drugs may decrease the rate of growth and cause developmental dysfunction, particularly in the nervous system.

As noted earlier, it is important to identify the precise period in embryonic development during which exposure occurred in order to address the specific organ system or systems that may be affected by a drug. If gestational age is calculated based on menstrual history, then 2 weeks must be subtracted to determine the correct embryonic age.

Finally, although less than 2% of known congenital anomalies are caused by drugs and medications used during pregnancy, the Food and Drug Administration (FDA) has established guide-

Table 27-1   Organogenesis

Number of days after fertilization	Organ system formation
<17	None; "all or nothing effect"
15-25	Central nervous system differentiates
20-30	Axial skeleton, musculature, and limb buds appear
25-40	Eyes, heart, and lower limbs differentiate
56	Organogenesis almost complete
>60	Fetal period of increased growth begins

lines with which to determine whether a specific drug can be used during pregnancy. In 1980, the FDA created five categories of drugs based on their potential for causing birth defects (see the box below). All medications must be labeled with information about teratogenicity. When human studies cannot be completed, animal studies may provide some guidance. If product information is unavailable to the physician, there are various other sources of information about medication use during pregnancy (see the box on p. 210). It is important that information be checked on all drugs when recommending and prescribing their use during pregnancy.

TERATOGENIC CLASSIFICATION OF DRUGS

Category A

Controlled studies have failed to demonstrate fetal risk (e.g., levothyroxine)

Category B

Animal studies demonstrate no fetal risk, but human studies have not been performed *or* animal studies demonstrate fetal risk that was *not* confirmed in controlled studies in humans (e.g., ampicillin)

Category C

Animal studies demonstrate fetal risk, and no controlled studies have been performed in humans *or* animal and human studies are not available (e.g., clonidine)

Category D

There is evidence of fetal risk, but benefits of drug use outweigh risks of use during pregnancy (e.g., diphenylhydantoin)

Category X

There is evidence of fetal risk, and risks of drug use outweigh benefits of use during pregnancy (e.g., isotretinoin)

❧ Patient Profile: Teratogenicity associated with seizure medications

A 26-year-old woman (gravida 1, para 0000) at 8 weeks' gestation comes to her obstetrician for prenatal care. Her medical history includes a 15-year history of a seizure disorder, for which she takes diphenylhydantoin (Dilantin). Her last seizure occurred 14 months ago.

QUESTION 1: DOES THE USE OF DIPHENYLHYDANTOIN POSE A THREAT TO THE DEVELOPING FETUS?

Obstetricians commonly choose to manage the epileptic patient. Approximately 1 in 200 pregnancies is complicated by epilepsy. Unfortunately, almost every known antiseizure medication is associated with fetal malformation. The exact mechanism is unknown but may

---

SOURCES OF INFORMATION ABOUT MEDICATION USE DURING PREGNANCY

Texts

Catalog of teratogenic agents, ed 7. Shepard TH: Baltimore, 1992, The Johns Hopkins University Press.

Drug use in pregnancy. Niebyl JR: Philadelphia, 1988, Lea & Febiger.

Drugs in pregnancy and lactation. Briggs GG, Freeman RK, Yaffe SJ: Baltimore, 1994, Williams & Wilkins.

Handbook for prescribing during pregnancy. Berkowitz RL, Coustan DR, Mochizuki TK: Boston, 1981, Little, Brown.

Physician's desk reference, ed 49. Huff B, editor: Oradell, N.J., 1995, Medical Economics Company.

Computerized databases

MEDLINE - National Library of Medicine, Bethesda, Md. 800-638-8480

REPROTOX- Reproductive Toxicology Center, Washington, D.C. 202-293-5946

TERIS - Teratogen Information System, Seattle, Wash. 206-543-4365

TOXLINE - Toxicology Information Online, Bethesda, Md. 800-638-8480

---

be related to folate antagonism. Management plans for the epileptic patient should ideally be made preconceptionally. The goal of therapy is to eliminate polypharmacy as long as seizure activity can be controlled by a single agent. A multidisciplinary approach that includes obstetrics, maternal-fetal medicine, and neurology may be extremely beneficial in decreasing multiple exposures.

The use of diphenylhydantoin during the embryonic period of development has been associated with characteristic anomalies initially recognized in 1964. The fetal hydantoin syndrome is characterized by craniofacial and limb abnormalities, including cleft lip and palate, a broad, depressed nasal bridge, low-set ears, a wide mouth with prominent lips, epicanthal folds, and hypertelorism. Limb defects include hypoplasia of distal phalanges and nails.[10,11,13] It is estimated that 1 in 10 fetuses exposed to diphenylhydantoin develops the fetal hydantoin syndrome, and an additional 1 in 3 develops various minor craniofacial and digital anomalies. Intrauterine growth retardation and mental retardation have also been associated with diphenylhydantoin use.

Carbamazepine (Tegretol) is another commonly prescribed anticonvulsant medication that was once considered safe for use during pregnancy. Today the literature supports the existence of a carbamazepine syndrome associated with use of the drug during pregnancy. Like diphenylhydantoin, teratogenic effects of carbamazepine use are manifested primarily as craniofacial and limb abnormalities. Craniofacial abnormalities include epicanthal folds, upslanting palpebral fissures, and a short nose with a long philtrum. Limb defects include distal phalanx and fingernail hypoplasia. Growth reduction, mental retardation, and developmental delay are also associated with carbamazepine use.[12,20] Neural tube defects are associated with carbamazepine use during pregnancy, with a risk as high as 1%.[20]

Trimethadione (Tridione) is another anticonvulsant medication used to treat absence seizures. Its use during pregnancy is associated with a syndrome called *trimethadione syndrome*. Craniofacial malformations include cleft palate, unusual upslant of the eyebrows (V-shape), a prominent forehead, a short upturned nose with a broad and low nasal bridge, backward-sloped ears, and epicanthal folds. Associated findings include cardiac septal defects, growth deficiency, mental retardation, developmental delay, hearing loss, and speech problems.[7,8,13]

Valproic acid (Depakene) is an anticonvulsant drug whose use in pregnancy is associated with meningomyelocele, spina bifida, and craniofacial abnormalities.[14,19] The risk of neural tube defects in fetuses of mothers who use valproic acid during pregnancy is thought to be approximately 1%.[14] Although the main risk of valproic acid use is neural tube defects, craniofacial abnormalities have also been described, including epicanthal folds connecting with an infraorbital crease, a broad nasal bridge with a short nose and anteverted nostrils, and hypertelorism. Cardiovascular defects and long, overlapping fingers and toes with hyperconvex fingernails have also been associated with valproic acid use during pregnancy.

Phenobarbital use during pregnancy appears not to increase the risk of fetal malformation. Although several epidemiologic studies of children exposed to phenobarbital during pregnancy indicated a higher than expected rate of cardiovascular defects and facial clefts, other studies have not confirmed these findings. Neonatal withdrawal with increased irritability is an associated finding that occurs approximately 1 week postpartum.

Management of the epileptic patient requires the careful consideration of maternal seizure history and fetal well-being. Maternal serum α-fetoprotein screening is recommended between 15 and 18 weeks' gestation. A targeted fetal ultrasound examination should be performed to evaluate possible structural anomalies. Amniotic fluid assessment of α-fetoprotein should be offered for patients exposed to valproic acid and carbamazepine, especially if the ultrasound imaging is suboptimal. The patient described in this patient profile should be appropriately counseled concerning the risks of diphenylhydantoin use to her developing fetus and the need for close surveillance throughout pregnancy.

❧ Patient Profile: Teratogenicity associated with anticoagulation medications

A 34-year-old woman (gravida 3, para 2002) at 12 weeks' gestation seeks prenatal care. Her medical history is complicated by rheumatic heart disease, for which she underwent mechanical mitral valve replacement. She is now taking warfarin (Coumadin) for anticoagulation.

QUESTION 1: SHOULD WARFARIN USE BE CONTINUED DURING PREGNANCY? WHAT, IF ANY, ARE THE POTENTIAL EFFECTS ON THE FETUS?

Warfarin is a category D drug that inhibits the action of vitamin K. It is contraindicated during pregnancy because of its ease of placental transfer and well-established teratogenicity. The fetal warfarin syndrome is caused by first-trimester use of warfarin. Characteristics of the syndrome include stippling in uncalcified epiphyseal areas, such as the proximal femur and axial skeleton, and nasal hypoplasia as a result of maldevelopment of the nasal septum.[9,24,25] Approximately 15% to 25% of fetuses are affected if exposed during the first trimester.

First-trimester spontaneous abortion is a common complication of warfarin use. Second- and third-trimester use can cause central nervous system dysfunction, microcephaly, mental retardation, optic atrophy, cataracts, and blindness. Intrauterine growth retardation, stillbirth, and neonatal death also occur more frequently with exposure to warfarin.[9] These fetal abnormalities are now thought to be caused by hemorrhage in the fetus and placenta.

Heparin, a category C drug that binds antithrombin III, is the drug of choice when anticoagulation is necessary during pregnancy. Because of its high molecular weight and negative charge, heparin does not cross the placenta and cause malformation.

The patient described in this profile should have the warfarin stopped as heparinization is initiated. She should be counseled that her fetus is at risk of developing fetal warfarin syndrome. Follow-up ultrasound examination may be used to evaluate growth abnormalities and may help detect effects of the warfarin. However, not all of these effects are visible on ultrasound. Maternal bone demineralization and thrombocytopenia are possible complications of prolonged heparin use during pregnancy (usually with use for 3 months or longer).[6] Maternal platelet counts should also be periodically assessed.

❧ Patient Profile: Teratogenicity associated with antihypertensive medications

A 34-year-old woman (gravida 1, para 0000) comes to her obstetrician for her first prenatal visit at 10 weeks' gestation. Physical examination in the sitting position reveals a repeated blood pressure of 170/102 mm Hg.

QUESTION 1: WHAT MEDICATIONS ARE RECOMMENDED FOR THE TREATMENT OF HYPERTENSION DURING PREGNANCY?

The treatment of chronic hypertension during pregnancy requires the judicious use of medications and close maternal and fetal surveillance. For many years, methyldopa (Aldomet) and hydralazine (Apresoline) have been the drugs of choice in the treatment of hypertension during pregnancy. The use of these catagory C drugs during pregnancy does not appear to cause an increased rate of congenital malformation. Diuretic medications, such as thiazide, are not generally recommended during pregnancy because of the associated risks of neonatal hemolysis and thrombocytopenia.[18]

Propranolol (Inderal) and other β-agonists are not associated with congenital malformation but have been associated with neonatal respiratory depression, fetal bradycardia, and fetal hypoglycemia in a small number of cases.[23] However, in general, β-blockers are well tolerated and safe during pregnancy. Calcium channel blockers, such as nifedipine (Procardia), have been shown to pose no teratogenic threat to the developing human fetus.

Angiotensin-converting enzyme (ACE) inhibitors have become a widely prescribed form of antihypertensive pharmacotherapy; however, they should not be used during pregnancy. Although it appears that use of ACE inhibitors during the first trimester does not increase the risk of fetal malformation, use later in pregnancy has been associated with fetal death. This class of drugs appears to cause intrauterine growth retardation, renal dysplasia, oligo-hydramnios, and Potter syndrome. Loose skin, joint contractures, pulmonary hypoplasia, and death may result.[21] The effect of the ACE inhibitors is on systemic and renal hemodynamics.

When a patient who seeks prenatal care is taking ACE inhibitors for chronic hypertension, the medication should be discontinued and replaced with methyldopa, hydralazine, or nifedipine. Management should generally include serial ultrasound evaluation of fetal growth and development and antenatal testing to assess fetal well-being.

❧ Patient Profile: Teratogenicity associated with cold medications

A 19-year-old woman (gravida 2, para 1001) at 14 weeks' gestation comes to her obstetrician with an upper-respiratory infection, including rhinorrhea and cough.

QUESTION 1: WHAT MEDICATIONS ARE RECOMMENDED FOR THE TREATMENT OF UPPER-RESPIRATORY INFECTIONS DURING PREGNANCY?

The presentation of the pregnant patient to her physician for evaluation of upper-respiratory complaints is both a common occurrence and a challenging problem. The symptomatic patient is usually uncomfortable and seeks treatment for rhinorrhea, cough, sore throat, and fever. The physician, on the other hand, is concerned not only about the treatment of the patient but also about the effects of drugs on the fetus. The judicious use of medications for the patient with an upper-respiratory illness is extremely important. Many patients must be counseled throughout pregnancy to contact their physicians before self-treating any condition, especially the common cold, with any of the many over-the-counter medications available today.

Acetaminophen is a non-narcotic analgesic for which no increased risk of teratogenicity in the developing fetus has been shown. This medication can safely be used to treat headaches and generalized aches associated with respiratory infections.

Cough remedies with antitussive, decongestant, and expectorant properties can be combined with codeine, guaifenesin, dextromethorphan, phenylpropanolamine, and pseudoephedrine. Although guaifenesin and phenylpropanolamine have not been associated with any congenital anomalies, the use of codeine early in pregnancy has been associated with both cardiac defects and cleft lip and palate.[1] Cough remedies with codeine are therefore not recommended for use early in pregnancy.

Pseudoephedrine and pseudoephedrine in combination with triprolidine have been used to treat upper-respiratory complaints. However, a 1992 case-control study found a significantly higher rate of gastroschisis in fetuses of mothers who recalled using pseudoephedrine during the first trimester.[26] Until further studies have been completed, it is recommended that pseudoephedrine not be used during the first trimester.

For the patient who requires antibiotic therapy during pregnancy to treat more serious upper-respiratory infections, such as sinusitis or pneumonia, the use of β-lactamase agents, such as penicillin derivatives, and cephalosporins in the penicillin-allergic patient is recommended.

❦ Patient Profile: Teratogenicity associated with alcohol and illicit drugs

A 24-year-old woman (gravida 2, para 1001) at 21 weeks' gestation comes to the clinic for prenatal care. The nurse notes that the patient's breath smells of alcohol, and physical examination reveals needle marks in her right forearm. Upon further questioning, the patient says that she has used cocaine, heroin, and alcohol daily.

QUESTION 1: WHAT ARE THE EFFECTS OF MATERNAL DRUG ADDICTION ON THE FETUS? HOW IS THIS PATIENT BEST MANAGED?

The management of the patient exposed to street drugs can be very difficult. It is most important to realize that the illicit drug user seldom abuses one drug alone. Abuse of multiple drugs is the rule rather than the exception.

The developing fetus depends on maternal hepatic transformation of consumed ethanol to rid itself of this known teratogen. The abuse of alcohol during pregnancy has long been known to cause fetal alcohol syndrome (Figure 27-1). This syndrome occurs in approximately 2% to 8% of infants born to alcoholic women. Findings characteristically associated with fetal alcohol syndrome are listed in the box at right. These findings are usually associated with maternal consumption of greater than 3 oz of absolute alcohol daily during pregnancy. A lesser quantity consumed has been associated with so-called *fetal alcohol effects;* the affected child exhibits some of the characteristics of the fetal alcohol syndrome, but to a lesser degree. If genetic causes are excluded, alcohol abuse during pregnancy is the most common identifiable cause of mental retardation in the United States.

Cocaine is a central nervous system stimulant that when abused by pregnant women has been associated with various genitourinary, cardiovascular, and central nervous system abnormalities, including disruptive brain anomalies, segmental intestinal atresia, congenital heart defects, prune-belly syndrome, and urinary tract and facial anomalies.[2,3] Limb reduction anomalies have also been associated with cocaine abuse during pregnancy. The effects of cocaine appear to be secondary to acute vasoconstrictive effects, which may interrupt blood flow. The consequence is destruction of normally developed embryonic structures.

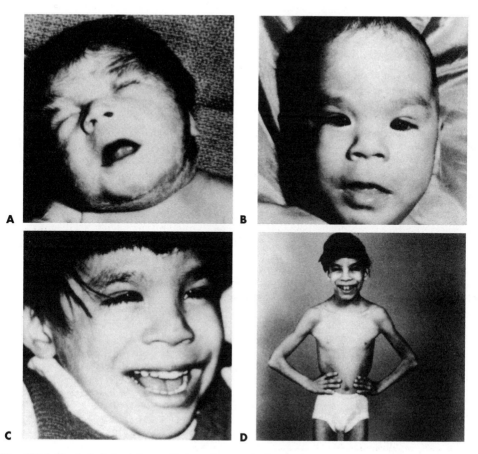

Fig. 27-1 Fetal alcohol syndrome. Patient photographed at birth (**A**), at 8 months (**B**), at 4½ years (**C**), and at 8 years (**D**). Note the short palpebral fissures, short nose, hypoplastic philtrum, thin upper-lip vermilion, and flat midface. (From CIBA Foundation Symposium: *Mechanisms of alcohol damage in utero,* London, 1984, Pitman Publishing.)

FINDINGS ASSOCIATED WITH FETAL ALCOHOL SYNDROME

Intrauterine growth retardation

Central nervous system abnormalities
Mild to moderate mental retardation
Developmental delay
Hypotonia

Congenital heart defects

Craniofacial abnormalities
Short palpebral fissures
Epicanthal folds
Poorly developed philtrum with thin
  upper lip
Maxillary hypoplasia

Opiates are a class of drugs that includes heroin, meperidine, fentanyl, propoxyphene, and methadone. Heroin abuse during pregnancy has not been associated with any increased risk of fetal structural defects but has been associated with intrauterine growth retardation, preterm labor and delivery, and fetal death. Neonatal withdrawal is common and includes a combination of central nervous system, metabolic, respiratory, and gastrointestinal dysfunctions.

In the patient who admits to drug abuse or is identified as a drug abuser, as in this patient profile, pregnancy may be an ideal time for intervention.[15] Management requires an experienced multidisciplinary team skilled at treating the drug-addicted patient. Hospitalization for drug withdrawal and initiation of methadone therapy is often helpful for both the mother and the fetus. Regularly scheduled appointments to include psychosocial counseling, toxicology screening, and fetal surveillance are recommended. Ultrasound evaluation with fetal echocardiography should be completed to detect structural anomalies, fetal growth deficiency, and cardiac lesions. Finally, it should be remembered that the drug-addicted patient is at increased risk of acquiring the human immunodeficiency virus, hepatitis, subacute bacterial endocarditis, and sexually transmitted diseases. Management should include consideration of these important medical problems.

REFERENCES

1. Bracken MB, Holford TR: Exposure to prescribed drugs in pregnancy and association with congenital malformations, *Obstet Gynecol* 58:336, 1981.
2. Chasnoff IJ, Burns WJ, Schnoli SH, Burns KA: Cocaine use in pregnancy, *N Engl J Med* 313:666, 1985.
3. Chouteau M, Namerow PB, Leppert P: The effect of cocaine abuse on birth weight and gestational age, *Obstet Gynecol* 72:351, 1988.
4. Clarren SK, Smith DW: The fetal alcohol syndrome, *N Engl J Med* 298:1063, 1978.
5. Day NL, Jasperse D, Richardson G et al: Prenatal exposure to alcohol: effect on infant growth and morphologic characteristics, *Pediatrics* 84:536, 1989.
6. De Swiet M, Dorrington Ward P, Fidler J et al: Prolonged heparin therapy in pregnancy causes bone demineralization, *Br J Obstet Gynæcol* 90:1129, 1983.
7. Feldman GL, Weaver DD, Lovrien EW: The fetal trimethadione syndrome, *Am J Dis Child* 131:1389, 1977.
8. German J, Kowal A, Ehlers KH: Trimethadione and human teratogenesis, *Teratology* 3:349, 1970.
9. Hall JG, Pauli RM, Wilson KM: Maternal and fetal sequelae of anticoagulation during pregnancy, *Am J Med* 68:122, 1980.
10. Hanson JW, Myrianthopoulos NC, Sedgwick Harvey MA, Smith DW: Risks to the offspring of women treated with hydantoin anticonvulsants, with emphasis on the fetal hydantoin syndrome, *J Pediatr* 89:662, 1976.
11. Hanson JW, Smith DW: The fetal hydantoin syndrome, *J Pediatr* 87:285, 1975.
12. Jones KL, Lacro RV, Johnson KA, Adams J: Pattern of malformations in the children of women treated with carbamazepine during pregnancy, *N Engl J Med* 320:1661, 1989.
13. Kelly TE: Teratogenicity of anticonvulsant drugs: review of the literature, *Am J Med Genet* 19:413, 1984.
14. Lindhout D, Schmidt D: In-utero exposure to valproate and neural tube defects (letter), *Lancet* 1:1392, 1986.
15. MacGregor SN, Keith LG, Bachicha JA, Chasnoff IJ: Cocaine abuse during pregnancy: correlation between prenatal care and perinatal outcome, *Obstet Gynecol* 74:882, 1989.
16. Monga M, Creasy RK: Cardiovascular and renal adaptation to pregnancy. In Creasy RK, Resnik R, editors: *Maternal-fetal medicine: principles and practice*, ed 3, Philadelphia, 1994, WB Saunders.
17. Paul M: Occupational and environmental reproductive hazards: a guide for clinicians, Baltimore, 1993, Williams & Wilkins.
18. Redman CWG: Treatment of hypertension in pregnancy, *Kidney Int* 18:267, 1980.
19. Robert E, Guibaud P: Maternal valproic acid and congenital neural tube defects, *Lancet* 2:934, 1982.

20. Rosa FW: Spina bifida in infants of women treated with carbamazepine during pregnancy, *N Engl J Med* 324:674, 1991.
21. Rosa FW, Bosco LA, Graham CF et al: Neonatal anuria with maternal angiotensin-converting enzyme inhibition, *Obstet Gynecol* 74:371, 1989.
22. Rosett HL, Weiner L, Lee A et al: Patterns of alcohol consumption and fetal development, *Obstet Gynecol* 61:539, 1983.
23. Rubin PC: Current concepts: beta-blockers in pregnancy, *N Engl J Med* 305:1323, 1981.
24. Shaul WL, Hall JG: Multiple congenital anomalies associated with oral anticoagulants, *Am J Obstet Gynecol* 127:191, 1977.
25. Stevenson RE, Burton M, Ferlauto GJ, Taylor HA: Hazards of oral anticoagulants during pregnancy, *JAMA* 243:1549, 1980.
26. Werler MM, Mitchell AA, Shapiro S: First-trimester maternal medication use in relation to gastroschisis, *Teratology* 45:361, 1992.

CHAPTER 28

Embryology and Experimental Teratology

THOMAS W. SADLER

For many years, teratologists have known that early periods of embryonic development are the most susceptible to teratogenic insult.[17] From the middle of the second week to the end of the eighth week after fertilization, most major structural defects are induced. The third and fourth weeks are particularly critical, and insults at this time result in malformations of the central nervous system, heart, and urogenital organs that may be severe or lethal. Since most women do not realize that they are pregnant before this critical period, prevention of birth defects is impossible without preconceptional planning and management. Such planning is essential for women in high-risk groups, including those with insulin-dependent diabetes, phenylketonuria, a previous infant with a birth defect, potentially harmful workplace exposures, and other factors. Those who use recreational drugs, such as alcohol and tobacco, are also at high risk.

❧ Patient Profile: Prevention of birth defects

A young woman is concerned about planning her first pregnancy. Her sister, who is diabetic, has had a child with a neural tube defect and, although the patient herself is not diabetic, she worries about having a baby with an abnormality. She would like to know whether there is anything she can do to protect her baby and when her baby might be most susceptible to a harmful exposure.

QUESTION 1: WHY IS THE EMBRYO SO SENSITIVE TO TERATOGENIC INSULT DURING THE THIRD AND FOURTH WEEKS AFTER FERTILIZATION?

At the end of the second week, the embryo begins the process of organ formation by establishing three layers of germ cells that will form the entire organism. At first, the embryo is in the form of a slipper-shaped disc consisting of two cell layers: a dorsal layer, the epiblast; and a ventral layer, the hypoblast (Figure 28-1). All three germ layers are derived from the epiblast by a process known as *gastrulation*, in which cells of this layer turn inward

218

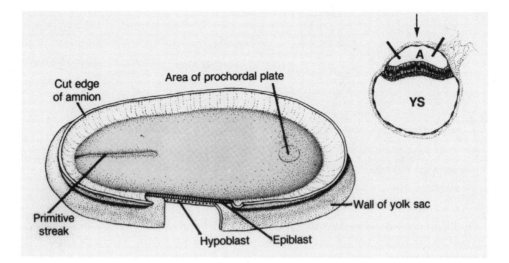

Fig. 28-1 Dorsal view of a 14-day embryo (postfertilization) at the beginning of gastrulation, the process during which the three germ layers of the embryo are formed. The embryo is a two-layered disc consisting of an epiblast layer, facing the amnion (*A*), and a hypoblast layer, facing the yolk sac (*YS*). The primitive streak forms in the caudal portion of the disc, and epiblast cells migrate through this structure to form mesoderm and endoderm. Cells that remain in the epiblast form ectoderm. (From Sadler TW: *Langman's medical embryology,* ed 6, Baltimore, 1990, Williams & Wilkins.)

through a groove, known as the *primitive streak,* and migrate between the original epiblast and the hypoblast (Figures 28-2 and 28-3). The streak forms at the caudal end of the disc and provides cells for succeeding segments as it regresses from the cervical to the sacral region. In each region, the first cells migrating inward become endoderm (the gut and its derivatives, including the lungs, liver, gallbladder, and pancreas) and the next become mesoderm (blood, skeleton, and supporting tissues). Those that remain in the epiblast form ectoderm (the skin and central nervous system). Even before the first cells turn inward, their fate has been assigned and organ and tissue patterns have been established.[8] Thus, exposure to teratogens at this time may have severe effects on pattern formation and stem cell populations. For example, loss of midline cells in the presumptive forebrain region as gastrulation is initiated results in hypotelorism. If the loss of cells is substantial, synophthalmia and holoprosencephaly result. Such defects may be produced by exposure to high concentrations of alcohol[14] or by diabetes.[2]

As the primitive streak moves caudally, establishing cell populations for tissue and organ formation in each region, some cells turn inward at the midline and move cranially. These cells form the head process of the notochord (see Figure 28-3), which signals the overlying epiblast in this region to become the neural plate. Directly above the notochord, in the center of the plate, the neural groove forms and the right and left cranial neural folds are established (Figure 28-4). Soon the folds elevate, and their lateral edges move toward the midline, where they fuse.

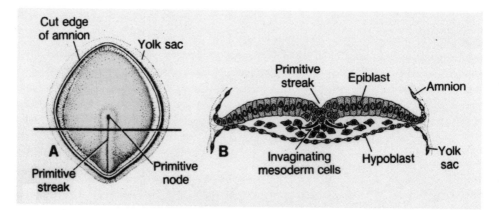

Fig. 28-2   Diagrams of 16-day embryos, showing the process of gastrulation. Epiblast cells migrate toward the primitive streak (**A**) and then turn inward (**B**). The first cells to migrate displace the hypoblast and become endoderm, whereas succeeding cells form mesoderm. The primitive node (Hensen's node), a small elevation at the cranial end of the primitive streak, is a source of retinoic acid, which signals pathways that control this morphogenetic process. Cells that migrate through this region remain in the midline and form the notochord. (From Sadler TW: *Langman's medical embryology*, ed 6, Baltimore, 1990, Williams & Wilkins.)

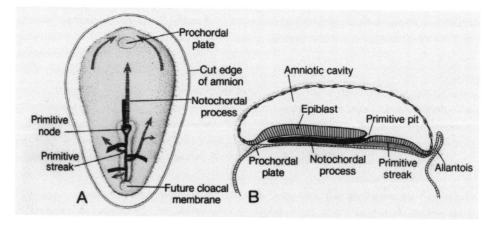

Fig. 28-3   Diagrams of 17-day embryos, showing the paths of cell migration during gastrulation (**A**) and formation of the notochordal process (**B**). Cells that enter the primitive streak through the primitive node remain in the midline and coalesce to form the notochord. This structure extends from the level of the prochordal plate (future opening of the oral cavity) to the caudal end of the neural tube and is responsible for inducing development of the neural plate, which forms the central nervous system. (From Sadler TW: *Langman's medical embryology*, ed 6, Baltimore, 1990, Williams & Wilkins.)

Fusion begins in the cervical region and progresses cranially and caudally in zipper-like fashion. Fusion occurs in an additional site in the forebrain and progresses caudally, to unite with the site initiated in the cervical area, and cranially, to close the cranial-most portion of the neural tube. The development of neuroectoderm for neural folds destined to form the spinal cord is also induced by the notochord, which is lengthened by the addition of midline cells as the primitive streak moves caudally. Closure of these folds proceeds continuously from the cervical region to the lumbosacral area (Figure 28-4).

Neural tube closure (neurulation) takes place during nearly the entire fourth week of development and, because of the complexity of events required for its orchestration, is

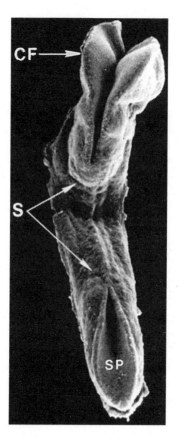

Fig. 28-4 Scanning electron micrograph of a mouse embryo undergoing closure of the neural tube. Closure begins in the cervical region and progresses cranially, to close the cranial folds (*CF*), and caudally, to close the spinal cord area (*SP*). Closure occurs in secondary sites in the forebrain and midbrain, which eventually unite with the cervical site. Segmented blocks of mesoderm called *somites* (*S*) form along the sides of the neural tube from occipital regions caudally and represent the primordia of the vertebral column. (From Sadler TW: *Langman's medical embryology*, ed 6, Baltimore, 1990, Williams & Wilkins.)

exquisitely sensitive to genetic and environmental insult. These insults result in spina bifida cystica and spina bifida occulta, meningoceles, encephaloceles, anencephaly, and other defects.

Furthermore, all along the edge of the neural folds, neuroectoderm cells undergo an epithelial to mesenchymal transformation to form neural crest cells. These cells migrate from the neural folds to form most of the face and cranial vault, ganglia of cranial and spinal nerves, melanocytes, neuroblasts for sympathetic and parasympathetic systems, cells for septation of the outflow tract of the heart, and other structures. These stem cells are extremely vulnerable to insult and usually respond by dying or failing to migrate to their appointed positions. Consequently, damage to this stem cell population may result in facial clefts, transposition of the great vessels, congenital megacolon, or other birth defects.[8] The vulnerability of the population may be due in part to a lack of enzymes necessary to scavenge free radicals that are produced by many toxicants (alcohol, retinoic acid, and many other cytotoxic agents) that kill cells.[4]

QUESTION 2: WHAT FACTORS CONTROL EMBRYONIC DEVELOPMENT DURING THE THIRD AND FOURTH WEEKS?

During the third week and part of the fourth week of development, the hemochorial placenta is not present, and in fact, the embryo does not have a beating heart and circulatory system until the middle of the fourth week.[8] Therefore, the placenta is not present as a barrier, and "placental transport," as it is described in the literature, cannot take place. During this time, the embryo depends on the trophoblastic shell that surrounds it to supply its basic needs. This shell ingests serum proteins from blood in lacunar lakes in the uterine decidua, breaks them down by proteolytic digestion, and passes free amino acids and small peptides to the embryo. Since the embryo is glycolytic, glucose is a key substrate, and even brief periods of hypoglycemia are not well tolerated, particularly by the central nervous system and heart. In fact, in laboratory animals, glucose concentrations two times higher than normal produce no apparent adverse effects, whereas levels decreased by as little as 40% are detrimental.[11]

Cellular and molecular factors that control pattern formation during gastrulation and neurulation are rapidly being identified. Homeobox genes, protooncogenes, genes encoding growth factors (particularly members of the TGF-β family), and retinoic acid receptors are also being documented as key factors in early developmental events. *Homeobox genes* are transcription factors that are expressed in many species, contain a conserved sequence called the *homeodomain*, and regulate key embryologic processes, such as patterning of the digits, segmentation in the hindbrain, and organization of the cranial nerves.[7] Protooncogenes, such as members of the *Wnt(int)* family, signal formation of the cerebellum and forebrain and patterning of the spinal cord.[1] Abnormalities in expression of these genes and others, such as *engrailed* and *sonic hedgehog*, in this signaling pathway may result in caudal regression.

A key agent in signaling many of these genes is retinoic acid (vitamin A). This molecule is critical for patterning the digits and central nervous system.[15] So delicate is the balance between this signal and its transmitted effects that both hypo- and hypervitaminosis A result in severe birth defects affecting nearly every organ system.[6] Furthermore, synthetic retinoids, such as isotretinoin (Accutane; 13-*cis*-retinoic acid) and etretinate (Tegison) are also teratogenic, especially during the third and fourth weeks of development.[13]

As genes responsible for morphogenesis are identified, it is becoming clear that mutations in these critical genes result in abnormal phenotypes. In fact, genes responsible for several mutant mouse strains have now been linked to specific human syndromes. For example, a mutation in *PAX3*, which causes neural tube and coat color defects in mice, is responsible for Waardenburg syndrome in humans.[16] This syndrome is characterized by partial albinism (white forelock), deafness, a broad mandible, and, occasionally, cleft lip and palate and Hirschsprung disease. All of these defects are related to abnormal neural crest cell development. In addition, a mutation in the homeobox gene *MSX2* is responsible for an autosomal dominant form of craniosynostosis.[5]

QUESTION 3: ARE THE THIRD AND FOURTH WEEKS AFTER FERTILIZATION THE ONLY CRITICAL PERIODS OF DEVELOPMENT?

The embryo is also vulnerable to genetic and environmental insults during other weeks of development. The major period of susceptibility to insults resulting in structural birth defects is the middle of the second week to the end of the eighth week of development, which comprises the embryonic period. During this time, primordia for all organ systems are established. After the eighth week, the conceptus enters the fetal period, when organ and tissue differentiation occurs and gross structural defects are produced only by physical factors, such as amniotic bands and oligohydramnios. During the embryonic period, most organs have a peak period of sensitivity to teratogenic insult that usually coincides with the period of rapid cell proliferation at the initiation of organogenesis. However, this generalization is by no means axiomatic, and structures such as the palate (which has four peak periods of sensitivity), mandible, and thyroid have multiple periods of susceptibility.[9]

QUESTION 4: CAN THE EMBRYO RECOVER FROM A TERATOGENIC INSULT?

The degree to which recovery is possible after the embryo receives a teratogenic insult is not clear. More than likely, resistance to an insult is a better measure of whether a teratogen will have an adverse affect. For example, even in laboratory animals with multiple implantation sites, administration of a teratogen to the mother does not affect all embryos equally. Furthermore, even if all embryos in a litter are exposed in vitro to equal concentrations of a teratogen, the response among embryos varies. Similarly, two women may have identical workplace exposures, but one may have an affected child and the other a normal offspring. Thus, the genome of the fetus, as well as that of the mother, plays a role in determining the outcome of exposure to a teratogen. This concept is well illustrated by results showing that fetuses deficient in the enzyme epoxide hydrolase, which normally eliminates toxic metabolites of anticonvulsant drugs, are more susceptible to the fetal hydantoin syndrome than infants with normal enzyme activity. Fetuses deficient in the enzyme are homozygous for the recessive allele of the gene.[3]

Even after an insult, the embryo has some potential for repair and recovery. Most teratogens produce malformation by causing excessive cell death, but because cells of the embryo have high proliferative rates, there is the potential to replace cells that are lost. However, there must be a threshold beyond which recovery is impossible. Furthermore, laboratory investigations suggest that the potential for recovery is greater after exposure to teratogens that have more general effects than after exposure to those that target specific cell populations.[10,12] It appears that generalized effects allow for synchronous repair among all tissues and cells, whereas effects on a targeted cell population result in asynchronous repair and growth. The result is dysmorphology in the structure or structures derived from the targeted cell population.

QUESTION 5: ARE THERE WAYS OF PREVENTING BIRTH DEFECTS?

In most cases, women do not visit their obstetricians until after the critical period in gestation (from the middle of the second week to the eighth week after fertilization) when birth defects are induced. Therefore, it is imperative that planning for a healthy baby begin before conception. At this time, every attempt should be made to encourage avoidance of teratogenic exposure in the workplace; abstinence from recreational drugs, such as alcohol, cocaine, and tobacco; and avoidance of exposure to teratogenic pharmaceutical compounds, such as isotretinoin and etretinate. If metabolic disease is present, such as diabetes or phenylketonuria, stabilization of the metabolic condition before conception is essential. A healthy diet is important and should include 0.4 mg of folic acid per day to aid in prevention of neural tube defects.

REFERENCES

1. Augustine K, Liu ET, Sadler TW: Antisense attenuation of *Wnt-1* and *Wnt-3a* expression in whole embryo culture reveals roles for these genes in craniofacial, spinal cord, and cardiac morphogenesis, *Dev Genet* 14:500, 1993.
2. Barr M, Hanson JW, Cuney K et al: Holoprosencephaly in infants of diabetic mothers, *J Pediatr* 102:565, 1983.
3. Beuhler BA, Delimont D, Van Waes M, Finnell RH: Prenatal prediction of risk of the fetal hydantoin syndrome, *N Engl J Med* 322:1567, 1990.
4. Davis WL, Crawford SA, Cooper OJ et al: Ethanol induces the generation of reactive free radicals by neural crest cells in vitro, *J Craniofacial Gen Dev Biol* 10:277, 1990.
5. Jabs EW, Muller U, Li X et al: A mutation in the homeodomain of the human *MSX2* gene in a family affected with autosomal dominant craniosynostosis, *Cell* 75:443, 1993.
6. Lammer E, Chen D, Hoar R et al: Retinoic acid embryopathy, *N Engl J Med* 313:837, 1985.
7. Lumsden A: The cellular basis of segmentation in the developing hindbrain, *Trends Neurosci* 13:329, 1990.
8. Sadler TW: *Langman's medical embryology*, ed 6, Baltimore, 1990, Williams & Wilkins.

9. Shenefelt RE: Morphogenesis of malformations in hamsters caused by retinoic acid: relation to dose and stage at treatment, *Teratology* 5:103, 1972.

10. Shum L, Sadler TW: Recovery by mouse embryos following teratogenic exposure to ketosis, *Diabetologia* 34:289, 1991.

11. Smoak IW, Sadler TW: Embryopathic effects of short-term hypoglycemia in the mouse, *Am J Obstet Gynecol* 163:619, 1990.

12. Snow MHL, Tam PPL: Is compensatory growth a complicating factor in mouse teratology? *Nature* 279:555, 1979.

13. Sulik KK, Alles AJ: Teratogenicity of the retinoids. In Saurat JH, editor: *Retinoids: 10 years on,* Basel, Switzerland, 1991, S Karger.

14. Sulik KK, Lauder JM, Dehart DB: Brain malformations in prenatal mice following acute maternal ethanol administration, *Int J Neurosci* 2:203, 1984.

15. Tabin C: Retinoids, homeoboxes, and growth factors: toward molecular models for limb development, *Cell* 66:199, 1991.

16. Tassabehji M, Read AP, Newton VE et al: Waardenburg's syndrome patients have mutations in the human homologue of the Pax-3 paired box gene, *Nature* 355:635, 1992.

17. Wilson JG: Current status of teratology—general principles and mechanisms derived from animal studies. In Wilson JG, Fraser FC, editors: *Handbook of teratology: general principles and etiology,* New York, 1977, Plenum.

PART EIGHT

THE FUTURE

CHAPTER 29

Prenatal Diagnosis Using Fetal Cells in the Maternal Circulation

MARY E. NORTON
DIANA W. BIANCHI

Standard prenatal genetic diagnosis currently involves either chorionic villus sampling (CVS) or amniocentesis. Both techniques are invasive and are accompanied by some risk of pregnancy loss. Although maternal serum biochemical screening can now detect a large percentage of Down syndrome fetuses, this test is neither optimally sensitive nor specific.[21,33] There is compelling evidence that fetal cells are present in the maternal circulation as early as 6 weeks of gestation,[26,28] and recent advances in molecular technology have made possible the isolation and analysis of such cells. Three criteria must be met for prenatal diagnosis to be made using this technique: (1) the fetal cells that are present must be distinguished from the more prevalent maternal cells; (2) the cells that are present must be enriched from their initial low concentrations; and (3) the fetal cells that are extracted must be analyzed using techniques that are sufficiently sensitive and specific. This noninvasive approach to prenatal diagnosis has been successful in identifying both chromosome and molecular genetic abnormalities.* Clinical studies are continuing to determine whether this technique is sensitive and specific enough to provide noninvasive prenatal diagnosis to all pregnant women.

❦ Patient Profile: Analysis of fetal cells isolated from the maternal circulation for the evaluation of aneuploidy

A 22-year-old woman (gravida 1, para 0000) seeks obstetric consultation at 8 weeks' gestation. She reports that her 10-year-old brother, born when her mother was 42 years old, has trisomy 21 (Down syndrome). Although she understands that her risk of having a child with Down syndrome is very small, she is quite anxious about this possibility. She has read a recent

---

*References 3, 8, 9, 18, and 34.

magazine article about a new noninvasive test that can be used to diagnose chromosome abnormalities, and she requests more information about testing for fetal chromosome abnormalities by isolating fetal cells from maternal blood.

QUESTION 1: ARE ENOUGH FETAL CELLS PRESENT IN THE MATERNAL CIRCULATION TO BE ISOLATED FOR PRENATAL DIAGNOSIS?

The presence of fetal cells in the maternal circulation was first reported in 1893 by a pathologist who identified trophoblasts in the lungs of women dying of eclampsia.[35] Although originally thought to be secondary to increased uterine manipulation or maternal trauma, the transplacental passage of fetal cells during the course of normal pregnancy has been found by many subsequent investigators.* Douglas and colleagues,[14] in 1959, identified large cells thought to be syncytiotrophoblasts in the broad ligament veins of pregnant women. Others have subsequently identified fetal lymphocytes and nucleated red blood cells (NRBCs) in the maternal circulation.†

To date, fetal cells isolated from maternal blood have not been successfully cultured or have not been responsive to commonly used mitogens.[45] It has therefore been necessary to analyze just the few isolated cells themselves, using techniques other than traditional metaphase cytogenetics, which requires dividing cells. This constraint has presented difficulties in both identifying the cells as definitely fetal and pursuing the ultimate goal of meaningful prenatal diagnosis.

Until the late 1980s, genetic analysis sophisticated enough to prove the fetal origin of a single cell among thousands or millions of maternal cells had not been available. However, the development of techniques such as polymerase chain reaction (PCR) and fluorescence in situ hybridization (FISH) has greatly improved the ability to pursue this type of noninvasive prenatal diagnosis. Most investigation has focused on isolating cells containing Y-specific gene sequences from women carrying male fetuses, since this is a simple way of conclusively proving the fetal origin of the cells. Such studies confirmed that fetal cells are present in the maternal circulation, although, as expected, at very low concentrations.[2,34]

Estimates of the ratio of fetal to maternal cells have varied widely. A number of factors, including gestational age, uterine manipulation, abnormal placentation, and abnormal pregnancy (e.g., aneuploid fetus), have been hypothesized to affect the number of fetal cells present.[4,15,38] Price and colleagues[34] estimated the ratio of fetal NRBCs to maternal NRBCs at $1{:}1 \times 10^7 - 1{:}1 \times 10^8$. Hall and Williams[22] estimated the ratio of fetal NRBCs to maternal NRBCs at $1{:}4.75 \times 10^6 - 1{:}6 \times 10^7$. Arinami and associates[1] estimated the average number of fetal leukocytes present in maternal blood at $1{:}5 \times 10^3 - 1{:}20 \times 10^3$. Thus, it appears that although fetal cells are probably present in the maternal circulation during most pregnancies, they are rare.

---

*References 2, 14, 20, 29, 32, and 37.
†References 2, 19, 23, 25, 34, and 43.

QUESTION 2: WHICH CELL TYPES ARE PRESENT, AND WHICH ONES ARE MOST USEFUL FOR PRENATAL DIAGNOSIS?

A number of cell types have been investigated as candidate fetal cells for use in prenatal diagnosis. The optimal cell type obviously must have a nucleus with DNA available for genetic analysis, must be consistently present in the maternal circulation, must be differentiable from maternal cells, and must originate from the current pregnancy.

Trophoblasts are an obvious candidate cell type because they are known to invade the uterus and thus might be expected to enter the maternal circulation. A number of investigators have attempted to isolate trophoblasts from the maternal circulation using a variety of monoclonal antibodies.[7,11,12,32] Although some of these investigators initially published promising results, their findings have been difficult to duplicate. Isolation techniques generally use monoclonal antibodies, and their success is largely dependent on the specificity of such antibodies. Although many of these antibodies were generated against placental tissue and were thought to be specific to trophoblastic cells, their use led to the isolation of many cells that morphologically appeared to be maternal leukocytes.[7,12] It is now believed that although these antigens are trophoblastic in origin, they can be adsorbed onto maternal cells and are therefore not useful in selectively identifying fetal cells.

Lymphocytes thought to be of fetal origin have been isolated by a number of investigators.[23,25,43] In these studies, maternal blood was sorted for the presence of cells expressing paternal HLA antigens. Lymphocytes are a well-known source of metaphases for cytogenetic analysis. However, lymphocytes presumably of fetal origin isolated from maternal blood have not been successfully cultured or have been unresponsive to mitogens.[44,45] Tharapel and colleagues[39] studied many cells in metaphase from maternal blood of pregnancies with known male or aneuploid fetuses; these metaphases were invariably 46,XX. Thus, fetal lymphocytes either were not present or were present but unresponsive to mitogens.

Another concern with fetal lymphocytes is that they might persist in the maternal circulation for many years. Several investigators have identified Y-specific material in the blood of women many years after they delivered male infants.[5,10,24,36] Thus, the concern is raised that isolated fetal lymphocytes could represent a previous, possibly even unrecognized pregnancy.[5]

Nucleated red blood cells have been the focus of some of the most successful work in this area. Bianchi and associates[2] first studied these red cell precursors, also known as *erythroblasts*.[2] Because most pregnancies are blood-group compatible, small numbers of fetal erythrocytes can circulate unchallenged by the maternal immune system. Although NRBCs are very rare in peripheral adult blood, they represent a much higher percentage of the nucleated cell population in the fetus.[13] Thus, any NRBCs present in maternal blood are likely to be fetal cells. In addition, NRBCs have a defined half-life and therefore would not be expected to persist into a later pregnancy.

A single group of investigators also reported the isolation of fetal granulocytes from maternal blood. Using a density-gradient centrifugation, fetal granulocytes that hybridized to a Y-chromosome–specific probe were identified in eight women, seven of whom gave birth to male infants.[42] Other investigators have not yet confirmed these findings.

QUESTION 3: HOW ARE THE FETAL CELLS ISOLATED AND ANALYZED?

To isolate the rare fetal cell from maternal blood, features unique to the fetal cells must be recognized. The distinguishing features chosen depend on the cell type that is targeted. Most investigators have relied on monoclonal antibodies that recognize fetal antigens. In lymphocyte studies, these have been primarily paternal-specific HLA antigens. As mentioned previously, some groups have also generated monoclonal antibodies against trophoblastic cells.[7,32] However, these have not been found to be specific and are present on maternal leukocytes as well.[7]

Nucleated red blood cells have the advantage over lymphocytes of being more specifically a fetal cell type. Studies using NRBCs have taken advantage of differences in cell size and granularity and have used antibodies to the transferrin receptor (CD71), the thrombospondin receptor (CD36), and glycophorin-A (GPA).[6,37,40] The transferrin receptor, CD71, is expressed by all cells that actively incorporate iron. Thus, it is present on erythroid precursors but not on mature RBCs. The thrombospondin receptor, CD36, is also expressed during the early stages of erythroid differentiation and agglutinates fetal, but not adult, erythrocytes. Glycophorin-A is a cell-surface protein unique to the erythroid cell line.[30] While neither CD71 nor CD36 is fetal cell or erythrocyte specific, GPA antibodies are red cell specific and thus promote the isolation of fetal NRBCs from maternal blood.[6]

Monoclonal antibodies are used in conjunction with a variety of separation techniques that sort for the presence or absence of a given antigen. Investigators have used density gradients and various devices, including a flow-activated cell sorter (FACS), magnetic-activated cell sorter (MACS), and immunomagnetic beads.* Density gradients take advantage of differences in cell size or volume, while the other techniques rely at least in part on binding to monoclonal antibodies. Antibodies can be fluorescently labeled and incubated with the cell suspension of interest. The FACS can then sort selectively for the cells labeled with the antibody and its fluorescent tag. Immunomagnetic beads and the MACS both use antibodies attached to magnetic beads. Target cells will bind the antibody-bead complex and can then be isolated with a magnetic device. In magnetic-activated cell sorting, the cell suspension is passed over a separation column with a magnetizable matrix that is placed into an extremely strong magnetic field. Unlabeled cells flow through the matrix, and labeled cells stick to the column and are eluted after being removed from the magnetic field.

QUESTION 4: AT WHAT GESTATIONAL AGE SHOULD MATERNAL BLOOD BE SAMPLED?

The optimal timing of testing maternal blood for fetal cells is not known. Bianchi and colleagues[3] specifically addressed this issue by summarizing several of their studies in which they sorted for CD71-positive cells and then used PCR for Y-specific sequences. In 12 pregnancies with male fetuses, Y-specific sequences could be isolated from maternal

---

*References 2, 19, 31, 32, and 40.

blood before 16 weeks, while patients studied at later gestational ages revealed no Y-specific material. The authors concluded that fetal NRBCs were unlikely to be present after 16 weeks' gestation. Ganshirt-Ahlert and associates,[19] however, found that NRBCs could be isolated during all three trimesters, and Simpson and associates[38] likewise found fetal cells to be present at least through 18 weeks' gestation, with no decrease in frequency after the sixteenth week. Other studies have shown fetal cells to be present as early as 6 weeks' gestation.[26,28] It is likely that NRBCs are present in increased numbers earlier in pregnancy, since the percentage of nucleated erythrocytes versus non-nucleated erythrocytes progressively decreases as the fetus matures.[13]

QUESTION 5: DO FETAL CELLS PERSIST FROM PREVIOUS PREGNANCIES?

Lymphocytes can have lifespans of many years. This knowlede has prompted the concern that fetal lymphocytes isolated from maternal blood could represent a previous, possibly even unrecognized pregnancy. This possibility is especially worrisome given the fact that early spontaneous abortion frequently occurs as a result of chromosome abnormalities. A number of investigators have reported the detection of Y-chromosome DNA in the blood of women as long as 27 years after they gave birth to male infants.[5,10,24,36] Bianchi and colleagues[5] hypothesize that pregnancy establishes a long-term low-grade chimeric state in the human female. Such concerns have prompted the recommendation that CD34-positive and CD38-positive lymphocyte stem cells be depleted from maternal samples before antenatal genetic diagnosis.[5] This difficulty is also one reason that current investigation has focused on other cell lines, specifically NRBCs. Few data are available regarding the half-life of fetal erythroblasts, but in the adult it appears that the maturation time from a multipotential stem cell to a reticulocyte is only about 5 days.[16] This short half-life makes it much less likely that fetal NRBCs from a previous pregnancy would lead to diagnostic error.

QUESTION 6: CAN ANALYSIS OF FETAL CELLS ISOLATED FROM MATERNAL BLOOD PROVIDE DEFINITIVE GENETIC DIAGNOSIS?

Ideally, the aim of isolating fetal cells from maternal circulation is to provide definitive genetic testing. Prospective clinical studies to determine the potential for such testing are continuing. Because the isolated fetal cells have not been responsive to mitogens, it has been necessary to perform genetic analysis on the few individual cells present. This limitation has necessitated testing with either FISH or PCR, neither of which provides a full cytogenetic diagnosis. Isolation of fetal cells from maternal blood currently is most likely to provide screening for the common aneuploidies (47,+13; 47,+18; 47,+21; 47,XXY; 45,X) and other genetic disorders for which the molecular defect is known. The test has already been used to diagnose fetal aneuploidies by in situ hybridization of DNA probes to fetal nucleated erythrocytes in maternal blood.[3,8,18,34] The DNA probes can recognize the presence or absence of specific chromosomes of interest (e.g., chromosome 13, 18, or 21). However, the probes are not capable of indicating whether a small portion of a chromosome is missing or rearranged. In addition, limitations in the number of fluorescent tags available as labels means that not all the chromosomes can be studied at once. Thus, abnormalities involving chromosomes other than 13, 18, 21, X, and Y, and chromosome rearrangements, would not be recognized with this technique.

Polymerase chain reaction, on the other hand, can be used to determine the presence or absence of specific gene sequences, either normal or abnormal. It can therefore be used to determine the presence of Y-specific sequences and thus fetal sex. In addition, PCR can probe for specific genetic defects. Camaschella and colleagues[9] have used PCR to detect paternally derived fetal hemoglobin Lepore sequences in maternal blood. Lo and associates[27] have used PCR to determine the fetal RhD status of Rh-negative mothers. However, use of PCR in the setting of a rare fetal cell among many maternal cells is difficult using current methods. In addition, PCR does not allow abnormalities in chromosome number (e.g., the trisomies) to be identified.

Ultimately, isolation of fetal cells from the maternal circulation may be used most commonly as a screening test for the clinically important aneuploidies. Isolated cells could be probed using FISH, with a threshold ratio of aneuploid cells to normal cells used to indicate a positive screen. Possibly in conjunction with biochemical or ultrasound screening, this test could form the basis for offering definitive cytogenetic testing via CVS or amniocentesis. Obviously, determination of the ultimate role of this exciting new technology awaits large clinic trials to establish its degree of efficiency in detecting fetal genetic abnormalities. The NIH is sponsoring such a trial, which began in 1994 and is expected to last 3½ years.

REFERENCES

1. Arinami I, Hamada H, Hamaguchi H et al: Fetal cells in maternal blood: frequencies measured by the polymerase chain reaction (PCR) and in situ hybridization, *Am J Hum Genet* 49(suppl):A1131, 1991.
2. Bianchi DW, Flint AF, Pizzimenti MF et al: Isolation of fetal DNA from nucleated erythrocytes in maternal blood, *Proc Natl Acad Sci U S A* 87:3279, 1990.
3. Bianchi DW, Mahr A, Zickwolf GK et al: Detection of fetal cells with 47,XY,+21 karyotype in maternal peripheral blood, *Hum Genet* 90:368, 1992.
4. Bianchi DW, Stewart JE, Garber MF et al: Possible effect of gestational age on the detection of fetal nucleated erythrocytes in maternal blood, *Prenat Diagn* 11:523, 1991.
5. Bianchi DW, Sylvester S, Zickwolf GK et al: Fetal stem cells persist in maternal blood for decades postpartum, *Am J Hum Genet* 53(suppl):A251, 1993.
6. Bianchi DW, Zickwolf GK, Yih M: Erythroid-specific antibodies enhance detection of fetal nucleated erythrocytes in maternal blood, *Prenat Diagn* 13:293, 1993.
7. Bruch JF, Metezeau P, Garcia-Fonknechten N et al: Trophoblast-like cells sorted from peripheral maternal blood using flow cytometry: a multiparametric study involving transmission electron microscopy and fetal DNA amplification, *Prenat Diagn* 11:787, 1991.
8. Cacheux V, Milesi-Fluet C, Druart L et al: Detection of 47,XYY trophoblast fetal cells in maternal blood by fluorescence in situ hybridization after using immunomagnetic lymphocyte depletion and flow cytometric sorting, *Fetal Diagn Ther* 7:190, 1992.
9. Camaschella C, Alfarano A, Gottardi E et al: Prenatal diagnosis of fetal hemoglobin Lepore-Boston disease on maternal peripheral blood, *Blood* 75:2102, 1990.

10. Ciaranfi A, Curchod A, Odartchenko N: Survie de lymphocytes fœtaux dans le sang maternel post-partum, *Schweiz Med Wochenschr* 107:134, 1977.

11. Covone AE, Johnson PM, Mutton D: Trophoblast cells in peripheral blood from pregnant women, *Lancet* 2:841, 1984.

12. Covone AE, Kozma R, Johnson PM et al: Analysis of peripheral maternal blood samples for the presence of placental-derived cells using Y-specific probes and McAb H315, *Prenat Diagn* 8:591, 1988.

13. De Waele M, Foulon W, Renmans W: Hematologic values and lymphocyte subsets in fetal blood, *Am J Clin Pathol* 89:742, 1988.

14. Douglas GW, Thomas L, Carr M et al: Trophoblast in the circulating blood during pregnancy, *Am J Obstet Gynecol* 78:960, 1959.

15. Elias S, Price J, Dockter M: First trimester prenatal diagnosis of trisomy 21 in fetal cells from maternal blood, *Lancet* 340:1033, 1992.

16. Erslev AJ: Production of erythrocytes. In Williams WJ, Beutler E, Erslev AM, Lietman MA, editors: *Hematology*, New York, 1990, McGraw-Hill.

17. Ganshirt-Ahlert D, Borjesson-Stoll M, Burschyk M et al: Noninvasive prenatal diagnosis: triple density gradient, magnetic activated cell sorting and FISH prove to be an efficient and reproducible method for detection of fetal aneuploidies from maternal blood, *Am J Hum Genet* 51:A48, 1992.

18. Ganshirt-Ahlert D, Borjesson-Stoll M, Burschyk M: Detection of fetal trisomies 21 and 18 from maternal blood using triple density gradient and magnetic cell sorting, *Am J Reprod Immunol* 30:194, 1993.

19. Ganshirt-Ahlert D, Burschyk M, Garritsen HSP: Magnetic cell sorting and the transferrin receptor as potential means of prenatal diagnosis from maternal blood, *Am J Obstet Gynecol* 166:1350, 1992.

20. Goodfellow CF, Taylor PV: Extraction and identification of trophoblast cells circulating in peripheral blood during pregnancy, *Br J Obstet Gynæcol* 89:65, 1982.

21. Haddow JE, Palomaki GE, Knight GJ et al: Prenatal screening for Down syndrome with use of maternal serum markers, *N Engl J Med* 327:588, 1992.

22. Hall JM, Williams SJ: Isolation and purification of CD34+ fetal cells from maternal blood, *Am J Hum Genet* 51:A257, 1992.

23. Herzenberg LA, Bianchi DW, Schroder J et al: Fetal cells in the blood of pregnant women: detection and enrichment by fluorescence-activated cell sorting, *Proc Natl Acad Sci U S A* 76:1453, 1979.

24. Hseih T-T, Pao CC, Hor JJ et al: Presence of fetal cells in maternal circulation after delivery, *Hum Genet* 92:204, 1993.

25. Iverson GM, Bianchi DW, Cann HM et al: Detection and isolation of fetal cells from maternal blood using the fluorescence-activated cell sorter (FACS), *Prenat Diagn* 1:61, 1981.

26. Liou JD, Pao CC, Hor JJ et al: Fetal cells in the maternal circulation during first trimester in pregnancies, *Hum Genet* 92:309, 1993.

27. Lo YM, Bowell PJ, Selinger M et al: Prenatal determination of fetal RhD status by analysis of peripheral blood of rhesus negative mothers, *Lancet* 341:1147, 1993.

28. Lo YM, Patel P, Baigent CN et al: Prenatal sex determination from maternal peripheral blood using the polymerase chain reaction, *Hum Genet* 90:483, 1993.

29. Lo YM, Wainscot JS, Gilmer MDG: Prenatal sex determination by DNA amplification from maternal peripheral blood, *Lancet* 2:1363, 1989.

30. Loken MR, Civin CI, Bigbee WL: Coordinate glycosylation and cell surface expression of glycophorin A during normal human erythropoiesis, *Blood* 69:1959, 1987.

31. Miltenyi S, Muller W, Weichel W et al: High gradient magnetic cell separation with MACS, *Cytometry* 11:231, 1990.

32. Mueller UW, Hawes CS, Wright AE et al: Isolation of fetal trophoblast cells from peripheral blood of pregnant women, *Lancet* 336:197, 1990.

33. Phillips OP, Elias S, Shulman LP et al: Maternal serum screening for fetal Down syndrome in women less than 35 years of age using alpha-fetoprotein, hCG, and unconjugated estriol: a prospective 2-year study, *Obstet Gynecol* 80:353, 1992.

34. Price J, Elias S, Wachtel SS et al: Prenatal diagnosis using fetal cells isolated from maternal blood by multiparameter flow cytometry, *Am J Obstet Gynecol* 165:1731, 1991.

35. Schmorl G: *Pathologisch-anatomische untersuchungen uber puerperal eklampsie*, Leipzig, Germany, 1893, Vogel.

36. Schroder J, Thlikainen A, de la Chapelle A: Fetal leukocytes in the maternal circulation after delivery, *Transplantation* 17:346, 1974.

37. Simpson JL, Elias S: Isolating fetal erythroblasts from maternal blood with identification of fetal trisomy by fluorescent in situ hybridization, *Prenat Diagn* 12:S34, 1992.

38. Simpson JL, Elias S: Isolating fetal cells from maternal blood: advances in prenatal diagnosis through molecular technology, *JAMA* 270:2357, 1993.

39. Tharapel AT, Jaswaney VL, Dockter ME et al: Can fetal cells in maternal blood be selected through cytogenetic means? *Am J Hum Genet* 45(suppl):271, 1989.

40. Wachtel S, Elias S, Price J: Fetal cells in the maternal circulation: isolation by multiparameter flow cytometry and confirmation by polymerase chain reaction, *Hum Reprod* 6:1466, 1991.

41. Walknowska J, Conte FA, Grumbach MM: Practical and theoretical implication of fetal/maternal lymphocyte transfer, *Lancet* 1:1119, 1969.

42. Wessman M, Ylinen K, Knuutila S: Fetal granulocytes in maternal venous blood detected in in situ hybridization, *Prenat Diagn* 12:993, 1992.

43. Yeoh SC, Sargent IL, Redman CWG: Detection of fetal cells in maternal blood, *Prenat Diagn* 11:117, 1991.

44. Youssef M, Shulman LP, Tharapel AT: Failure to document fetal cells in maternal circulation using the Selypes-Lorencz "air-culture" cytogenetic technique, *Hum Genet* 85:133, 1990.

45. Zilliacus R, De la Chapelle A, Schroder J et al: Transplacental passage of foetal blood cells, *Scand J Hæmatol* 15:333, 1975.

CHAPTER 30

Preimplantation Embryo Analysis

MELISSA H. FRIES

Couples at risk for genetic disorders are currently offered invasive fetal testing, such as chorionic villus sampling or amniocentesis, to determine whether their pregnancy is affected. Such procedures are performed on an established pregnancy and carry low but distinct risks for procedure-related pregnancy loss. If an affected fetus is identified, the parents may choose to terminate the pregnancy, which can be physically difficult and emotionally wrenching. Preimplantation embryo analysis is a technique used to obtain genetic information about a particular embryo before it is implanted into the uterus. Preimplantation embryo analysis is intended to preclude the need for pregnancy termination of affected fetuses by identifying affected embryos before pregnancy implantation so that only unaffected embryos are implanted. Although largely an investigational procedure now, the technique holds great promise for future application in the identification of genetic disorders.

❧ Patient Profile: Preimplantation embryo analysis for cystic fibrosis

A 27-year-old Caucasian woman (gravida 1, para 1000) and her husband seek genetic counseling because they were identified as carriers of the ΔF508 mutation for cystic fibrosis (the most common cystic fibrosis mutation) after the birth of their first child, who died of complications of this disease. They deeply desire to have more children but feel that the 25% risk of recurrence is too great to warrant another pregnancy. They are strongly opposed to pregnancy termination on religious grounds and are not comfortable with the option of artificial insemination using noncarrier sperm. They have heard of preimplantation embryo analysis and wish to assess its appropriateness for themselves.

QUESTION 1: WHICH GENETIC CONDITIONS CAN BE DIAGNOSED BY PREIMPLANTATION EMBRYO ANALYSIS?

Human preimplantation embryo analysis has been accomplished by Handyside and colleagues[5] for sex determination in cases of X-linked disorders, in which male fetuses (who may receive an affected X chromosome from their carrier mothers) are at risk of being affected. Female fetuses (who may receive an affected X chromosome from their carrier mothers but who have an additional normal X chromosome from their fathers) are not at risk. Thus, disorders such as hemophilia A, Duchenne muscular dystrophy, Pelizaeus-Merzbacher disease (a neurodegenerative disorder that causes rotatory nystagmus and early death), and Lesch-Nyhan disease (an incapacitating neurologic disorder characterized by severe mental retardation and self-mutilation), all of which are inherited in an X-linked recessive pattern, could be prevented by the identification and selective transfer of only female embryos.[8] Conditions such as Rett syndrome (a neurologic disorder manifested by loss of previously achieved developmental milestones and continual hand wringing) that appear to affect only females could be prevented by the selective transfer of only male embryos.[12]

Sex determination is necessary for preimplantation embryo analysis if the gene for a particular X-linked condition has not been isolated and cloned (identified). However, if a gene and the specific

---

SOME DISORDERS POTENTIALLY DIAGNOSABLE BY PREIMPLANTATION EMBRYO ANALYSIS

Cystic fibrosis

A pulmonary disorder of varying severity; common in the Caucasian population

Lesch-Nyhan disease

An incapacitating neurologic disorder characterized by severe mental retardation and self-mutilation

Tay-Sachs disease

A neurodegenerative disorder that leads to mental retardation and early death; common in people of Ashkenazi Jewish and French Canadian ancestry[8]

Fragile X syndrome

A common cause of mental retardation; seen predominantly in males[9]

Gorlin syndrome

A condition characterized by basal cell nevi, jaw cysts, distinctive facies, and mild developmental delay

Ornithine transcarbamylase deficiency

A metabolic abnormality of the urea cycle that leads to severe neonatal hyperammonemia and death

Multiple endocrine neoplasia, type II

A disorder characterized by pheochromocytoma and medullary carcinoma of the thyroid

Hemophilia A

A bleeding disorder caused by deficiency of clotting factor VIII

mutations are known (from previous analysis of the parents and usually a previous affected child), then theoretically any such condition could be diagnosed by preimplantation analysis. The disorders listed in the box on p. 237 have been diagnosed in single-cell assay, a technology that could be used for preimplantation analysis. At present, only births of infants who have undergone preimplantation biopsy for sex selection and for cystic fibrosis have been reported in the literature.[4-6]

Chromosome abnormalities could potentially be diagnosed by preimplantation analysis, using a technique called fluorescence in situ hybridization (FISH).[11] This technique involves the use of specific fluorescently labeled probes for chromosomes X, Y, 13, 18, and 21. The probes are hybridized to the biopsied cell and enable the number of each of these chromosomes to be counted in that particular cell. Thus, an embryo with Down syndrome (three chromosome 21s) could be identified. However, this technique has been performed only experimentally, and its utility remains to be proved. Routine chromosome assessment is not yet possible using preimplantation analysis.

QUESTION 2: HOW ARE EMBRYOS OBTAINED FOR ANALYSIS?

The analysis is performed in conjunction with in vitro fertilization programs. The woman is treated with gonadotropins for superovulation, and ova are harvested by standard methods, using sonographically guided transvaginal aspiration. Semen is obtained by noncoital ejaculation. Embryos may also be harvested by uterine lavage, but the yield of this method is also improved by ovulation induction, rather than spontaneous ovulation.[1] This method has the advantage of not requiring invasive harvesting techniques but may not result in complete garnering of all embryos and potentially could be associated with ectopic pregnancy.

QUESTION 3: HOW IS THE EMBRYO BIOPSY PERFORMED?

Embryo biopsy may be performed by using one of three techniques. The first and earliest technique involves analysis of the first polar body of the egg, before fertilization has occurred.[14] Because the woman is presumed to be a carrier but is not affected with the condition in question, she will have two alleles for the gene involved: one that is normal and one that is abnormal or mutant. Analysis of the genetic status of the first polar body can be performed to determine the status of the oocyte because if the polar body carries the mutant allele, the oocyte will be unaffected. However, if the polar body is normal, the oocyte would have the mutant allele and would not be used in fertilization. This technique has the theoretic advantage of not posing a threat to the early embryo. However, it is applicable only in the identification of known genetic disorders mapped close to the centromere. In all other disorders there is a risk for crossover of the homologous chromosomes before the separation of the primary oocyte and the first polar body, which would lead to an inaccurate diagnosis. The technique cannot be used for sex determination of embryos because both polar body and oocyte will contain an X chromosome. Such a biopsy is also technically difficult.

The second embryo biopsy technique, the one most often described, involves biopsy of the embryo at the four- to eight-cell stage after fertilization.[10,15] Harvested oocytes and sperm are incubated together, in the standard fashion for in vitro fertilization, and the culture is observed until cell division to a four- to eight-cell stage has occurred. At this point, the embryos are removed to be placed in separate cultures. Under micromanipulation, zona drilling is performed. In this technique, a dilute acid solution is used to form a hole in the surrounding zona pellucida, and a microneedle formed from finely drawn micropipettes is inserted through the hole. A single blastomere is aspirated, washed, and separately analyzed while the residual embryo remains in culture. If the analysis reveals that the embryo is not affected with the condition in question, the embryo can be transferred to the uterus for potential implantation. This process usually occurs 48 hours from the time of ovum harvest; embryo biopsy, analysis, and transfer can then be accomplished on the same day.

The third embryo biopsy technique involves biopsy of the trophoectoderm.[12,14] In this technique, the embryo is incubated until it reaches the blastocyst stage (approximately 4 days). At this time, the cells will separate into the inner cell mass, destined to become the body of the embryo, and the outer cell mass, or trophoectoderm, destined to become the placenta. Biopsy of the trophoectoderm comprises the removal of 10 to 15 cells, without affecting future placental growth. As in the second technique, the zona pellucida is drilled with dilute acid solution, and the cells that spontaneously herniate through the hole are aspirated with a micropipette. Such a technique has the distinct advantage of allowing a large number of cells to be obtained, which makes analysis easier. However, the incubated blastocyst is less likely to implant than the younger eight-cell embryo, making this a less attractive technique for in vitro fertilization programs. Blastocysts obtained by uterine lavage after superovulation and spontaneous insemination may not have altered implantation characteristics and thus might be analyzed successfully using this technique.[12]

QUESTION 4: HOW IS THE BIOPSY SPECIMEN ANALYZED?

Because of the very small number of cells obtained by embryo biopsy and the limited time available before the embryo must be transferred to the uterus if it is to implant, the use of standard culture methods for chromosome analysis is impossible. The tissue is instead analyzed by polymerase chain reaction (PCR). Polymerase chain reaction is a technique for amplifying a very small amount of DNA. It has been used successfully in the study of DNA obtained from single or very few cells. The technique involves the use of specific primers for the defined areas of DNA under study, such as specific Y chromosome genes *ZFY* or *SRY* (unique regions of DNA found only on the Y chromosome), to determine male sex, or X chromosome genes, such as *ZFX* (a distinctive region of DNA found uniquely on the X chromosome).[5] Polymerase chain reaction has also been used in the study of known genetic mutations, such as the $\Delta F508$ mutation in cystic fibrosis.[6] The primers are constructed to allow the amplification of only the region of DNA that they flank, thus targeting the specific gene or chromosome region in question. Polymerase chain reaction can amplify a single copy of a gene many thousands of times, facilitating its recognition by molecular biologic methods. Sex has also been determined using FISH, with probes specific for the X and Y chromosomes (see Question 1).[11]

QUESTION 5: HOW SAFE IS PREIMPLANTATION ANALYSIS FOR THE EMBRYO?

Extensive studies using a mouse model have indicated that embryos on which biopsy is performed at the four- or eight-cell stage of development are not compromised in their continued development.[15] This finding has also been established in human embryos at the eight-cell stage, although the number of pregnancies evaluated is very small.[7] Biopsy at the four-cell stage may retard subsequent cleavage of the embryonic cells, and improved growth has been observed if the embryo is allowed to divide to at least five cells before biopsy is performed.[6] None of the infants delivered after embryo biopsy has had any physical anomaly that could have been attributed to the biopsy.[4-6]

QUESTION 6: HOW SUCCESSFUL IS THE IN VITRO FERTILIZATION PROCESS IN ACHIEVING PREGNANCIES AFTER BIOPSY?

The successful continuing pregnancy rate after a single cycle of in vitro fertilization in infertile couples varies from center to center but may average 14% to 15% per cycle. Since most couples who seek preimplantation embryo analysis are not infertile, pregnancy rates per transfer may be higher for them. A recent report indicates that among 11 patients who had preimplantation embryo analysis and were treated through 16 cycles of in vitro fertilization, there were 13 embryo transfers, with seven positive pregnancy tests and six established pregnancies.[4]

QUESTION 7: HAVE ANY HEALTHY INFANTS BEEN BORN AFTER PREIMPLANTATION EMBRYO ANALYSIS?

Handyside and colleagues[5] have reported two successful twin pregnancies in which the embryos had undergone sex determination by preimplantation embryo analysis; they have also reported a liveborn infant who had been correctly diagnosed as being unaffected with the ΔF508 cystic fibrosis mutation after embryo biopsy.[6] Grifo and colleagues[4] have reported three deliveries of four infants (one set of twins) whose sex had been correctly determined by preimplantation embryo analysis; three pregnancies were continuing.[4]

QUESTION 8: HOW RELIABLE HAS PREIMPLANTATION ANALYSIS BEEN?

Of the infants born after preimplantation embryo analysis, all have been of the previously determined sex. Grifo and colleagues[4] reported a case of cystic fibrosis in which the diagnosis of a carrier but unaffected fetus was made. However, on chorionic villus sampling the fetus was in fact determined to be affected. This error was attributed to misinterpretation of the PCR results.[4] Single-cell PCR techniques, such as those used for preimplantation analysis, may be readily contaminated by even the most minute amounts of stray DNA. Thus, false-positive or false-negative results may be obtained unless extremely stringent measures are taken to minimize all possible contamination.

QUESTION 9: WHAT ARE THE MATERNAL RISKS OF PREIMPLANTATION EMBRYO ANALYSIS?

The risks for the mother are principally those of in vitro fertilization. These include the risk of ovarian hyperstimulation syndrome after superovulation, the risk of infection at the time of ovum harvest or embryo transfer, the risk of miscarriage, and the risk of multifetal pregnancy, with the associated risks of preterm labor and delivery, preeclampsia, and uterine atony and hemorrhage. Embryo biopsy in itself does not add to these risks. However, because of the experimental nature of preimplantation analysis and the risk of obtaining false-positive or false-negative results from PCR contamination, women who undergo preimplantation analysis and achieve successful pregnancies are still offered confirmatory prenatal diagnostic studies, such as amniocentesis or chorionic villus sampling.

QUESTION 10: HOW AVAILABLE IS PREIMPLANTATION ANALYSIS, AND WHAT ARE ITS COSTS?

Most centers that perform in vitro fertilization are unable to perform embryo biopsy. The cost of embryo biopsy may add approximately $2000 to $3000 to the cost of each cycle of in vitro fertilization.[12] However, this additional amount may be equivalent to the cost of a second-trimester pregnancy termination. Although early results are encouraging, preimplantation embryo analysis is currently considered to be an investigational technique, and its widespread use will require substantiation of its efficacy through greater numbers of pregnancies.

REFERENCES

1. Buster JE, Bustillo M, Rodi IA et al: Biologic and morphologic development of donated human ova recovered by nonsurgical uterine lavage, *Am J Obstet Gynecol* 153:211, 1985.
2. Chong SS, Kristjansson K, Van den Veyver IB et al: Preimplantation analysis for dystrophin gene deletions after single cell genome preamplification, *Am J Hum Genet* 3(suppl 53):1392, 1993.
3. Dokras A, Barlow DH, Jones E et al: Preimplantation diagnosis using single human blastomeres and trophoectoderm biopsies, *Am J Hum Genet* 3(suppl 53):1399, 1993.
4. Grifo J, Tang YX, Alikani M et al: First babies born in the USA after preimplantation genetic diagnosis of sex-linked diseases, *Am J Hum Genet* 3(suppl 53):7, 1993.
5. Handyside AH, Kontogianni EH, Hardy K et al: Pregnancies from biopsied human preimplantation embryos sexed by Y-specific DNA amplification, *Nature* 344:768, 1990.
6. Handyside AH, Lesko JG, Tarin JJ et al: Birth of a normal girl after in vitro fertilization and preimplantation diagnostic testing for cystic fibrosis, *N Engl J Med* 327:905, 1992.

7. Hardy K, Martin KL, Leese HJ et al: Human preimplantation development in vitro is not adversely affected by biopsy at the 8-cell stage, *Hum Reprod* 5:708, 1990.

8. Lesko JG, Snabes MC, Cota J et al: Preimplantation diagnosis of single human blastomeres for cystic fibrosis, Tay-Sachs, Lesch-Nyhan and hemophilia A disease, *Am J Hum Genet* 4(suppl 51):61, 1992.

9. Malter HE, Karickhofof L, Tucker M et al: Single cell analysis of the repeat expansion mutation associated with fragile X syndrome, *Am J Hum Genet* 3(suppl 53):1435, 1993.

10. Monk M, Handyside AH: Sexing of preimplantation mouse embryos by measurement of X-linked gene dosage in a single blastomere, *J Reprod Fertil* 82:365, 1988.

11. Munne S, Weier HUG, Grifo J et al: Simultaneous preimplantation genetic diagnosis of aneuploidy X, Y, 18, 13, and 21 by multiple probe in situ hybridization, *Am J Hum Genet* 3(suppl 53):92, 1993.

12. Simpson JL, Carson SA: Preimplantation genetic analysis, *N Engl J Med* 327:951, 1992.

13. Snabes MC, Subramanian S, Krisjansson K et al: Whole genome amplification in preimplantation genetic diagnosis, *Am J Hum Genet* 3(suppl 53):90, 1993.

14. Verlinsky Y: Biopsy of human gametes. In Verlinsky Y, Kuliev A, editors: *Preimplantation genetics*, New York, 1991, Plenum.

15. Wilton LJ, Shaw JM, Tounson AO: Successful single-cell biopsy and cryopreservation of preimplantation mouse embryos, *Fertil Steril* 51:513, 1989.

CHAPTER 31

Stem Cell Transplantation for the Treatment of Genetic Disease

JOSEPH M. WILEY

Several human genetic diseases are characterized by defective, deficient, or altered bone marrow hematopoietic stem cells.[1,46,61,62] The common characteristic of these diseases is that they all eventually result in the death of the patient. The first successful allogeneic bone marrow transplants (BMTs)* were performed in 1968 in patients with severe combined immune deficiency (SCID) syndrome and Wiskott-Aldrich (WAS) syndrome.[4,32] Since then, variations of the transplant procedure have been developed and applied to a wide variety of disorders.† Bone marrow transplantation has become an established part of the treatment of acquired or congenital diseases that cause single or multilineage bone marrow failure in children and young adults.[1,14,33,53] Some disorders, such as SCID, cause death very early in life, whereas others (e.g., sickle cell anemia) may cause substantial morbidity but only a modestly increased mortality rate during the first 20 to 30 years of life and an overall shortened average lifespan.[28,42,43] In general, these disorders can be divided into three categories of disease: immune deficiency disorders; marrow failure syndromes and hematopoietic gene defects; and congenital metabolic disorders (see the box on p. 240).

Many of these disorders can be palliated or treated effectively for varying periods of time, but no standard treatment other than BMT is truly curative. Bone marrow transplantation has been used quite successfully to treat these diseases and is the only known curative therapy for most of these disorders. Bone marrow transplantation, however, is associated with substantial morbidity and mortality. Careful consideration must be given to the risk-benefit ratio for this procedure when used to treat certain diseases. The risks of infection, preparative regimen toxicity, graft versus host disease (GVHD), and therapy-induced secondary cancers must be weighed against the likelihood of reversal of the disease phenotype.[9,72] The risk-benefit considerations may vary significantly, depending on the disease type.

---

*The abbreviation *BMT* is used throughout this chapter to refer to both "bone marrow transplant" and "bone marrow transplantation."

†References 1, 33, 43, 49, and 73.

CONGENITAL DISEASES CURABLE BY ALLOGENEIC BONE MARROW TRANSPLANTATION

Immunodeficiency states

Severe combined immune deficiency syndrome
Wiskott-Aldrich syndrome
Lymphohistiocytic disorders
Omenn syndrome

Hematopoietic disorders

Congenital aplastic anemia
Blackfan-Diamond anemia
Fanconi anemia
Homozygous β-thalassemia
Sickle cell anemia
Reticular dysgenesis
Dyskeratosis congenita
Osteopetrosis (osteoclast activity deficiency)

Leukocyte adhesion deficiency
Cartilage hair hypoplasia
CD11 and CD18 deficiencies
Chédiak-Higashi syndrome

Congenital metabolic disorders

Maroteaux-Lamy syndrome
Adrenoleukodystrophy
Metachromatic leukodystrophy
Hurler syndrome
Hunter syndrome
Fucosidosis
Gaucher disease
Farber disease
Wolman disease

Liquid bone marrow contains pluripotent hematopoietic progenitor cells that are capable of reconstituting hematopoiesis after myeloablative chemotherapy or radiotherapy.[70,74] Better understanding of the biology of blood cell production and the nature of the pluripotent progenitor cells, called *stem cells*, has led to marked improvement in the application of bone marrow (stem cell) transplants in genetic disorders. This review will discuss unique uses of stem cells and focus on the important issues facing obstetricians, general practitioners, and pediatricians. Some newer discoveries in stem cell biology will be described, and several of the more novel approaches that currently make use of these discoveries will be discussed.

Hematopoiesis

The study of hematopoiesis using suitable animal models and human in vitro cell cultures has greatly enhanced our understanding of bone marrow cellular and microenvironmental function.[10,18] The unifying premise of this study is the concept that a small percentage of bone marrow cells has a unique capacity for self-renewal and multilineage proliferation and differentiation. This group of cells is well demonstrated but incompletely defined; collectively the group is termed *stem cells*.[10,47,52] The existence of bone marrow stem cells has been conclusively demonstrated in animal marrow transplant studies and confirmed by large numbers of successful human bone marrow transplants.[32,42,78] Molecular studies performed at various lengths of time post-BMT demonstrate that post-transplant hematopoiesis is largely or exclusively donor in origin for an indefinite time period.[32,42,78] These studies confirm the theory that hematopoiesis is generated by a group of cellular-derived stem cells and that these cells are capable of fully reconstituting normal hematopoiesis in histocompatible recipients.

Bone marrow stem cells used in transplantation are usually obtained from multiple iliac crest aspirations performed with the aid of local or general anesthesia in the operating room. Bone marrow obtained in this manner from an allogeneic source (related donor or matched unrelated donor [MUD]) or from the patient (autologous donor) may be transplanted unmanipulated or may undergo a variety of in vitro procedures to deplete targeted cell populations deemed unnecessary or harmful to the recipient (e.g., tumor cells, T lymphocytes responsible for GVHD).[27,50,74] Recently, alternative sources of stem cells capable of self-renewal and marrow repopulation have been identified. These sources include peripheral blood, umbilical cord blood, and the fetal liver. The potential for ex vivo expansion of isolated stem cells also exists.[6,25,31,85] In addition, use of stem cell transplantation has expanded to include gene therapy and in utero prenatal treatment of genetic diseases.[17,19,21,29]

Biology of Human Bone Marrow–Derived Stem Cells

Human bone marrow is a large and complex organ with all of the genetic material required to produce human blood cells. The proliferation, differentiation, maturation, and release of these cells are well controlled by a variety of interactions involving contact among cells, regulation by stromal cells, and secretion of a variety of systemically and locally active cytokines.[15,18,51] Different stresses result in preferential expansion of certain bone marrow subsets. For example, anemia will stimulate the generation and proliferation of red cell precursors as long as adequate precursor molecules and substrate are available. A small subset of bone marrow cells has the capacity to self-renew and proliferate in response to these stresses and to generate multilineage differentiated cells. This compartment of the bone marrow is often referred to as the *progenitor compartment* and includes all of the colony-forming cells (CFCs) and lineage-specific and lineage-unrestricted stem cells.[16,47]

Within the progenitor compartment (Figure 31-1) is a group of cells called *pluripotent stem cells*. This subset of bone marrow cells has the ability to self-renew and to produce lymphoid, myeloid, erythroid, and megakaryocytic progenitors under the influence of specific factors and cytokines.[47,52] There are no known distinguishing morphologic, cytochemical, or immunologic features that specifically identify this subset of cells, but many characteristics have been described. Careful analyses in animal and human transplantation studies demonstrate trilineage production of donor blood cells in specimens obtained in short-term and long-term follow-up after BMT.[42,78] Many in vitro assays have been developed by tissue culture methods to study bone marrow progenitors and to determine their function and numbers.[11,12,16,22,76] In these assays, aliquots of blood, bone marrow, or other sources (e.g., cord blood, fetal liver) are placed in tissue culture media and supplemented by a variety of nutrients, growth factors, cytokines, and support cells. Proliferative capacity of the seeding population is measured by production of colonies in semi-solid media, increase in numbers of cells, and demonstration of other biologic characteristics of human blood cells. These assays

PROGENITORS

PRECURSORS

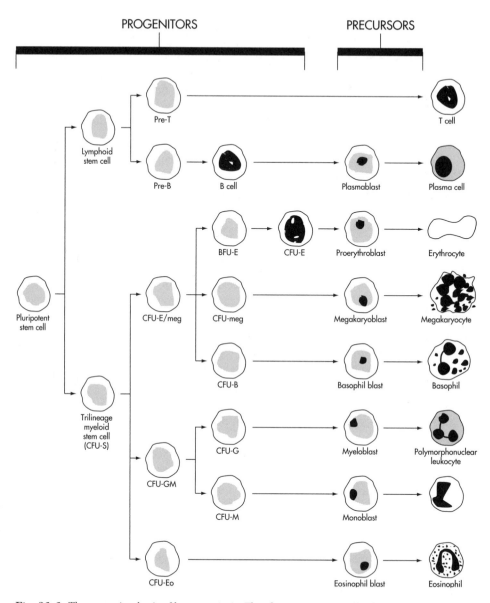

Fig. 31-1 The progenitor basis of hematopoiesis. The pluripotent stem cell exhibits self-renewal and stochastic differentiation into the committed progenitor pool. (From Williams D, Nathan D: *Semin Hematol* 28:115, 1991.)

are quite useful because they allow comparison of the progenitor content of bone marrow, peripheral blood, and human placental cord blood.[6,15,30,51] Assays have been developed that measure committed progenitors, uncommitted progenitors, lineage-restricted progenitors, and multilineage progenitors.

The proliferative capacity of bone marrow–derived or blood-derived hematopoietic cells is measured in the laboratory by placing these cells in various forms of in vitro assays and looking for colony production or cell proliferation. The measurement expressed as *CFUs in methylcellulose culture* describes the number of cells capable of proliferation in short-term culture conditions for the various lineages. Measurement of CFUs for erythroid (CFU-E) or granulocyte-macrophage (CFU-GM) allows an estimation of committed progenitors in short-term assay (7 to 10 days).[15] More immature progenitors give rise to mixed colonies of granulocyte, erythroid, myeloid, or megakaryocytic cells (CFU-GEMM or "CFU mix") in 14-day culture systems supported by a variety of stimulatory cytokines.[16] These culture assays describe a group of lineage-committed, mature progenitor cells that are responsible for the earliest phases of hematopoietic recovery after dose-intensive chemotherapy and bone marrow transplantation.[6] However, they are not true stem cells and lack the capacity for extended self-renewal or lymphoid differentiation. Cells that, after 28-day methylcellulose culture, are capable of self-renewal and formation of very large colonies with extensive replicating capacity are called *high–proliferative potential colony-forming cells (HPP-CFCs)*. Recent studies have demonstrated that these cells lack the ability to form lymphoid progenitors and are probably very immature myeloid progenitor stem cells capable of limited self-renewal.[12]

Long-term bone marrow cultures (LTBMCs) are systems for studying stromal cell and stem cell biology of hematopoietic cells placed in liquid culture with an adherent stromal support layer, continuous replacement of cytokines, or both. Stem cells responsible for establishing 8- to 14-week cultures are called *long-term culture–initiating cells (LTC-ICs)* and have the ability to generate trilineage hematopoiesis and to provide progenitors for lymphoid precursors.[22,56] These cells are characterized as very immature progenitors and under appropriate cytokine stimulation will develop lymphoid and myeloid progenitors.[22,56,78] Additional studies are needed to further refine LTBMC and to determine whether the LTC-IC can be classified as a true stem cell.

Monoclonal antibodies have been developed to characterize progenitor cells on the basis of expression of cell-surface molecules. The CD34 antigen (*CD* denotes "cluster designation," a term used to refer to a cluster of different antibodies that recognize the same epitope) recognized by a variety of mouse monoclonal antibodies (HPCA-1, HPCA-2, Ab-12.8, etc.) is present on most of the CFCs in blood and bone marrow and is present on the most immature progenitor cells.[3] Suspensions of bone marrow cells positively selected for CD34 are highly purified for progenitor cells. These cell suspensions represent less than 5% of the total nucleated cells present in bone marrow or peripheral blood yet contain most of the CFCs and LTC-ICs in the preparation.[3,6,30] These cell preparations have now been shown to produce complete hematopoietic engraftment in patients undergoing BMT.[7,67] Therefore, the

CD34 antigen marks a subset of bone marrow cells that contains virtually all of the proliferative component and probably also the stem cell component of bone marrow and peripheral blood.

Using a variety of methods, the CD34-positive fraction of bone marrow can be further purified to exclude cells with lineage-restricted antigens. The resultant cells are highly purified for immature progenitors and LTC-ICs.[3] One of the more promising applications of this technology is the in vitro expansion of the highly purified stem cells by the addition of cytokines and hematopoietic growth factors. Methods are currently available to isolate very immature progenitor cells with multipotential capability.[37,67] These cells can be used for culture, for infusion after chemotherapy, as targets for gene therapy (see below), and as a starting point for ex vivo expansion.[17,21,31,51] Investigators have studied a variety of methods of expanding hematopoietic stem cells in vitro through LTBMC.[25,31] More recently, the use of the ligand for the c-kit protooncogene (also known as *stem cell factor [SCF]*, *steel factor*, and *c-kit ligand*) has greatly enhanced the success of these experiments. Using stem cell factor and combinations of cytokines, several investigators have been able to demonstrate remarkable expansion of the progenitor compartment in vitro[11,76] and to maintain LTBMC independent of a stromal cell layer.[11,51,56,76] These studies carry promise for the ex vivo expansion of normal hematopoietic progenitors to be used in dose-intensive chemotherapy, stem cell transplantation, gene therapy, and other applications.

Allogeneic Transplantation of Human Bone Marrow Stem Cells

The first successful transplantation of allogeneic bone marrow cells was performed in 1968 for a patient with SCID.[32] The first complete correction of a congenital hematopoietic defect was accomplished in 1976.[59] Since then, thousands of bone marrow transplants have been performed for a variety of disorders. The concept of BMT is relatively straightforward, yet its application is very complex. The process requires a source of transplantable hematopoietic stem cells, a regimen to prepare the recipient to accept these cells and allow for their viable growth, and supportive care to manage complications and mediate sustained engraftment of transplanted stem cells. Successful transplantation is dependent on compatibility between donor and recipient. This compatibility is determined largely by a set of closely grouped alleles on chromosome 6 called *histocompatibility-linked antigens (HLAs)*.[2,42] Matching is required for the antigens A, B, and DR. These antigens are the gene products of these alleles expressed on the surface of most cells. There must be at least a 5/6 antigen match between donor and recipient to allow for successful BMT of non–T cell-depleted bone marrow. Specific choice of preparative treatments, source of stem cells, and supportive care requires careful analysis of the disease to be treated and the circumstances and associated risks of the available stem cell source.

❧ Patient Profile: Stem cell transplantation for aplastic anemia

A 3-year-old girl is brought to her physician for fatigue and pallor. Physical examination reveals pale skin with petechial lesions, no organomegaly, and mild gingivitis. A complete blood count demonstrates pancytopenia, and bone marrow aspiration and biopsy show severe aplastic anemia.* The child has three older siblings, ages 5, 9, and 16. HLA typing reveals that the 5-year-old sister and the 16-year-old brother are 6/6 HLA matches, and the mother is a 5/6 antigen match.

QUESTION 1: IS BONE MARROW TRANSPLANTATION THE BEST OPTION FOR THIS PATIENT? IF SO, WHAT IS THE BEST SOURCE OF STEM CELLS?

Bone marrow transplantation is the treatment of choice for children with complete stem cell defects. In severe aplastic anemia, BMT is clearly better than other therapies in children. Stem cells can be obtained from a histocompatible family donor (allogeneic), from the patient's own bone marrow (autologous), or in rare instances, from an identical twin (syngeneic). This patient has no identical twin, and the patient's own marrow is damaged. Therefore, an allogeneic donor is required for treatment. The relative likelihood of success and the risks of transplant-related complications dictate the choice of bone marrow source. This topic is discussed further in Question 3.

QUESTION 2: HOW WILL THE CHILD BE TREATED TO INCREASE THE LIKELIHOOD OF SUCCESS OF THE TRANSPLANT?

Patients will not simply improve with infusion of donor stem cells if there is remaining host immunity. Even in severe aplastic anemia, host immune function is fully capable of recognizing and rejecting allogeneic stem cell grafts. Therefore, except in SCID syndrome, BMT patients usually receive a treatment regimen, also called the *preparative regimen*. This is a group of treatments, delivered over several days, designed to allow for engraftment of donor marrow, to prevent host immune cells from rejecting donor stem cells, to eradicate host hematopoietic tissue to allow "space" for donor stem cell expansion, and to treat the underlying disorder.[74]

In genetic diseases, the focus is to ensure engraftment and to create space by eliminating damaged bone marrow cells. Therefore, a preparative regimen that is immunosuppressive and myeloablative will enhance engraftment potential by suppressing host immune rejection and

---

*Severe aplastic anemia is usually acquired but is thought to be, in some cases, a consequence of increased risk secondary to an undiscovered genetic defect. Although the patient described in this profile does not have classic genetic disease, her case demonstrates the features important in bone marrow transplantation.

providing a competitive advantage for infused donor stem cells. The use of postgraft immuno-suppression with cyclosporin A and other agents helps maintain a healthy graft. The dose intensity of the preparative regimen is sufficient to approximate eradication of host hema-topoiesis and usually results in substantial nonhematopoietic toxicity. Therefore, careful mea-sures to decrease infection risk, to ensure nutritional support, and to maintain electrolyte bal-ance are necessary during the post–marrow infusion period. The hospital stay may be extended, and transplant-related mortality ranges from 5% to 50%.

QUESTION 3: WHAT RISK DO THE DONOR STEM CELLS POSE TO THE RECIPIENT?

Allogeneic bone marrow is a source of stem cells that are healthy, normal, and fully capa-ble of bone marrow reconstitution.[2,74] The infused allogeneic bone marrow contains immuno-competent T lymphocytes that can mount an immune response to host HLA-associated anti-gens.[2,35,71,74] Unless the donor and recipient are genotypically identical (syngeneic), there will be antigenic differences that can cause potentially serious complications.

A problem in allogeneic bone marrow transplantation is the phenomenon of donor T lym-phocyte recognition of recipient (host) tissue. This phenomenon, known as *graft versus host disease (GVHD)*, is a major cause of morbidity and mortality after allogeneic transplant and is often the limiting factor in this type of transplant.[35] Graft versus host disease is a complex immunologic reaction of donor-derived immunocompetent lymphocytes directed against HLA-associated major and minor antigenic class differences in transplant recipients. Graft versus host disease is caused by the recognition of class I and class II HLA differences as well as non-HLA differences in the host by immunocompetent T cells in the graft. Graft ver-sus host disease is common despite careful HLA matching and occurs in 40% to 70% of allo-geneic BMTs. Increased risk of significant GVHD is associated with many factors, including advanced donor or recipient age, increased HLA mismatch, use of nonsibling familial donors, use of MUDs, and donor-recipient sex mismatch.[35,71] The risk of GVHD is substan-tially lower in sibling donor BMT, especially in younger patients with sex-matched, younger donors. Therefore, the 5-year-old sister who is a 6/6 antigen match is the best donor with respect to GVHD, with about a 10% risk of severe GVHD.

QUESTION 4: WHAT ARE THE MANIFESTATIONS OF GRAFT VERSUS HOST DISEASE?

Graft versus host disease has two major clinical manifestations: acute and chronic. Acute GVHD typically occurs within the first 75 to 100 days post-BMT. The incidence of acute GVHD is about 50%, with a range based on age and other factors.[20] The clinical syndrome usu-ally involves the skin first and may also involve the gut or liver. Systemic organ involvement correlates with a poorer outcome. Chronic GVHD is a biologically distinct syndrome that usually occurs 75 to 100 days or later after allogeneic transplant. The onset may occur after acute GVHD, as a progression of the disorder, after acute GVHD has improved, or de novo, with no prior acute GVHD. The risk of chronic GVHD increases with age and may involve multiple organ systems, including skin, liver, gut, eyes, oral mucosa, and lungs.[70,72] The occurrence of GVHD increases the risk of infection and pneumonitis and results in significant delay in recovery of immune function post-transplant.[70,82] Treatment consists of cyclosporin A, corticosteroids, and other immunosuppressive agents, such as antithymocyte globulin (ATG), OKT3 antibody, IL-1 and IL-2 receptor antagonists, and other, less studied agents.[35,71,74] It has been well demonstrated that GVHD is caused by an attack mediated by donor-derived T cells against recipient tissue.[71,72] Graft versus host disease can be ameliorated or completely prevented by depleting the donor graft of mature T cell phenotypes, but doing so creates a substantial risk for failure of sustainable donor marrow engraftment and for B cell lymphoproliferative disease. Therefore, in this instance, one of the HLA-matched siblings is the best donor.

QUESTION 5: WHAT MEASURES CAN BE TAKEN TO DECREASE THE RISK OF SEVERE GRAFT VERSUS HOST DISEASE?

Large-scale efforts to decrease the incidence of GVHD include systemic treatment with immunosuppressive agents, such as cyclosporin A, as prophylaxis or to treat GVHD, as well as in vitro manipulation of the donor marrow to remove T lymphocytes.[27,50] A greater than 2 log decrement in the number of infused donor T cells markedly reduces the incidence of severe acute and, to a lesser extent, chronic GVHD, making allogeneic transplant more tolerable in older patients, MUD transplants, and mismatched transplants.[5,27,28] However, T cell depletion increases the risk of graft failure, immune reconstitution delay, relapse (in leukemia and lymphoma), and B cell lymphoproliferative disease after BMT.[5,27,61] These methodologies are undergoing intense study and refinement to decrease the untoward effects of this process while making allogeneic transplant available to a greater number of recipients.

In the patient described in this profile, one of the siblings is the best donor. If other features, such as cytomegalovirus (CMV) status (see Question 6) and ABO compatibility, are equivalent, then the 5-year-old sibling is a slightly better donor than the older sibling, based on age. However, donor safety issues may lead the transplantation team to choose the 16-year-old, based on his size and the risk of blood loss from the bone marrow harvest.

QUESTION 6: WHAT OTHER SEVERE COMPLICATIONS ARE ASSOCIATED WITH BONE MARROW TRANSPLANTATION?

In addition to GVHD, infection poses a significant threat to the recipient. After treatment, the patient will have a 10- to 20-day period of severe pancytopenia, requiring hospitalization, reverse isolation, antibiotics, and a controlled environment.[70-72] With modern therapies, almost all patients survive this period until blood count recovery. A more pressing problem is the development of opportunistic infections during the 6-month or longer period of immunosuppression required to prevent or treat GVHD. Occurrence of GVHD increases the risk of both new infection with fungi, bacteria, or viruses and the reactivation of latent infection with DNA viruses.[74,82] In the past, CMV has been the major infectious cause of death after BMT, usually manifested by interstitial pneumonitis at 40 to 60 days post-transplant. If the recipient and donor are CMV IgG negative, then transfusion of only CMV-negative blood products prevents infection. A CMV-negative donor is, therefore, better if the patient is also CMV IgG negative. In CMV-positive patients, treatment or prophylaxis with ganciclovir, beginning at 3 to 4 weeks after BMT or after a positive urine or blood culture, also reduces risk.[36]

Bone Marrow Transplantation in Immune Deficiency States

The first successful allogeneic bone marrow transplants were performed in 1968 in patients with SCID and WAS.[4,32] Since then, additional variations of BMT (e.g., use of unrelated donors or haploidentical donors and T cell depletion)[48,60-62] have been pioneered in certain immune deficiency states. It is clear that the disorders listed in the box on p. 240 will all eventually result in death of the affected individuals despite aggressive supportive care. The only curative approach is the replacement of the deficient lymphoid stem cells. Accordingly, allogeneic BMT has now been successfully performed for patients with SCID, WAS, Chédiak-Higashi syndrome, and the lymphohistiocytic disorders.[73]

Severe combined immune deficiency syndrome is a lethal heterogeneous congenital disorder. Although the manifestations of SCID vary from patient to patient, most of those affected have no significant T cell or B cell immune function.[60,61] Approximately one third of patients with SCID have some mitogenic T cell response, and the remainder are completely anergic. These patients die very early in childhood from severe recurrent infections attributable to their immunodeficiency. Because of the severe deficiencies and low lymphocyte counts, it can be difficult to determine the HLA type of these patients. In some instances, maternal lymphocytes can cross the placenta and engraft in the fetus, further confounding studies of typing. The ability of allogeneic cells to engraft without rejection in these patients, however, allows infusion of phenotypically normal donor stem cells.[31,61] Patients with SCID have now been successfully treated with bone marrow infusion for many years.[61]

Wiskott-Aldrich syndrome is an X-linked recessive disorder characterized by eczema, thrombocytopenia with morphologically "dust-like" platelets, and a progressive T cell and B cell immunodeficiency.[4,13] Patients have a decreased response to T cell antigens and are at high risk for infection and early death. As in SCID, it was demonstrated as early as 1968 that infusions of HLA-compatible stem cells corrected the immunologic disorder. However, WAS requires lymphoid as well as myeloid engraftment because, despite correction of the lymphoid deficiency, the thrombocytopenia does not resolve with donor stem cell infusions.[13] In addition, some host reactivity exists, necessitating the use of a chemotherapeutic preparative regimen (with or without radiotherapy) and prophylaxis for GVHD. In patients with WAS, myeloablation is a prerequisite for successful BMT.[40]

✤ Patient Profile: Stem cell transplantation for severe combined immunodeficiency syndrome

A 1-month-old infant is brought to the physician for recurrent diarrhea, morbilliform rash, persistent oral thrush, and failure to thrive. After an extensive evaluation, immune studies demonstrate no T cell or B cell function, with falling maternal-derived serum immunoglobulins. All of these findings are consistent with the diagnosis of SCID. After treatment with IgG replacement and antimicrobial agents, the patient improves. An unaffected sibling is found to be HLA identical.

QUESTION 1: WHAT IS THE SUCCESS RATE OF BONE MARROW TRANSPLANTATION IN PATIENTS WITH SEVERE COMBINED IMMUNE DEFICIENCY SYNDROME?

Success rates for these patients vary, with most failures attributable to infections present before successful lymphoid engraftment. Earlier diagnosis and treatment lead to an improved success rate.[61] When the disease has been diagnosed in a previous child, it can be diagnosed prenatally in subsequent children by T cell determination using percutaneous umbilical blood sampling, or the diagnosis can be investigated during the first few days of life. Early BMT is clearly more efficacious because the treatment is given before the child develops serious or life-threatening infections. Over time, success rates have improved from 45% to 50% to about 75% to 80%. The rate is even higher if BMT is performed early in the first month of life.[60-62]

QUESTION 2: IS A PREPARATIVE REGIMEN NECESSARY BEFORE BONE MARROW TRANSPLANTATION IN A PATIENT WITH IMMUNE DYSFUNCTION?

Patients with SCID and no alloreactivity to HLA antigens do not require preparation before stem cell infusion. Only in the rare case of a patient with natural killer cell activity or alloreactivity and in cases in which initial or repeated marrow infusions fail is preparative treatment and immunosuppression required. In addition, these patients can be successfully engrafted with lower doses of bone marrow nucleated cells.[61] Therefore, if transplantation is performed during infancy, these children can be successfully treated with small amounts of marrow aspirate, associated with minimal peripheral T cell contamination.

QUESTION 3: WHAT IS THE NATURE OF IMMUNE FUNCTION RECOVERY?

Engraftment rates for T lymphoid stem cell function are high (90%) but are usually less than 50% for B cell function. Myeloid stem cell engraftment is unusual, and GVHD is uncommon.[31,61] Despite the lack of donor B cell engraftment, there is usually full reconstitution of T cell and B cell function.

❧ Patient Profile: Bone marrow transplantation when no HLA-matched relative can be identified

A male infant with confirmed WAS is referred for consideration of BMT. Human leukocyte antigen typing of the family reveals no match.

QUESTION 1: WHAT ARE THE PROSPECTS FOR BONE MARROW TRANSPLANTATION FOR THIS CHILD?

The child requires allogeneic BMT for long-term survival. Because there is no sibling or family match, alternative donors must be sought. Each parent shares a common haplotype with the child and could serve as a donor, but with substantial risk of GVHD even with T lymphocyte depletion. Another stem cell source could be identified through the unrelated bone marrow donor registry. The National Marrow Donor Program (NMDP) is a federally funded project whose aim is to develop a sizable registry of volunteer bone marrow donors.[5] Volunteers are screened for health problems, and initial blood screening is performed. At this time, HLA-A and HLA-B testing is performed and catalogued. Recently, the NMDP has been cataloguing HLA-D and HLA-DR types at the initial screening as well. There are several other registries that can be searched with computerized methods to compare and match catalogued donors with comparable HLA-A and HLA-B antigens. Search of these registries may lead to finding a potential donor for this patient.

QUESTION 2: WHAT IS THE LIKELIHOOD OF FINDING A DONOR, AND HOW LONG DOES A SUCCESSFUL DONOR SEARCH TAKE?

Finding an unrelated donor depends on several factors. First, the registry must contain enough volunteers to make a search statistically likely to be successful. Second, HLA antigens are clustered according to descent and race. Therefore, representation in the registry must be broad, not only in number but also in various ethnic groups, to ensure a likely match. Finally, after successful location of a potential donor or donors, subsequent testing must demonstrate compatibility. The donor must be healthy and must be HLA compatible with the recipient. An HLA antigen match is not the only feature determining the success of BMT, as evidenced by the rate of GVHD in related sibling donor transplants.[35,71] Testing of mixed lymphocyte reactions between potential donors and recipients or compatible DNA HLA typing must be completed to achieve the best match possible. In the case of multiple possible donors, CMV and infectious status, sex match, and ABO blood group compatibility should dictate the choice of donor. Because of these factors, the usual length of time to BMT with an unrelated donor is 4 to 6 months from the time of the initial search. Even then, the likelihood of finding a donor is highly variable due to ethnic HLA diversity. It is estimated that even with a registry of 1 million volunteers with common ethnic origin, only about 60% of patients will find a suitable donor.[5,27]

QUESTION 3: WHAT IS THE RISK OF GRAFT VERSUS HOST DISEASE WHEN A MATCHED UNRELATED DONOR IS USED?

All donors in the registry are over 18 years of age because of the small risks to the donor and the ethical issue of informed consent in minors. Despite HLA matching and compatible mixed lymphocyte culture, there are major differences likely in non-HLA antigens in unrelated donors. Therefore, the risk of GVHD is substantially higher in MUD-BMT, with the risk of severe GVHD being two to three times higher in this group.[5,27] The use of T cell depletion may decrease this risk but lead to higher risks of graft failure, recipient immune dysfunction, and B cell lymphoproliferative disease. Filipovich and colleagues[28] have demonstrated that children with MUD-BMT for immune deficiency syndromes generally do quite well despite these risks. Therefore, in otherwise fatal diseases the use of an MUD is appropriate. The development of improved methods of depleting T cells, treating and preventing GVHD, and diagnosing these disorders early will broaden the application of stem cell transplantation and improve the outcome for these patients. As gene defects are characterized, gene therapy may become another option for these patients (see p. 264).

Bone Marrow Transplantation in Genetic Hematopoietic Disorders

DISORDERS OF COMMITTED HEMATOPOIETIC PROGENITORS

Multiple bone marrow disorders of committed progenitors (e.g., thalassemia major, sickle cell anemia, Blackfan-Diamond anemia) or function (e.g., leukocyte adhesion disorders) are associated with a poor prognosis for a variety of reasons. Patients with red cell aplasia, Blackfan-Diamond anemia, and β-thalassemia major become RBC transfusion dependent. Despite the use of chelation therapy, these patients are at high risk for morbidity and subsequent mortality from iron overload.[1,43,49] Studies have demonstrated that BMT is the only potential cure for these disorders.[14,43,49] Timing of BMT is particularly crucial. In β-thalassemia major, the only one of these disorders with which there has been substantial experience, early BMT is associated with a markedly better outcome.

✤ Patient Profile: Stem cell transplantation for β-thalassemia major

An infant of Mediterranean descent is found at his 1-month checkup to be severely anemic. Careful workup demonstrates that the child has severely microcytic red blood cell indices. Hemoglobin electrophoresis demonstrates that he has only HbF and HbA$_2$. These findings are consistent with β-thalassemia major, and the child is started on transfusion therapy. When the child is 4 years old, his parents conceive another child. Prenatal testing demonstrates *thalassemia trait. At the infant's first birthday, his hemoglobin is normal and HLA testing reveals that he is an identical match for his affected brother.*

QUESTION 1: IS BONE MARROW TRANSPLANTATION A SUCCESSFUL AND SAFE THERAPY FOR β-THALASSEMIA?

Lucarelli and colleagues[49] report the results of several hundred BMTs performed to treat severe β-thalassemia. Success rates are excellent, with about 80% to 85% of transplants successful in these patients. Almost all survivors have hematopoiesis of donor origin, with correction of the hemoglobinopathy.

QUESTION 2: WHAT FACTORS GOVERN THE OUTCOME OF BONE MARROW TRANSPLANTATION IN PATIENTS WITH β-THALASSEMIA?

Lucarelli and colleagues[49] have reported outcome data for allogeneic BMT in patients with β-thalassemia. Bone marrow transplantation performed before the age of 15, before liver abnormalities had developed from iron overload, and in the absence of RBC alloimunization led to potential curative therapy in 90% to 94% of patients. This cure rate decreased to 80% when one risk factor was present and about 55% when two or more risk factors were present. These transplants were performed with preparative regimens that did not include radiation therapy, and morbidity was low in patients who had no risk factors. The major toxicities were GVHD and hepatic damage, the latter presumably related to toxicity of the preparative regimen on already hemosiderin-damaged livers. It is evident that early chelation therapy must be instituted in chronically transfused thalassemic patients. Therefore, until other definitive treatment is developed, allogeneic BMT performed early in the course of the disease is the only curative treatment for these patients. The use of MUDs in this disease has not been highly recommended.

SICKLE CELL ANEMIA

More recently, the use of BMT has been advocated for children with severe sickle cell anemia (SCA). Sickle cell disease is a single-gene defect that causes a single amino acid substitution of valine for glutamic acid at position 6 in the β chain. The result is a spectrum of disease, which has been widely reviewed.[1,43] Most children with SCA have a predictable course, with increased risk for infection and occasional severe crises involving multiple organ systems. A small percentage (5% to 15%) has much more severe disease, with cerebrovascular events in childhood and severe multiple painful or other organ crises.[1] This subgroup, currently defined only by clinical criteria, is at much higher risk for early mortality, despite supportive care and chronic transfusion therapy. Recent studies demonstrate that allogeneic BMT from HbAA or HbAS sibling donors can be performed successfully, with subsequent disappearance of disease stigmata.[43] National collaborative trials are under way, but this disease may be the ideal target for other strategies, such as in utero BMT or gene therapy.[57,63]

FANCONI ANEMIA

Fanconi anemia is a rare autosomal recessive disorder characterized clinically by a constellation of phenotypic abnormalities and characterized biologically by an abnormal sensitivity for chromosome breakage with clastogenic stress.[1] Most patients have the characteristic findings of limb anomalies and associated skeletal problems, but as many as 10% to 25% are phenotypically normal.[1] Bone marrow failure and an abnormally high rate of acute leukemias are characteristic hematologic problems. The underlying abnormality is not known, but the diagnosis is made by chromosome breakage analysis in which phytohemagglutinin-stimulated lymphocytes are exposed to diepoxybutane or other DNA-damaging agents (e.g., mitomycin C). Fanconi cells have an abnormally high number of chromosome breaks after this exposure, compared with normal bone marrow cells.[1,44] The treatment of the underlying bone marrow failure is similar to the therapy used for severe aplastic anemia. Eventually, standard therapies fail, and these patients either die from the complications of marrow failure or develop leukemia. Survival beyond the age of 40 is distinctly rare.

❧ Patient Profile: Stem cell transplantation for Fanconi anemia

A 6-year-old girl is brought to her pediatrician for new-onset bruising. At birth the child was noted to have bilateral hypoplastic thumbs. She subsequently developed many areas of melanin skin deposits as well as some areas of hypopigmentation. A blood count demonstrates thrombocytopenia, anemia, and mild leukopenia. Bone marrow aspirate and biopsy show severely hypoplastic marrow. Cytogenetic studies demonstrate markedly increased chromosome breakage with in vitro exposure to mitomycin C. The parents are told that the child has Fanconi anemia. The mother is currently 2 months pregnant.

QUESTION 1: WHAT TREATMENT IS AVAILABLE FOR CHILDREN WITH FANCONI ANEMIA?

The overall prognosis for this child is dismal: without BMT, she will eventually die from aplastic anemia or leukemic transformation. Treatment with androgens and corticosteroids may lead to temporary (months to years) improvement, but with substantial morbidity and eventual relapse. The use of allogeneic BMT offers the only possible cure for patients with Fanconi anemia.

QUESTION 2: ARE PATIENTS WITH FANCONI ANEMIA WHO UNDERGO BONE MARROW TRANSPLANTATION AT INCREASED RISK BECAUSE OF THEIR CHROMOSOME FRAGILITY?

The use of conventional BMT dose chemotherapy and radiation therapy preparative regimens in these children is associated with excessive morbidity and a lower event-free survival rate than newer approaches. Patients with Fanconi anemia generally develop more severe regimen-related mucosal damage and gastrointestinal problems. A newer approach, described by Gluckman and colleagues,[33] is to administer a total dose of 20 mg/kg of cyclophosphamide, followed by a low dose (5 Gy) of thoracoabdominal radiation. This approach has resulted in a 71% overall survival rate. The GVHD rate with this regimen has been similar to that of patients with severe aplastic anemia. Failure in related-donor BMT has been largely due to GVHD, with failure of engraftment occurring frequently in BMT with partially matched or unrelated donors. The use of antithymocyte globulin in the preparative regimen to suppress host alloreactivity may ameliorate these latter problems.[68]

QUESTION 3: WHO MIGHT BE A SUITABLE DONOR FOR THIS CHILD?

Currently, this child has no familial or sibling donor. A suitable donor might be obtained through the unrelated donor registry. However, the patient's mother is pregnant, and the fetus has a 25% chance of being HLA identical to the affected child. Chorionic villus sampling (CVS) could be performed in this instance for two related purposes. First, CVS will provide cells that can be tested for chromosomal fragility and thus establish the risk for Fanconi anemia in the unborn child. Second, HLA analysis can be performed on this villus material. If the fetus is HLA compatible and phenotypically normal, then placental cord blood collected at delivery could be used as a source of stem cells for the BMT.[44]

Human Cord Blood (Placental Blood) as a Source of Stem Cells

The use of human cord blood as a source of hematopoietic progenitor and stem cells in sibling allogeneic BMT has recently shown promise.[78] Although the number of actual transplants that have been done with cord blood is small, there is strong evidence that a single cord blood collection contains an adequate number of hematopoietic stem cells to reconstitute the bone marrow of pediatric allogeneic recipients (<40 kg) after myeloablative therapy.[6,30,79]

The use of cord blood has several advantages over allogeneic bone marrow obtained using standard methods. The risk to the donor is significantly lower than in allogeneic bone marrow harvesting. Using standard techniques to collect placental cord blood, a study by

Hows and colleagues[39] of 132 newborn infants demonstrated no significant risk to the delivered infant or to the mother. Cord blood is usually a discarded product, so its collection does not interfere with care of the mother or the child. Cord blood as a source of stem cells would, therefore, eliminate the need for anesthesia, the blood loss complications, the discomfort, and much of the cost usually associated with allogeneic bone marrow collection.

CORD BLOOD STEM CELLS

Studies of cord blood products demonstrate relatively high numbers of immature progenitors and proportionately higher numbers of LTC-ICs and HPP-CFCs.[6,26,55] On average, cord blood volume is 100 to 150 ml and contains 5 to 15×10^6 nucleated cells/ml. Progenitor cell content is exceptionally high, with 50% to 90% of the CFU content and an equivalent percentage of CD34-positive cells usually obtained in autologous bone marrow collections.[6] In vitro expansion experiments demonstrate that cord blood progenitor cells have a greater capacity for expansion and proliferation than bone marrow progenitors.[18,22,32,51] Finally, cord blood progenitors appear to have higher transfection efficiency than bone marrow progenitors in gene therapy experiments, suggesting a more efficient delivery system for target genes.[55] This advantage highlights cord blood as an inexpensive, easily obtainable source of progenitor cells and true stem cells for use in further study of gene therapy strategies.

RISK OF GRAFT VERSUS HOST DISEASE IN CORD BLOOD STEM CELL TRANSPLANTATION

Cord blood lymphocytes appear to have a more immature phenotype, appear to be naïve in their immune response, and are significantly less responsive to allogeneic targets.[26,55] Clinically, human cord blood allogeneic transplants have resulted in significantly lower rates of GVHD, correlating with these in vitro responses.[79,80] Therefore, human cord blood is an excellent source of hematopoietic progenitor cells. A broad range of transplant applications deserve further study.

There are several potential and theoretic problems with the use of human cord blood in allogeneic BMT. The most disadvantageous feature of cord blood as a source of stem cells for hematopoietic reconstitution after myeloablative chemotherapy is the limited number of progenitors available. Human cord blood has not been studied extensively as a potential means of hematopoietic reconstitution in larger children (>40 kg) or in adults, so this small number of progenitors remains an unknown and potentially limiting feature of this product.[79,80] Current studies of in vitro expansion using long-term stromal or liquid culture techniques and applications of newer cytokines may help overcome this difficulty and broaden the application of stem cell transplantation using cord blood.

In addition to absolute cell dose, there are additional concerns regarding engraftment potential of cord blood. In a report by Wagner and colleagues[80] of 26 human transplants performed with cord blood as a source of progenitor cells, four of twenty-two evaluable allogeneic pairs failed to engraft. Questions remain regarding the reason for this failure, but conceivably, the mononuclear cell composition of cord blood may contain fewer T cells responsible for facilitating engraftment; further study is needed.

COLLECTION AND STORAGE OF CORD BLOOD FOR USE IN BONE MARROW TRANSPLANTATION

Several methods of collecting placental cord blood have been described.[26,34] Each method has its proponents, but all these methods lead to adequate collection of cord blood for study. To collect cord blood for use in clinical transplantation, there are additional considerations. The blood must be collected in a way that minimizes risk to the mother and newborn. The process should also be carried out in a way that causes the least inconvenience for the mother and for the delivery room staff. The method of collection must introduce little or no risk of contamination by bacteria, must minimize the risk of contamination by maternal blood, and must maximize the number and ensure the viability of mononuclear cells in the specimen.

Two major collection methods have evolved during the past decade. The first was proposed by Rubinstein and colleagues,[66] from the newly formed Unrelated Cord Blood Registry. In this method, the child is delivered, and the cord cross-clamped and cut close to the infant. As soon as the placenta is delivered, it is moved to an adjacent room, where the placental vein is cleaned with antiseptic and entered through venipuncture. Cord blood is aspirated into syringes that contain anticoagulant (usually heparin) and then removed to the stem cell laboratory for aliquoting, in vitro testing for pathogenic and progenitor cell content, and cryopreservation or packaging for transport. In the second method, proposed by Gluckman and colleagues,[34] as soon as the baby is delivered the cord is clamped close to the infant and cut. Then the cut end of the cord is wiped clean with antiseptic. After the cord is lowered into a sterile container prepared with heparin, it is unclamped and blood collection is assisted by gravity and by maternal uterine contractions. When the placenta has been fully delivered, blood is needle-aspirated from all sizable veins, and the two fractions are transported to the laboratory for further testing.

Both methods have produced satisfactory results. Choice of technique depends on many factors, including individual patient factors and the skill and experience of the personnel collecting the specimen. Observance of quality control measures, performance of progenitor assays, and careful screening for infectious agents are vital components of the process. Paramount to the process is securing consent from the mother before the procedure is performed. This consent should be obtained using local institutional protocol and a consent form reviewed by the institutional investigative review board.

Appropriate indications for cord blood collection include possible use as a source of stem cells for a family member undergoing BMT, use for approved research studies, and use in association with the Unrelated Cord Blood Registry.

Bone Marrow Transplantation for the Treatment of Storage Disorders

Several inherited enzymatic deficiencies are characterized by a variety of systemic and central nervous system (CNS) abnormalities that result in significant morbidity and early death (see the box on p. 240).[46] The enzymatic deficiencies in these patients lead to an accumulation of toxic substances that interfere with cellular function. Prominent manifestations include bone marrow failure, hepatosplenomegaly, and, in some disorders, progressive CNS deterioration with demyelination.[38,46] Experimental animal models and clinical experience have demonstrated that myeloablative chemotherapy followed by infusion of genotypically normal allogeneic bone marrow cells leads to the development of circulating and tissue monocytes and macrophages with near-normal or normal enzyme levels.[38,45,46,64] These cells provide a source of normal enzyme to tissue and to the CNS. Systemic symptoms have been noted to resolve with near-normal circulating levels of enzyme. For most patients, CNS symptoms stabilize but rarely improve. In some cases, despite normal blood enzyme levels after BMT, CNS symptoms continue to worsen.

Most of the disorders listed in the box on p. 240 have been treated with BMT, with varying degrees of success. With some diseases, such as metachromatic leukodystrophy (MLD), the disease course and prognosis are unpredictable. In others, such as adrenal leukodystrophy (ALD), the presence at the time of BMT of any neuropsychologic progression is a bad prognostic sign. Experience has led to the application of BMT only in patients with minimal or undetectable CNS disturbance.[46]

❧ Patient Profile: Stem cell transplantation for adrenoleukodystrophy

A 7-year-old boy with ALD is referred for consideration of BMT. He was diagnosed at age 5 with progressive memory loss. Testing demonstrated visual processing deficits, and he subsequently developed behavioral problems. Very long chain fatty acid (VLCFA) determination demonstrated elevation greater than two standard deviations above the normal range. There were no familial matches, and an unrelated donor search was successful in locating a donor after 6 months. Bone marrow transplantation was performed, and moderate GVHD occurred but was well controlled with immunosuppressive therapy. At 6 months, he was taken off immunosuppression, with normal counts and normal VLCFA. However, neurologic deterioration continued, and seizures and motor dysfunction occurred during the next several years.

QUESTION 1: HOW COULD THIS NEUROLOGIC DETERIORATION HAVE BEEN PREVENTED?

This case illustrates the need for earlier diagnosis, better treatment, and more rapid availability of alternative sources of stem cells. In some storage diseases, such as ALD, toxic compounds accumulate in the central nervous system, damaging cellular components. These neural cells progressively die over the course of months to years, with corresponding progression of neurologic deterioration. This deterioration occurs despite normalization of plasma enzyme levels after BMT. The frustration of obtaining this result after treatment for these disorders, coupled with the morbidity of BMT, especially unrelated donor BMT, has prompted the exploration of newer technologies, such as the use of cord blood from unrelated donors and in vitro expansion of stem cells. Additional studies have been conducted to investigate new avenues of stem cell therapy, such as prenatal transplantation.

In Utero Stem Cell Transplantation

Several human genetic defects strike very early in child development. Many of these disorders are hematopoietic in origin, such as β-thalassemia and Chédiak-Higashi syndrome, while others are enzymatic deficiencies that result in tissue deposition of toxic compounds. Several of these diseases, such as disorders of mucopolysaccharide metabolism, including Hurler syndrome, Hunter syndrome, ALD, and MLD, have been corrected by allogeneic BMT.[46,69] However, in many disorders, suitable donors are not available or the disease progression is so rapid that by the time the disorder is diagnosed the disease process has already caused substantial target-organ damage. This is especially true for disorders such as late infantile MLD, ALD, and SCID.

❧ Patient Profile: In utero stem cell transplantation

A pregnant woman (gravida 4, para 3002) is referred because of a previous child with severe late infantile MLD. The child died before age 10 because no familial or unrelated donor could be found, and the disease progressed early. The mother is currently 6 weeks pregnant. There are two unaffected children, ages 6 and 9, who are doing well.

QUESTION 1: SHOULD PRENATAL DIAGNOSIS BE ATTEMPTED?

The availability of molecular techniques, including the polymerase chain reaction (PCR) technique, has led to the discovery and subsequent cloning and sequencing of many of the genes responsible for inborn errors of metabolism and for congenital bone marrow disorders.[45,46,64] In addition, many storage diseases have characteristic biochemical markers present in somatic cells and plasma. Chorionic villus sampling, in this case, could be used to diagnose MLD during the first trimester by determining arylsulfatase levels. The choice must be made by the family, but the option should be offered. In addition, since previous HLA testing has been performed in the two unaffected siblings, HLA testing of the fetus by CVS would be informative to determine whether a bone marrow donor already exists for the potentially affected fetus.

QUESTION 2: WHAT OPTIONS ARE AVAILABLE FOR THIS FAMILY?

Until recently, CVS simply provided expectant mothers and families with reasonably reliable information regarding whether the child would be affected. The only choice the family had to make was whether to prepare for the care needs of the child or to abort the pregnancy. Recent advances in understanding and developments in stem cell biology are making a third option available to these families.

Studies by Zanjani and colleagues[84-86] in preimmune fetal sheep have demonstrated that first-trimester sheep embryos have little ability to recognize or reject allograft or xenograft bone marrow cells. In a series of experiments, they demonstrated that unseparated or CD34-positive selected adult human bone marrow stem cells could be safely infused intraperitoneally or via percutaneous umbilical blood sampling in these animals. Despite species differences, presence of human hematopoiesis was prolonged in nearly half of the sheep and remained stable in sheep bone marrow during the first year after birth. Although these data are preliminary, they suggest that the first-trimester embryo is immunologically naïve and will accept and support stable chimerism with infused donor stem cells. Other investigators have confirmed these findings.[65,68]

QUESTION 3: IF A SIBLING OR OTHER SUITABLE DONOR CAN BE IDENTIFIED FOR AN AFFECTED FETUS, WHEN CAN BONE MARROW TRANSPLANTATION BE PERFORMED?

Bone marrow transplantation could logistically be performed anytime during this child's first year of life. Bone marrow transplantation for this disorder would require the completion of a preparative regimen and a prolonged hospital stay. In addition, there is a risk for regimen-related toxicity and late effects.[9,71] Another option, in utero stem cell transplantation, has several theoretic advantages. First, the normal hematopoietic stem cells (from sources such as bone marrow, cord blood, and fetal liver) are infused early in the course of the disease, before significant target-organ damage has occurred. Second, CVS and molecular techniques are reliable means of evaluating potential candidates who have no other curative or therapeutic options. Third, stem cells are now relatively easy to obtain from a variety of sources and can be purified, concentrated, and given as small-volume infusions. Finally, normal stem cells can be isolated from the fetus or young infant to determine efficacy and degree of chimerism and the need for additional infusions or standard BMT. Using this process, the child receives no preparative therapy, has few, if any, long-term effects, and avoids prolonged hospitalization. In addition, this procedure costs considerably less than conventional BMT.

QUESTION 4: WHAT IS KNOWN ABOUT ENGRAFTMENT AND THE RISK OF GRAFT VERSUS HOST DISEASE IN THE FETUS?

Evidence to date suggests that, although the preimmune fetus will allow engraftment, there is still a substantial risk of GVHD. This complication in the fetus leads to substantial morbidity and increased risk of fetal loss. The limited clinical experience to date was reported by Cowan and Golbus[19] at the 1993 meeting of the American Society of Hematology. Their experience with 13 in utero transplants reveals the many problems associated with this approach. Most of the children treated had confirmed evidence of a genetic disorder (five had β-thalassemia, two had SCID, two had MLD, and four had other disorders). They received stem cells from a variety of sources, including haploidentical parental marrow (n=6), fetal liver (n=6), fetal thymus (n=4), or sibling marrow (n=1). Only four had documented engraftment, and there were two fetal losses. However, engraftment in four patients is encouraging, although these data were reported too early for clinical benefit to be determined. In animal models, GVHD has been a problem with adult marrow, and T cell depletion, which compromises engraftment potential, has been necessary. However, the decreased potential of cord blood to cause GVHD makes unrelated-donor cord blood an attractive alternative stem cell source, and studies are in progress. Much work still needs to be done in this area, but the possibility that this will become a viable therapeutic option in years to come is exciting.*

Applications of Gene Therapy in Pediatrics

The treatment of potentially lethal congenital disorders is unique to pediatrics. Many of these defects are single-gene mutations carried in hematopoietic stem cells and can be cured by allogeneic BMT from phenotypically normal sibling donors or unrelated HLA-matched donors.[46,64,69] Because of family size at diagnosis and the potential for siblings to be similarly affected, it may not be possible to find a suitable donor for all affected individuals. The use of T cell–depleted haploidentical parental donors and MUDs can obviate this need, but at the cost of greater morbidity and mortality. A potential avenue of therapy is the collection of autologous hematopoietic stem cells from bone marrow or stimulated peripheral blood, with ex vivo manipulation to correct the genetic defect, followed by reinfusion of the altered hematopoietic stem cells.[17,21,24,59] Several techniques have been successful in transducing hematopoietic progenitor cells with DNA material, including retroviral gene insertion, electroporation, and homologous recombination.[59] These techniques allow insertion of target genetic material into cells that are deficient in the candidate gene. Problems with these techniques include poor gene transfection efficiency, lack of functional transcription after insertion, damage of genetic material, and possible contamination with helper viruses.[17,59]

❦ Patient Profile: Gene therapy for adenosine deaminase deficiency

A 1-month-old infant is evaluated by his pediatrician for oral candidiasis and failure to thrive. Immune workup reveals SCID. Further characterization indicates complete deficiency of the enzyme adenosine deaminase (ADA). Supportive care is started. An exhaustive family and unrelated donor registry search fails to identify a suitable donor.

---

*References 19, 29, 77, 84, and 85.

QUESTION 1: WHAT OPTIONS, BESIDES SUPPORTIVE CARE, ARE AVAILABLE TO THIS INFANT?

The ADA deficiency leads to accumulation of deoxyadenosine in these patients, which causes lymphocytopenia and severe immunodeficiency. Therapy is available with conjugated ADA given systemically, but this is palliative. Recently, techniques have been developed to insert the functional ADA gene into lymphoid progenitors in autologous bone marrow or peripheral blood stem cells.[23] Other techniques have been used in selected CD34-positive cells in an attempt to purify stem cells before gene transfection.[8] Patients treated thus far have markedly improved, creating optimism about the use of gene therapy for this disorder.

QUESTION 2: DOES GENE THERAPY REQUIRE AN APPROACH SIMILAR TO THAT USED FOR BONE MARROW TRANSPLANTATION?

Certainly if a patient received preparative therapy followed by infusion of true pluripotent stem cells corrected by gene transfection, BMT would be curative. Unfortunately, gene transfection efficiency is usually low.[59] In addition, the true pluripotent stem cell would have to be transduced for this therapy to be curative. The use of preparative therapy is obviously complicated by regimen-related toxicity and infectious risks.[9,72,74] A few studies have examined the possibility of inserting selected marker genes into stem cells.[17,54,59] Some of these marker genes, such as the gene for the multiple drug resistance (MDR) membrane pump, could be used to select these cells by treating the recipient with drugs that damage the nontransfected cells but give the genetically altered cells an advantage.[54] In this type of transplant, a patient receives a transfusion of marked stem cells from a donor, from autologous bone marrow, or from peripheral blood stem cells that have also been corrected for the target gene. The recipient is then treated with a drug, such as Taxol, to which resistance is conferred by the MDR phenotype. A few sequential treatments would, theoretically, lead to an advantage for hematopoietic recovery driven by the transfected, normal cells at the expense of the untransfected cells. The toxicity of such treatment could be considerably lower than that of conventional BMT, with similar results.

Gene therapy strategies and treatments are new and under intense study. However, strategies already exist for a variety of diseases, including Krabbe disease, ADA deficiency, SCID, Gaucher disease, Fanconi anemia, and a host of others.* Further studies will determine the future of this promising approach.

The Future of Stem Cell Transplantation

The application of BMT in human disease is widening in scope as well as in the nature of the approach. Identification of alternative sources of hematopoietic stem cells, including

---

*References 8, 23, 33, 41, 58, and 81.

purified marrow products, peripheral blood stem cells, placental cord blood stem cells, and ex vivo expansion of these products, will usher in a new era of cellular therapy and transplantation therapy for human diseases, especially for children. With improvements in molecular techniques, it will be possible to select appropriate candidates for treatment and offer them more refined therapeutic techniques. It is likely that the field of pediatric BMT will be the leader in the application of gene therapy as well as in the development of new methods of achieving tolerance in transplant recipients. These advances will lead to higher cure rates in an expanded group of patients, with lower morbidity and cost. These procedures, which only a few years ago seemed to be mere fantasies, are now entering clinical trials and will result in even greater understanding of stem cell biology and in the application of stem cell transplantation in the treatment of human genetic disease.

REFERENCES

1. Alter BP, Young NS: The bone marrow failure syndromes. In Nathan DG, Oski FA, editors: *Hematology of infancy and childhood*, Philadelphia, 1993, WB Saunders.
2. Anasetti C, Beatty PG, Storb R. et al: Effect of HLA incompatibility on graft-versus-host disease, relapse, and survival after marrow transplantation for patients with leukemia or lymphoma, *Hum Immunol* 29:79, 1990.
3. Andrews RG, Singer JW, Bernstein ID: Monoclonal antibody 12.8 recognizes a 115-kd molecule present on both unipotent and multipotent hematopoietic colony-forming cells and their precursors, *Blood* 67:842, 1986.
4. Bach FH, Albertini RJ, Joo P et al: Bone marrow transplantation in a patient with Wiskott-Aldrich syndrome, *Lancet* 2:1364, 1968.
5. Beatty PG, Clift RA, Mickelson EM et al: Marrow transplantation from related donors other than HLA-identical siblings, *N Engl J Med* 313:765, 1985.
6. Bender JG, Unverzagt K, Walker DE et al: Phenotypic analysis and characterization of CD34+ cells from normal human bone marrow, cord blood, peripheral blood, and mobilized peripheral blood from patients undergoing autologous stem cell transplantation, *Clin Immunol Immunopathol* 70:10, 1994.
7. Bernstein ID: Antigen CD34+ marrow cells engraft lethally irradiated baboons, *J Clin Invest* 81:951, 1988.
8. Blaese RM, Culver KW, Chang L et al: Treatment of severe combined immunodeficiency disease due to adenosine deaminase deficiency with CD34+ selected autologous peripheral blood cells transduced with human ADA gene. Amendment to clinical research project, Project 90-C-195, January 10, 1992, *Hum Gene Ther* 4:521, 1993.
9. Bozzola M, Giorgiani G, Locatelli F et al: Growth in children after bone marrow transplantation, *Horm Res* 39:122, 1993.
10. Brandt J, Baird N, Lu L et al: Characterization of a human hematopoietic progenitor cell capable of forming blast cell containing colonies in vitro, *J Clin Invest* 82:1017, 1988.
11. Briddell RA, Broudy V, Bruno E et al: Further phenotypic characterization and isolation of human hematopoietic progenitor cells using a monoclonal antibody to the c-kit receptor, *Blood* 79:3159, 1992.
12. Brochstein JA, Gillo AP, Ruggiero M et al: Marrow transplantation from human leukocyte antigen-identical or haploidentical donors for correction of Wiskott-Aldrich syndrome, *J Pediatr* 119:907, 1991.
13. Broxmeyer HE, Hangoc G, Cooper S: Clinical and biological aspects of human umbilical cord blood as a source of transplantable hematopoietic stem and progenitor cells, *Bone Marrow Transplant* 1(suppl 9):7, 1992.
14. Camitta BM, Thomas ED, Nathan DG et al: A prospective study of androgens and bone marrow transplantation for treatment of severe aplastic anemia, *Blood* 53:504, 1979.
15. Caracciolo D, Clark S, Rovera G: Differential activity of recombinant colony-stimulating factors in supporting proliferation of human peripheral blood and bone marrow myeloid progenitors in culture, *Br J Hæmatol* 72:306, 1989.
16. Carow CE, Hangoc G, Broxmeyer HE: Human multipotential progenitor cells (CFU-GEMM) have extensive replating capacity for secondary CFU-GEMM: an effect enhanced by cord blood plasma, *Blood* 81:942, 1993.
17. Chertkovj L, Jiang S, Lutton JD et al: The hematopoietic stromal microenvironment promotes retrovirus-mediated gene transfer into hematopoietic stem cells, *Stem Cells (Dayt)* 11:218, 1993.

18. Cicuttini FM, Loudovaris M, Boyd AW: Interactions between purified human cord blood haemopoietic progenitor cells and accessory cells, *Br J Hæmatol* 84:365, 1993.

19. Cowan MJ, Golbus M: In utero hematopoietic stem cell transplants for inherited diseases, *Am J Pediatr Hematol Oncol* 16:35, 1994.

20. Deeg HJ, Cottler-Fox M: Clinical spectrum and pathophysiology of acute graft versus host disease. In Burakoff SJ, Deeg HJ, Ferrara J, Atkinson K, editors: *Graft-vs.-host disease*, New York, 1990, Dekker.

21. Dick J, Karnel-Reid S, Murdoch B, Doedens M: Gene transfer into normal human hematopoietic cells using in vitro and in vivo assays, *Blood* 78:624, 1991.

22. Durand B, Eddleman K, Migliaccio AR et al: Long-term generation of colony-forming cells (CFC) from CD34+ human umbilical cord blood cells, *Leuk Lymphoma* 11:263, 1993.

23. Einerhand MP, Bakx TA, Kukler A, Valerio D: Factors affecting the transduction of pluripotent hematopoietic stem cells: long-term expression of a human adenosine deaminase gene in mice, *Blood* 81:254, 1993.

24. Einerhand MP, Bakx TA, Kukler A, Valerio D: Transduction and culture of purified hemopoietic progenitor cells, *Bone Marrow Transplant* 1(suppl 9):158, 1992.

25. Emerson SG, Palsson BO, Clarke MF: The construction of high efficiency human bone marrow tissue ex-vivo, *J Cell Biochem* 45:268, 1991.

26. Falkenburg JH, van-Luxemburg-Heijs SA, Zijlmans JM, et al: Separation, enrichment, and characterization of human hematopoietic progenitor cells from umbilical cord blood, *Ann Hematol* 67:231, 1993.

27. Filipovich AH: Progress in broadening the uses of marrow transplantation: donor availability, *Vox Sang* 51(suppl 2):95, 1986.

28. Filipovich AH: Bone marrow transplantation from unrelated donors for congenital immunodeficiencies, *Bone Marrow Transplant* 11(suppl 1):78, 1993.

29. Flake AW, Zanjani ED: In utero transplantation of hematopoietic stem cells, *Crit Rev Oncol Hematol* 15:35, 1993.

30. Fritsch G, Buchinger P, Printz D: Use of flow cytometric CD34 analysis to quantify hematopoietic progenitor cells, *Leuk Lymphoma* 10:443, 1993.

31. Gabutti V, Timeus F, Ramenghi U et al: Expansion of cord blood progenitors and use for hematopoietic reconstitution, *Stem Cells (Dayt)* 11(suppl 2):105, 1993.

32. Gatti RA, Meuwissen HJ, Aller HD et al: Immunological reconstitution of sex-linked lymphopenic immunological deficiency, *Lancet* 2:1366, 1968.

33. Gluckman E, Devergie A, Dutreix J: Radiosensitivity in Fanconi anæmia: application to the conditioning regimen for bone marrow transplantation, *Br J Hæmatol* 54:431, 1983.

34. Gluckman E, Wagner J, Hows J et al: Cord blood banking for hematopoietic stem cell transplantation: an international cord blood transplant registry, *Bone Marrow Transplant* 11:199, 1993.

35. Glucksberg H, Storb R, Fefer A et al: Clinical manifestation of graft-versus-host disease in human recipients of marrow from HLA-matched sibling donors, *Transplantation* 18:295, 1974.

36. Goodrich JM, Mori M, Gleaves CA et al: Early treatment with ganciclovir to prevent cytomegalovirus disease after allogeneic bone marrow transplantation, *N Engl J Med* 325:1601, 1991.

37. Haylock D, To L, Dowse T et al: Ex vivo expansion and maturation of peripheral blood CD34+ cells into the myeloid lineage, *Blood* 80:1405, 1992.

38. Hobbs JR, Hugh-Jones K et al: reversal of clinical features of Hurler's disease and biochemical improvement after treatment by bone marrow transplantation, *Lancet* 2:709, 1981.

39. Hows JM, Marsh JC, Bradley BA et al: Human cord blood: a source of transplantable stem cells? *Bone Marrow Transplant* 1(suppl 9):105, 1992.

40. Kapoor N, Kirkpatrick D, Blaese RM et al: Reconstitution of normal megakaryocytopoiesis and immunologic function in Wiskott-Aldrich syndrome by marrow transplantation following myeloablation and immunosuppression with busulfan and cyclophosphamide, *Blood* 57:692, 1991.

41. Karlsson S, Correll PH, Xu L: Gene transfer and bone marrow transplantation with special reference to Gaucher's disease, *Bone Marrow Transplant* 11(suppl 1):124, 1993.

42. Katz F, Malcolm S, Strobel S et al: The use of locus-specific minisatellite probes to check engraftment following allogeneic bone marrow transplantation for severe combined immunodeficiency disease, *Bone Marrow Transplant* 5:199, 1990.

43. Kirkpatrick DV, Barrios NJ, Humbert JH: Bone marrow transplantation for sickle cell anemia, *Semin Hematol* 28:240, 1991.

44. Kohli-Kumar M, Shahidi NT, Broxmeyer HE et al: Hæmopoietic stem/progenitor cell transplant in Fanconi anemia using HLA-matched sibling umbilical cord blood cells, *Br J Hæmatol* 85:419, 1993.

45. Krivit W, Freese D, Chan KW, Kulkarni R: Wolman's disease: a review of treatment with bone marrow transplantation and considerations for the future, *Bone Marrow Transplant* 1(suppl 10):97, 1992.

46. Krivit W, Shapiro EG: Bone marrow transplantation for storage diseases. In Forman SJ, Blume KG, Thomas ED, editors: *Bone marrow transplantation*, Boston, 1993, Blackwell.

47. Lansdorp PM, Dragowska W, Mayani H: Ontogeny-related changes in proliferative potential of human hematopoietic cells, *J Exp Med* 178:787, 1993.

48. Lenarsky C, Parkman R: Bone marrow transplant for the treatment of immune deficiency states, *Bone Marrow Transplant* 6:361, 1990.

49. Lucarelli G, Galimberti M, Polchi P et al: Marrow transplantation in patients with advanced thalassemia, *N Engl J Med* 322:417, 1990.

50. Matthay K, Wara DW, Ablin AJ, Cowan MJ: Haploidentical bone marrow transplantation using soybean agglutinin-processed, T-depleted marrow, *Transplant Proc* 19:2678, 1987.

51. Mayani H, Dragowska W, Lansdorp PM: Cytokine-induced selective expansion and maturation of erythroid versus myeloid progenitors from purified cord blood precursor cells, *Blood* 81:3252, 1993.

52. Mayani H, Dragowska W, Lansdorp PM: Lineage commitment in human hematopoiesis involves asymmetric cell division of multipotent progenitors and does not appear to be influenced by cytokines, *J Cell Physiol* 157:579, 1993.

53. McGlave PB, Haake R et al: Therapy of severe aplastic anemia in young adults and children with allogeneic bone marrow transplantation, *Blood* 70:1325, 1987.

54. Mickisch GH, Aksentijevich I, Schoenlein PV et al: Transplantation of bone marrow cells from transgenic mice expressing the human *MDR1* gene results in long-term protection against the myelosuppressive effect of chemotherapy in mice, *Blood* 79:1087, 1992.

55. Migliaccio AR, Baiocchi M, Durand B et al: Aspects of the biology of the neonatal hematopoietic stem cell, *Stem Cells (Dayt)* 11(suppl 2):56, 1993.

56. Migliaccio G, Migliaccio AR, Druzin M: Long-term generation of colony-forming cells in liquid culture of CD34+ cord blood cells in the presence of recombinant human stem cell factor, *Blood* 79:2620, 1992.

57. Miller JL, Donahue RE, Sellers SE et al: Recombinant adeno-associated virus (rAAV) mediated expression of a human globin gene in human progenitor derived erythroid cells, *PNAS* 91:10183, 1994.

58. Moritz T, Keller DC, Williams DA: Human cord blood cells as targets for gene transfer: potential use in genetic therapies of severe combined immunodeficiency disease, *J Exp Med* 178:529, 1993.

59. Nienhius AW, Kevin TM, Bodine DM: Gene transfer into hematopoietic stem cells, *Cancer* 67(suppl 10):2700, 1991.

60. O'Reilly RJ, Dupont B, Pahwas S et al: Reconstitution in severe combined immunodeficiency to transplantation of marrow from an unrelated donor, *N Engl J Med* 297:1311, 1977.

61. O'Reilly RJ, Freidrich W, Small TN: Transplantation approaches for severe combined immunodeficiency disease, Wiskott-Aldrich syndrome, and other lethal, genetic, combined immunodeficiency disorders. In Forman SJ, Blume KG, Thomas ED, editors: *Bone marrow transplantation*, Boston, 1993, Blackwell.

62. Parkman R: Bone marrow transplantation for genetic diseases, *Pediatr Ann* 20:677, 1991.

63. Plavec I, Papayannopoulou T, Maury C, Meyer F: A human beta-globin gene fused to the human beta-globin locus control region is expressed at high levels in erythroid cells of mice engrafted with retrovirus-transduced hematopoietic stem cells, *Blood* 81:1384, 1993.

64. Rappeport JM, Barrenger JA, Ginns EI: Bone marrow transplantation in Gaucher's disease, *Birth Defects* 22:101, 1986.

65. Roodman GD, Vandeberg JL, Kuehl TJ: In utero bone marrow transplantation of fetal baboons with mismatched adult marrow: initial observations, *Bone Marrow Transplant* 3:141, 1988.

66. Rubinstein P, Rosenfield RE, Adamson JW, Stevens CE: Stored placental blood for unrelated bone marrow reconstitution, *Blood* 81:1679, 1993.

67. Shpall EJ, Jones RB, Bearman SI et al: Transplantation of enriched CD34-positive autologous marrow into breast cancer patients following high-dose chemotherapy: influence of CD34-positive peripheral-blood progenitors and growth factors on engraftment, *J Clin Oncol* 12:28, 1994.

68. Srour EF, Zanjani ED, Cornetta K et al: Persistence of human multilineage, self-renewing lymphohematopoietic stem cells in chimeric sheep, *Blood* 82:3333, 1993.

69. Storb R, Etzioni R, Anasetti C et al: Cyclophosphamide combined with antithymocyte globulin in preparation for allogeneic marrow transplants in patients with aplastic anemia, *Blood* 80(suppl 1):669a, 1992.
70. Sullivan KM, Agura E, Anasetti C et al: Chronic graft-versus-host disease and other late complications of bone marrow transplantation, *Semin Hematol* 28:250, 1991.
71. Sullivan KM, Parkman R: The pathophysiology and treatment of graft versus host disease, *Baillieres Clin Hæmatol* 12:775, 1983.
72. Sullivan KM, Sanders JE, Anasetti C et al: Long-term complications of bone marrow transplantation. In Buckner CD, Gale RP, Lucarelli G, editors: *Advances and controversies in thalassemia therapy: bone marrow transplanatation and other approaches,* New York, 1989, Alan R. Liss.
73. Sullivan JL, Woda BA: Lymphohistiocytic disorders. In Nathan DG, Oski FA, editors: *Hematology of infancy and childhood,* Philadelphia, 1993, WB Saunders.
74. Thomas ED, Storb R: Technique for human marrow grafting, *Blood* 36:507, 1970.
75. Touraine JL, Raudrant D, Rebaud A et al: In utero transplantation of stem cells in humans: immunological aspects and clinical follow-up of patients, *Bone Marrow Transplant* 1(suppl 9):121, 1992.
76. Tsujino Y, Wada H, Misawa M et al: Effects of mast cell growth factor, interleukin-3, and interleukin-6 on human primitive hematopoietic progenitors from bone marrow and cord blood, *Exp Hematol* 21:1379, 1993.
77. Van-Zant G, Thompson BP, Chen J: Differentiation of chimeric bone marrow in vivo reveals genotype-restricted contributions to hematopoiesis, *Exp Hematol* 19:941, 1991.
78. Varma A, El-Awar FY, Palsson BO et al: Can Dexter cultures support stem cell proliferations? *Exp Hematol* 20:87, 1992.
79. Wagner JE: Umbilical cord blood stem cell transplantation, *Am J Pediatr Hematol Oncol* 15:169, 1993.
80. Wagner JE, Kernan NA, Broxmeyer HE, Gluckman E: Allogeneic umbilical cord blood transplantation: report of results in 26 patients, *Proc Am Soc Hematol* 330a, 1993.
81. Walsh CE, Nienhuis AW, Samulski RJ et al: Phenotypic correction of Fanconi anemia in human hematopoietic cells with a recombinant adeno-associated virus vector, *J Clin Invest* 94:1440, 1994.
82. Weiner RS, Bortin MM, Gale RP et al: Interstitial pneumonitis after bone marrow transplantation, *Ann Intern Med* 104:168, 1986.
83. Weinthal J, Nolta JA, Yu XJ et al: Expression of human glucocerebrosidase following retroviral vector-mediated transduction of murine hematopoietic stem cells, *Bone Marrow Transplant* 8:403, 1991.
84. Zanjani ED, Ascensao JL, Flake AW et al: The fetus as an optimal donor and recipient of hemopoietic stem cells, *Bone Marrow Transplant* 10(suppl 1):107, 1992.
85. Zanjani ED, Ascensao JL, Tavassoli M: Liver-derived fetal hematopoietic stem cells selectively and preferentially home to the fetal bone marrow, *Blood* 81:399, 1993.
86. Zanjani ED, Pallavicini MG, Ascensao JL et al: Engraftment and long-term expression of human fetal hemopoietic stem cells in sheep following transplantation in utero, *J Clin Invest* 89:1178, 1992.

Index